THE FOOD DOCTOR ULTIMATE DIET

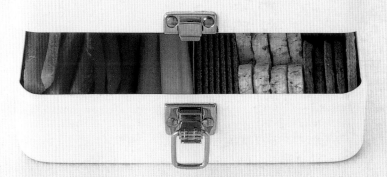

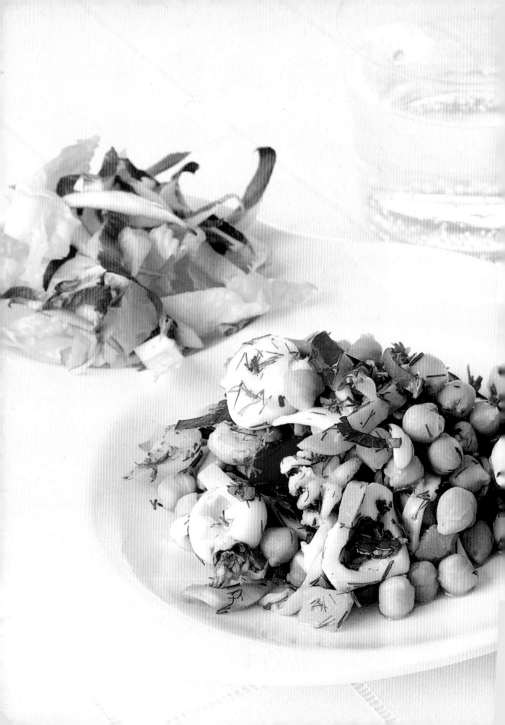

THE FOOD DOCTOR™ ULTIMATE DIET

Ian Marber MBANT Dip ION

Recipes by Rowena Paxton Dip ION

For more information on The Food Doctor, visit
www.thefooddoctor.com

LONDON, NEW YORK, MELBOURNE,
MUNICH AND DELHI

DK LONDON
Editorial assistant Ariane Durkin
Senior art editors Isabel de Cordova, Susan Downing
Managing editor Dawn Henderson
Production editor Jenny Woodcock
Production controller Elizabeth Cherry
Creative technical support Sonia Charbonnier
Project editors Susannah Steel, Jennifer Lane,
Janice Anderson
Project designers Jo Grey, Mark Cavanagh
Photography Sîan Irvine, Francis Loney

DK DELHI
Editorial Manager Glenda Fernandes
Design Manager Romi Chakraborty
Project Editor Ankush Saikia
DTP Coordinator Sunil Sharma
DTP Designer Pushpak Tyagi

First published in Great Britain in 2009 by
Dorling Kindersley Limited, 80 Strand, London WC2R 0RL
A Penguin Company

2 4 6 8 10 9 7 5 3 1

Copyright © 2009 Dorling Kindersley Limited, London
Text copyright © 2009 Ian Marber

The Food Doctor Ultimate Diet first published by DK in 2008

The Food Doctor Diet Club first published by DK in 2007;
The Food Doctor Everyday Diet Cookbook first published by DK
in 2006; The Food Doctor Everyday Diet first published by DK
in 2004; The Food Doctor Diet first published by DK in 2003

Note to readers: Do not attempt the Seven-day diet if you are pregnant, or are 16 years old or younger. Always consult your health practitioner before starting a nutrition programme if you have any health concerns.

A CIP catalogue record for this book
is available from the British Library

ISBN 978-1-4053-3908-7

Colour reproduced by MDP, UK
Printed and bound in Hong Kong
by Sheck Wah Tong Printing Press Ltd

Discover more at
www.dk.com

Contents

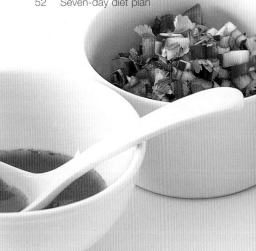

30-day diet plan

Plan for life

Recipes

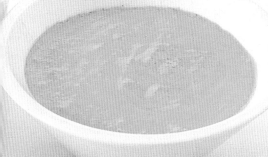
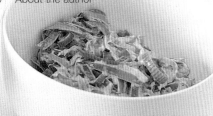

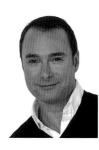

Introduction

In this age of diet-related health issues and celebrity obsession, we are all under pressure to "eat well". It's the driving force that motivates millions of us to look at what we're eating.

The greatest problem we face when it comes to weight issues is how to sort out the truth from information and advice that is commercially driven. Newspapers are full of features about weight loss, miracle nutrients, scientific breakthroughs and food labelling. They also carry horror stories of diet-related diseases and shortened life spans. Despite all this, we don't seem to make changes to our diet until we feel pressured to lose weight.

Social pressure

If you do eat well, then surely the outward manifestation of that is being slim, isn't it? I feel that the influence of social pressure goes further than that: if people are slim, we believe that they are "good", in control of their lives and thus to be admired. In our society, that's a mark of success.

Conversely, if you are overweight, does this signify that you are a bad person, out of control, to be scorned and pitied?

So what about the vast majority of us who try to eat well, or have dieted forever, but simply can't lose weight unless we eat next to nothing and exercise furiously? The millions of people who have battled with their weight for years – or even those of us who aren't obese, but feel we should just be a little slimmer – are understandably influenced by the pressure generated by the marketing and media aspects of the food industry.

It is always distressing to see people in my clinic whose feelings of self worth are directly tied in to what they weigh. To them, fat is bad, slim is good, and they experience these thoughts at some level every day. Therefore, when the next diet or wonder food is trumpeted, it's entirely understandable that they will leap at it, even if the diet may go against their natural instincts.

Marketing tactics

Imagine a business that had to create something new every single day, without exception, and present new ideas and products to its customers accordingly. If it didn't, it would risk losing the customers to a rival who is offering them what they want. That's what marketing and the media, in all its forms, constantly have to do. We buy magazines, read features, follow the diets, lose weight. If a diet is too successful, other publications will investigate how safe it is and bring any doubts about the diet to their readers' attention – and so another media source brings its influence to bear on what we think. This leaves us wanting a replacement for that diet and, sure enough, there is bound to be one. And if the media can attach a celebrity to a new diet, so much the better.

This constant bombardment of potentially conflicting information confuses the issues. Add in the social pressures to be slim and, all of a sudden, anyone who wants to lose weight just doesn't know what to eat anymore.

Food manufacturers and supermarkets have a duty of care to their shareholders to maximize profits and minimize costs. Some trade ethically, others less so, but still within the letter of the law (especially when it comes to food labelling).

These days, we are told that we lead very busy lives and are too busy to cook for ourselves, so we can now buy ready meals and snacks that the food industry terms "meal solutions". This is ironic, as one could argue that it's convenience foods that have partially created the "meal problem" in the first place. The marketing and labels are cleverly presented to appeal

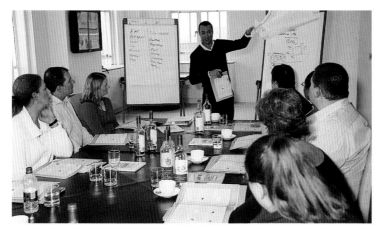

Telling it as it is
My job is to explain the basic science behind what happens to food after you eat it so that you can make better food choices.

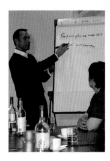

not only to the time-poor, but also to those of us who want fresh food that won't add to any weight problems. Better still, if the food has an aura of aiding weight loss, it has an increased value to us and we buy it more often. Take a moment to reflect on the ready foods you buy – diet or otherwise – which you could actually make yourself for next to nothing. I have found that even my busiest clients can make time to prepare simple, basic meals and snacks that form the foundation of a successful food plan.

Our metabolic rate

With all that in mind, how does The Food Doctor Diet differ? My plan works because you gain a healthy understanding of the real value of food and eat regularly; other diets ultimately fail because they are about deprivation. But what does this mean in terms of how our bodies work?

I believe that our lifestyles and history of dieting (be it in the extreme, or just too frequently) affect our metabolic rate, so any initial success at weight loss will be followed by a natural physiological response in our bodies: as our inbuilt metabolic rate senses famine, the weight loss slows or stops. We feel we must be doing something wrong, blame ourselves, and perpetuate any feelings of low self-worth we may have. We try harder by eating a little less or exercising a little harder, and thus trying to cheat our metabolism. It can't be done, but we are influenced to such a degree that we feel it can. So, it's back on the diet treadmill again – though, in the long run, we lose everything except the weight.

The science of energy

Energy cannot be created or destroyed; it merely changes its state. This is the basic law of energy. Thus the food we eat becomes glucose, which is used as fuel to make energy, and if our cells make full use of that glucose, no energy is changed into fat. It seems logical that if you eat more than you need, the surplus will be stored as fat and, conversely, eating less will force stored fat to be released. In practice, this doesn't always work as planned because of how we think and feel (our desires and goals cannot be separated from our physiology) and because of the numerous influences on our metabolism. Our metabolism dictates the speed at which we function. If you imagine this in terms of a car, its "metabolism" is a combination of the size of the car, the engine and the availability and quality of the fuel used.

When glucose levels in the blood exceed the body's needs (due to the amount of food we eat), they are first stored away in a water-based solution called glycogen. If glucose requirements increase, glycogen is released to meet the need and the water in which it was held is excreted. This reduction in hydration is one of the reasons why we lose weight quickly and urinate more when we first start a diet that does not provide optimum levels of fuel from food. In order to succeed with The Food Doctor Diet plan, we need to have a good understanding of some basic truths. So, a reduction in energy intake (i.e., food) will result in weight loss. The problem is that we don't cut our intake by, say, five per cent: offered the choice of a diet that could enable you to lose excess weight – say, two stone (12.7kg) – in a year, or one that promises the same results in two months, which one would you go for? If you are someone who has battled with weight issues for many years, then it's natural that you'd want to try the quickest diet.

When we take in too few calories, or expend too much energy, many things occur. If we eat too little, which is the only way that quick weight-loss promises can be fulfilled, then we alert our metabolic rate to potential famine, and it begins to behave accordingly. It will slow down the release of fat and trigger the adrenal glands to produce energy to make up the shortfall. However, we need a certain amount of energy to help us move around, so if you are a particular size, eating too little results in energy having to be released from elsewhere in the body to meet requirements. Fat isn't always the first choice as it's not easy to break down, and I have found that it is often people's adrenaline levels that increase instead.

Glucose-raising agents (GRA)

Bear in mind that it's not just eating food that raises our glucose levels. When we encounter stress, the adrenal glands are stimulated to secrete adrenaline, which may temporarily provide us with the energy we need to react to the situation. It's like the battery in the car, providing a separate source of energy that works independently of fuel levels. As there are countless stress triggers in modern life, this reaction is frequent, and it is common for the adrenal glands to be over-stimulated. Think of the mornings when you haven't eaten, but feel energetic and capable; by rights, you should feel tired and lethargic. Adrenaline is a wild card and we can't regulate it like we do with food.

Fat cells do not give up their contents easily: if we have too much adrenaline, our energy requirements are met, so the fat cells can often take this as a sign to stop releasing their stores. If the process of fat being released to be converted back into glucose is hindered or even halted by

---

The Food Doctor theory

Food converted into glucose is used by cells to make energy. Too much glucose is stored as fat, but on my plan you use up all the glucose as energy.

food
▽
glucose
▽
blood
▽
cells
▽   ▽
energy or fat

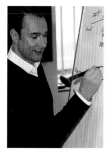

adrenaline being released, the total energy intake is now in excess of 100 per cent, so some of the food we eat must be stored as fat. Until the signal for the adrenal glands is switched off, this situation can perpetuate. The problem is that the signal isn't always reliable, as adrenal glands can become overly responsive due to almost constant stimuli. A major trigger of adrenaline is a result of low levels of glucose in the blood – something that can be regulated on The Food Doctor Diet plan.

Caffeine also provides short-term energy by blocking the action of a chemical called adensine in the brain. The pituitary gland senses a problem and tells the adrenal glands to secrete adrenaline to combat this block, leading to excess glucose and a subsequent low in energy levels.

So if you eat too little, are anxious or stressed or drink excess amounts of caffeine, you no longer lose weight. You then eat even less – and end up feeling fatigued, denying yourself food, developing cravings, and perpetuating metabolic issues: the moment you cut your calorie intake, you cut your metabolic rate. Thus the metabolism slows down into famine mode and tries to hold on to its fat.

How to eat well

The Food Doctor Diet plan minimizes the influence that GRAs create in several ways. Firstly, food groups are combined in the right proportions. When eaten alone, carbohydrates such as bread and potatoes are like a thin, runny fuel, which is converted into energy quickly. However, this energy runs out equally quickly, so we need to eat sooner. (If you're dieting and eating mainly carbohydrates, you apply willpower because you don't want to eat too much food, possibly triggering an adrenaline release.)

Complex carbohydrates create the equivalent of a thicker liquid, as they have a higher content of fibre that is harder to break down. Eaten alone, however, even complex carbohydrates are potentially too available (that is, too runny), so the energy is used relatively quickly and we feel hungry again. The simple addition of protein and fat at every meal means that

---

Why other diets fail

REDUCED CALORIE INTAKE	=	Less energy released, disrupted metabolic rate, raised adrenaline levels
RESULT	=	Unsustainable diet regime, fatigue, hunger cravings, slow or no further weight loss

Why The Food Doctor Diet works

SMALL REGULAR MEALS	=	Energy released consistently, active metabolic rate, reduced need for adrenaline
RESULT	=	High energy levels, no hunger cravings, steady weight loss

the energy produced is like a thick and gooey fuel, so it's released in a measured way. This gives steady glucose levels to feed cells evenly, and we have sufficient energy until the next intake of food.

Secondly, portion size is vital: eating the perfect amount of food in the right proportions to create the glucose we need – no more than that – and then eating again within three hours starts the process of retraining the metabolism to understand that you are in a time of just enough and not too much, and certainly not too little to trigger the famine mode. In short, you take in fuel in the morning, use it up, re-fuel mid-morning and again at lunch, snack time and lastly at dinner. Frequent, consistent meals of the ideal ratio and size will trigger weight loss that can be sustained.

Thirdly, using fresh food with maximum nutrient content means that you'll have a decreased risk of common diseases, better sleep and digestion and more energy. Lots of other things will change too, and not necessarily what you'd expect: you'll have better skin, hair and nails, your moods will improve and you will feel more in control of what and how to eat.

This book contains everything you need to know about the Food Doctor Diet. Follow the 7-day or the 30-day plan to establish good digestive health and kick-start your weight loss. If you wish to continue with a daily plan after completing the 7-day diet, you can go straight into week two of the 30-day diet. The Plan for Life, a long-term healthy eating plan, shows you how to apply my ten principles and change the way you eat, forever.

The truth is simple, and it works. Aside from the obvious issue of weight loss, my plan will benefit you in ways that most diets cannot match: you'll regulate your metabolic rate; you won't worry about passing fads; you'll eat well forever and never feel deprived; and you'll be in the best of health. Good luck!

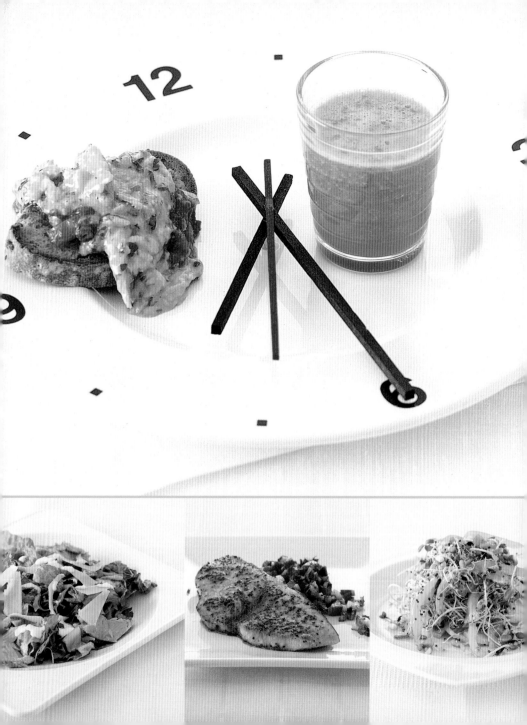

The 10 Principles

The 10 Food Doctor principles, my essential guidelines on how to eat, are based on some fascinating concepts. This chapter will show you how poor food choices and long-term or crash dieting can affect your insulin levels and metabolic rate. You can then, more importantly, discover why The Food Doctor Diet is the answer.

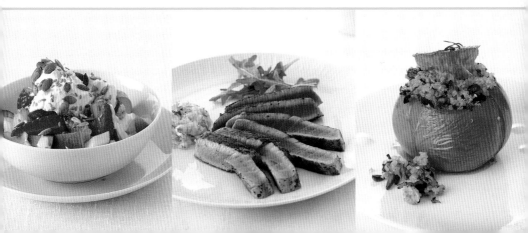

Principle 1
Eat protein with complex carbohydrates

The first Food Doctor principle is based on the fact that some foods are converted into glucose quickly while other foods take longer to be broken down. By understanding how to combine the right foods in the correct proportions, you will remain full of energy and still be able to lose weight.

Understanding the speed at which different foods are broken down into glucose for the body to use as fuel is crucial to The Food Doctor plan. Simple carbohydrates are quickly converted into glucose once they are digested, while protein and complex carbohydrates take longer to be broken down. The glycaemic index (GI) is a measure of how high blood-glucose levels rise after different foods have been digested. So if you eat only foods that have a slow conversion rate – in other words, a low GI score (*see pp.18–21*) – your body receives a steady supply of energy and prevents excess glucose being as fat.

Rather than having to remember the individual GI value of every food, there is an easier way to follow this principle. If you learn to combine the right proportions of protein and fibrous vegetables for every meal and snack, then this plan should work for you. The best way to begin to understand this concept is to look at the food on your plate and ask yourself, "Where is the protein?"

Complete proteins

Proteins contain amino acids, which are, in effect, the building blocks of the body. There are 22 amino acids in total, of which eight are classed as essential for adults as they cannot be generated by the body and must come from your diet. These essential amino acids, known as complete proteins, contain all the elements the body needs to generate the remaining amino acids. Examples of complete proteins are fish, tofu and eggs.

THE FOOD DOCTOR EQUATION

ANIMAL OR VEGETABLE
COMPLETE PROTEIN

STARCHY OR VEGETABLE
COMPLEX CARBOHYDRATES

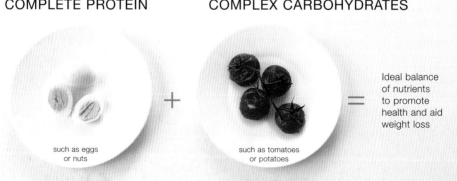

+   =   Ideal balance of nutrients to promote health and aid weight loss

such as eggs or nuts

such as tomatoes or potatoes

The right combination?

protein 0%

complex carbohydrates 90%
of which starch 80%, vegetables 10%

simple carbohydrates 0%

vegetable fat 10%

low in fibre

Wholewheat pasta with tomato sauce

Although this meal looks healthy, there is no source of protein and the fibre content is low. The proportion of vegetable carbohydrates to starchy carbohydrates in the form of wholewheat pasta is also far too low.

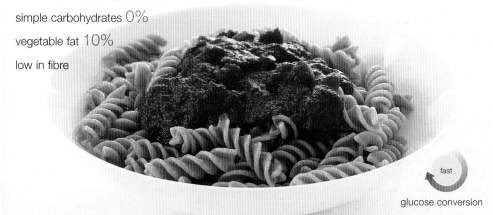

fast

glucose conversion

protein 40%

complex carbohydrates 50%
of which starch 10%, vegetables 40%

simple carbohydrates 0%

vegetable fat 10%

high in fibre

Salmon with broccoli, mangetout and wholewheat pasta

Fish provides the correct amount of protein in this meal, while the proportion of complex vegetable carbohydrates to complex starchy carbohydrates is balanced and the fibre content is substantial.

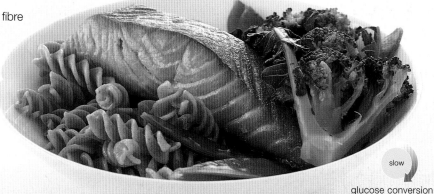

slow

glucose conversion

Complex versus simple carbohydrates

In the same way that there are two types of protein – complete and incomplete – there are also two types of carbohydrate. A complex carbohydrate is so-called because its natural form has not been interfered with or changed in any way, or, if it has been processed at all, it is by a minimal amount. In contrast, a simple carbohydrate has been processed into a refined product and its fibre is lost. For example, if wheat grain is gently processed into wholemeal bread, it remains a complex carbohydrate. If the grain is polished further, it becomes a refined product, white bread, which is classed as a simple carbohydrate. The same is true of brown rice and pasta compared to white rice and pasta, or an unsweetened muesli mix compared to a sugared, processed cereal.

When we think of carbohydrates we tend to think of starchy foods such as bread or potatoes, forgetting that fruits and vegetables are also carbohydrates. Complex vegetable carbohydrates are usually dense or green and leafy, such as broccoli and spinach. Some fruits, however, can be classed as simple carbohydrates if they have a low fibre content to start with. Since these fruits contain relatively little fibre to slow down the conversion rate to

The correct proportions?

Lunch proportions

This lunchtime meal shows the ideal ratio of protein to complex carbohydrates. The size of chicken breast you should eat must be a little smaller than the palm of your hand, while vegetables should make up the largest proportion of complex carbohydrates on your plate. This balance of foods should supply you with enough nutrients and energy until your mid-afternoon snack.

40% complex carbohydrates
as vegetables

40% protein
as chicken

20% complex carbohydrates
as brown rice

glucose, and are naturally high in sugar *(see pp.32–33),* they are broken down quickly inside the body. Examples of these fruits include watermelon and honeydew melon.

Correct ratios

By choosing the correct proportions of complete protein and complex carbohydrates, you can benefit from the energy generated by the slow release of glucose created from each meal or snack right up until it's time to eat again. And as complex carbohydrates contain plenty of fibre, each meal or snack helps to promote good digestive health, as well as energy and weight loss.

How do I get the proportions right?

Rather than having to weigh all your food, the portion of protein you should eat is a little smaller than the size of the palm of your hand. A piece of, say, chicken breast this size will supply 30–40 per cent of the total amount of food on your plate – the right protein requirement for an average person. However, we all require slightly differing amounts of protein and I have found that as much as 40–50 per cent protein works for me; you may thrive on less, or perhaps more. Complex carbohydrates complete the meal, although vegetables must, without fail, make up at least 60 per cent of these carbohydrates.

Dinner is different

There is just one exception to the rule about meal proportions. If you eat later on in the evening, I suggest that you avoid starchy carbohydrates altogether, since you won't use the energy they create. This means adding extra protein and vegetables to your evening meal so that the ratios are nearer to 50 per cent protein and 50 per cent vegetables.

I also recommend keeping a little portion of food back from your meal to snack on later – even if it's just a mouthful or two – to avoid those late night cravings with which you may be familiar.

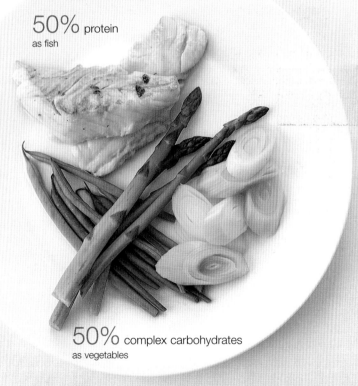

50% protein
as fish

50% complex carbohydrates
as vegetables

Protein profiles

The proteins that I recommend you should eat on the Plan for Life are all lean proteins, and are what is known as "complete". Remember that complete proteins cannot be generated by the body and must therefore come from your diet. The lean protein foods in the ideal category (*see chart, below*) contain all the essential amino acids.

Can I eat red meat?

I do not consider red meat to be a lean protein as it contains a higher proportion of saturated fats than, for example, skinless poultry. Saturated fats are not ideal for overall digestive health as they may promote the proliferation of unfriendly bacteria and yeasts in the intestines. However, red meat is classed as a complete protein and it is a good source of minerals, so eating red meat two or, if absolutely necessary, three times a week is a good way of maintaining some variety and interest in your choice of proteins.

Can I eat too much protein?

There is controversy as to whether you can eat too much protein, not least because diet plans based on 100 per cent protein plans do lead to weight loss – although the long-term cost to overall health is not yet fully understood. Too much protein can lead to a situation in which minerals are released from the bones to counteract the acidity of the blood. This is a natural occurrence when excess protein is eaten and can lead to reduced bone density. In addition, kidney damage is a risk for some individuals as the kidneys must cope with the added strain of breaking down large amounts of protein. Pure-protein diets are, by nature, low in fresh produce, so fibre and antioxidant intake is low as well.

A pure-protein diet is precisely the opposite of The Food Doctor plan, which has been designed to enhance digestive health and includes only about 40 per cent protein to meet most people's dietary requirements.

WHAT IS THE GLYCAEMIC INDEX?

The Glycaemic Index (GI) is, in effect, a list of the sugar content of foods. As a general rule, proteins and fats have low GI scores because the body takes longer to break them down into glucose. Carbohydrates have higher scores as they are broken down more rapidly.

Carbohydrates fall into two categories: simple and complex. Simple carbohydrates have had their fibre removed, while the fibre of complex carbohydrates remains intact. For example, apple juice is a simple carbohydrate because it is converted rapidly from food to glucose, but a whole apple remains a complex carbohydrate. The quicker the conversion, the higher the GI score (*see pp.20–21*). So the juice has a high score and the fruit has a low score.

	MEAT & POULTRY
Ideal choice These foods are all complete proteins and are therefore the best choice.	Duck eggs Hens' eggs Quails' eggs Calves' liver Lambs' liver Skinless chicken Skinless turkey Veal
Good choice You can include these food choices frequently as part of a healthy diet.	
Adequate choice Eat these foods occasionally.	Bacon Mince Beef Pork chops Ham Lamb chops

Why is fish so good for you?

Fish really does offer the best of both worlds. Not only is it an ideal source of protein, it is also rich in omega-3 essential fats. These fats have many functions in the body, but in terms of weight loss research has shown that such fats promote rather than hinder weight loss. Omega-3 fats also have an important role in promoting cardiovascular health, reducing the risk of Type 2 diabetes and enhancing brain function.

DAIRY	VEGETARIAN	FISH			
	Chick-peas	Anchovy	Gurnard	Marlin*	Sea bream
	Lentils	Bluefish*	Haddock	Monkfish	Skate
	Nuts (raw)	Bream	Hake	Orange roughy	Sprat*
	Quinoa	Brill	Halibut*	Perch*	Swordfish*
	Quorn	Carp*	Herring*	Plaice	Trout*
	Pumpkin seeds	Cod	Hoki	Red mullet*	Tuna*
	Sesame seeds	Dover sole	Lemon sole	Salmon*	Turbot
	Sunflower seeds	Eel*	Mackerel*	Sardine*	Whitebait*
	Tofu	Grey Mullet*	Mahi Mahi*	Sea bass	Whiting
Low-fat cottage cheese Low-fat live natural yoghurt	Baked beans (unsweetened)				
Full-fat yoghurt Hard cheese					

*Also a good source of omega-3 fats

Carbohydrate profiles

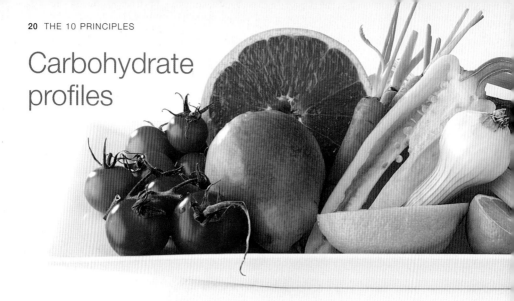

	GRAIN-BASED FOODS	**FRUITS**	
Ideal choice The complex carbohydrates at this level are ideal choices because they supply high levels of energy for longer *(see p.16)*. They are all broken down slowly into glucose by the body so they have a low GI score.	Barley Oatmeal Wholegrain rye bread	Apples Apricots (fresh) Blackberries Cranberries Grapefruit Lemons Limes	Pears Plums Strawberries
Good choice The foods in this category have a medium GI score and so they provide reasonably good levels of energy at a fairly steady rate.	Brown rice Couscous Granola bars containing nuts Pumpernickel bread Wholemeal bread Wholewheat pasta and spaghetti	Blueberries Cherries Grapes Loganberries Mangoes Oranges Papayas	Peaches Pineapples Tangerines
Adequate choice These carbohydrates are either refined, low in fibre, high in sugar or a combination of all three. As a result, they have a high GI score and provide only short-term energy.	Bagels Biscuits Breadsticks Breakfast cereals Croissants Doughnuts French bread Melba toast Muffins White bread White pasta and spaghetti White rice	Bananas Dried fruit Figs Fruit juices Prunes	

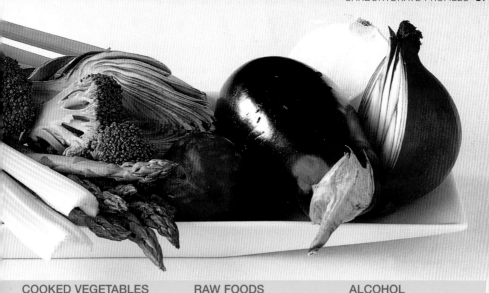

COOKED VEGETABLES

Artichokes
Asparagus
Broccoli
Brussels sprouts
Cabbage
Cauliflower
Greens
Kale

Leeks
Onions
Pak choi
Peppers
Spinach
String beans

Carrots
Courgettes
Kidney beans
Pumpkin
Turnips
Yellow squash

Aubergines
Parsnips
Peas
Potatoes (baked,
  boiled, mashed)
Squash

Sweet potatoes
Yams

RAW FOODS

Bean-sprouts
Mushrooms
Raw sprouted seeds and beans
Tomatoes
Various salad leaves

Avocados
Beetroot
Carrots
Celeriac
Olives

ALCOHOL

Beer
Spirits
Wine

Principle 2
Stay hydrated

We all know how important it is to drink plenty of water, and you should aim to drink at least six generously sized glasses or more of water a day. Water is also the best thirst-quencher; other beverages can only quench your thirst in proportion to the amount of water they contain.

There can be no doubt that keeping your fluid intake consistently high is imperative in order to aid weight loss. So does that mean drinking plain water only throughout the day? Many people ask me whether the water in tea, coffee, canned drinks, alcohol, juices and soups can count towards this fluid intake.

Regular tea and coffee contain caffeine, which has a mild diuretic effect and reduces overall hydration. So these drinks do not count towards your required fluid intake. Canned drinks, most of which are carbonated and probably sugared too, also don't count. Soups and juices do, but nothing beats water. Drink at least a litre and a half of water a day in addition to other liquids.

Limit your alcohol intake

Alcohol can have a detrimental effect on any weight-loss programme. Alcohol is a fermented product and as such can affect the levels of beneficial bacteria in the intestines. It's also defined as a simple sugar, so it affects glucose levels quite rapidly – added to which it also acts as a dehydrating element.

The final blow is that alcohol reduces your resolve. In other words, even if you are following all ten principles and succeeding in your weight-loss plan, after a glass of alcohol your thoughts may wander to sugary, fatty foods, which can undermine all your good efforts. Having said that, alcohol is a part of life and can be an enjoyable social pastime, so there is a way to slot it into The Food Doctor plan. I suggest that you drink alcohol no more than three times a week and that you limit yourself to two glasses of wine or two measures of spirits without mixers, which are highly sugared. If you have been used to drinking alcohol most days of the week, cutting down to a

maximum of two or three times a week is an important first step. Wine is the best choice – although stay away from sweet wines – followed by pure vodka mixed with plenty of mineral water, ice and a squeeze of fresh lime juice (avoid lime cordial as this is also highly sugared). I do not recommend beers, stouts, lagers, or cider, all of which contain yeast, if not sugar, and can be detrimental to your overall digestive health.

Avoid salt

Excess salt intake can contribute to thirst, and the most likely sources of salt in the modern diet are ready-made meals. Since my weight-loss plan does not include such foods, your salt intake will automatically reduce. Stop adding salt in cooking or to your food, and use herbs (either dried or fresh), freshly ground black pepper or sugar-free mustards to flavour foods instead.

ALCOHOL: THE GOLDEN RULES

1 Never drink alcohol on an empty stomach. Drinking alcohol with food is preferable, so have your first drink when you start your meal to reduce the absorption of alcohol.

2 Drink alcohol no more than three times a week – preferably less.

3 Mix spirits with water and ice, not mixers or fruit juices.

4 Do not drink alcohol on two consecutive days.

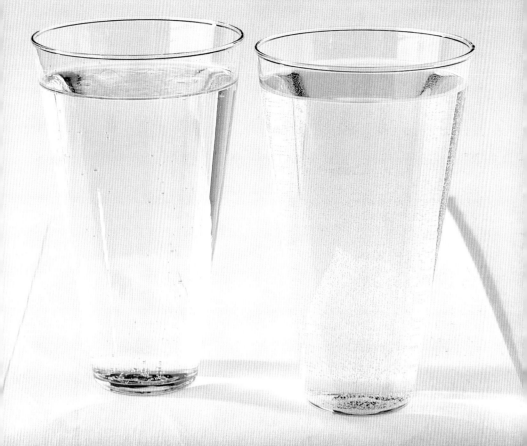

Tap or bottled water?

With regard to weight loss, there is little difference between choosing tap, bottled mineral or filtered water to drink as long as you ensure that you drink at least one litre of plain water a day in addition to juices and soups (totalling at least one and a half litres a day). This figure should be increased when you are exercising or during hot weather.

Still, rather than sparkling, water is my preferred choice of bottled mineral water as the gas contained in sparkling water can encourage bloating and discomfort in the gut.

Principle 3
Eat a wide variety of food

If you have a long-term weight issue, it's very possible that some foods have, over time, become off-limits in your mind, while you have grown to consider other foods "safe". This often tends to limit the range of foods you buy to just those that you feel most comfortable eating.

When I ask new clients to keep a food diary of their eating habits for a few days, all too often I am struck by the fact that they eat the same food nearly every day. In fact, for 90 per cent of the time most of us tend to buy the same small percentage – as little as 10 per cent – of foods available to us. We invariably shop, select and order food almost as if we are on autopilot, buying identical products week in, week out. Likewise, many weight-loss plans focus purely on a small group of foods. Perhaps in the past you have found that such dieting plans initially seem to work well when you eat the same food every day? Yet this strategy eventually makes any plan hard to follow, since you inevitably become bored and seek out foods from the so-called "forbidden list" that you know will satisfy you instead.

Why variety is important

It's vital that we eat a wide variety of foods in order to benefit from the wonderful array of nutrients that food offers. And in order to encourage a healthy relationship with food, I suggest that you be brave and try one new food every week. Some of the ideal foods listed in the proteins and carbohydrates charts (see pp.18–21) may be new to you, in which case I hope that you will try them. Similarly, although some of the ingredients listed in the recipe section may not be familiar to you, please do try them: you may develop a taste for exciting new flavours and enjoy broadening your experience of foods.

So next time you are in the supermarket or at your local food market, buy something you have never tried before. You might want to flick through a recipe book first to look for something that appeals to you, or ask your shopkeeper how to cook what you have bought.

I am sure that once you begin to try a range of new foods you will enjoy eating many of them. and add them regularly to your usual shopping list, thus making the meals you eat more varied and interesting.

The issue of grains

You may notice that grain-based foods do not feature heavily in the Diets, and nor do they appear much in the long-term Plan for Life. The reason is that some grains contain elements that can easily aggravate the sensitive lining of the digestive tract.

FOOD INTOLERANCE

There is much discussion these days about how many wheat and dairy products people should eat. While I don't think that avoiding either food is altogether necessary for everyone, there is a strong case for becoming aware of just how much of one food you might be eating and whether it is causing inflammation in your intestines (see box, p.26). You may have a food intolerance if you suffer from any of the following symptoms:

- Bloating
- Irritable bowel syndrome (IBS)
- Dark circles under the eyes
- Excessive flatulence
- Runny nose
- Fatigue

Do you buy the same food every week?

It's all too easy to become rooted in our shopping habits and repeatedly buy the same foods that we know and rely on. Ideally, however, we should all aim to eat one new food a week, be it a vegetable, fruit, grain, legume or herb.

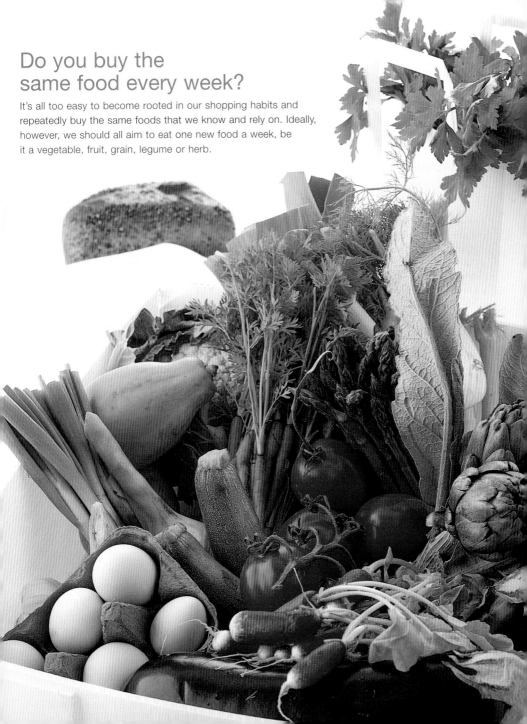

Gluten grains

Wheat, rye, barley and oats are known as gluten grains because they all contain "gliadin" in varying amounts. Gliadin is a substance found in gluten grains that can irritate the lining of the intestinal tract. Gluten is a sticky substance that helps to trap the air in bread, ensuring that it expands and has the correct feel. In recent years, grains have been cross-bred to produce new variants with a higher gluten content. If you look at the grain family tree (*see below*), you will notice that wheat, barley, oats and rye are closely related, and rice slightly less so, while corn, millet and cane sugar are from the other side of the family.

Over the years, I have worked with many clients who have benefited enormously from minimizing their intake of grains, especially those containing gluten. Having said that, grains are included in small amounts in both the Diets and the Plan for Life because they are good sources of fibre and are rich in B vitamins, both of which aid weight loss. So do eat some wheat products, but keep the amounts as low as you can. Where possible, try to vary your grains. For example, buy 100 per cent rye bread one week, yeast-free soda bread the next and wholegrain brown bread the week after that.

White pasta, made from refined wheat, is often served and eaten in large quantities. If you want to eat pasta, have a few strands as part of a meal – much as you would have some potatoes or a spoonful of rice. Avoid eating a whole bowl of pasta, even if it's just a starter. When you shop, buy wholewheat pasta, which is a complex carbohydrate, or try products made from corn or rice flour (a word of warning: they do not have the same consistency as wheat pasta and are more likely to be soft than *al dente*).

WHEAT AND WEIGHT PROBLEMS

There does seem to be a link between wheat intake and weight problems for some people. Wheat contains around 45 per cent gliadin, the substance that can cause irritation and lead to mild inflammation of the lining of the gut. If you think that wheat may be linked to any digestive problems you have, visit an appropriate nutrition professional for advice. Even if you do not have a food intolerance, vary your intake of grains weekly.

THE RELATIONSHIP OF MAJOR CEREAL GRAINS

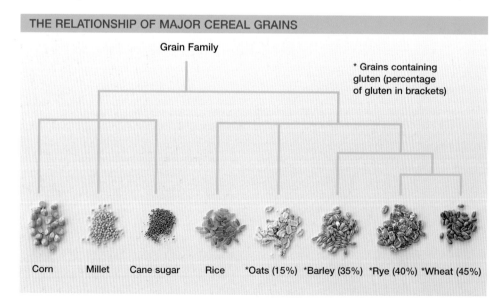

Grain Family

* Grains containing gluten (percentage of gluten in brackets)

Corn   Millet   Cane sugar   Rice   *Oats (15%)   *Barley (35%)   *Rye (40%)   *Wheat (45%)

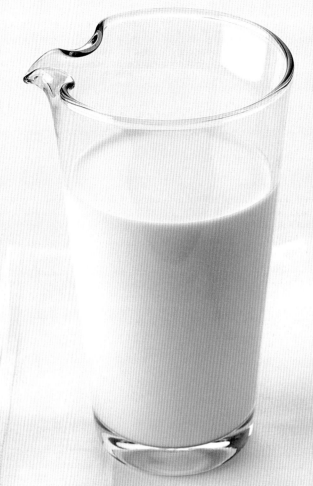

How much dairy should I have?

Many diets exclude dairy products but, as my aim is to encourage you to eat a wide variety of foods, I suggest that you include dairy products from time to time. If you are concerned about the possibility of food intolerance from dairy products, you need to vary the dairy products you eat at home, so that day to day you don't have too much of, say, cows' milk. If you follow this advice, you needn't be worried about avoiding dishes with cows' milk when you dine out.

Principle 4
Fuel up frequently

You are probably becoming used to the idea that if you eat the right amount of food combinations that are broken down into glucose slowly, you will create a consistent supply of energy and still be able to lose weight. But it's not just the foods and amounts that are important, it's the timing too.

Eating little and often is a crucial element of my plan. By eating the right foods and snacks at regular intervals through the day, you should be able to keep your energy levels constant so that you can function well without food cravings – the downfall of so many dieters.

The benefits explained

In the same way that you need to eat proteins with complex carbohydrates to maximize the benefits of a healthy diet and minimize the frequency of insulin production, so fuelling up frequently ensures that a

ENERGY TIMELINE

The pink line on this energy timeline depicts the range of highs and lows that a typical person will experience through the day. Set against those peaks and troughs is the stabilizing green line of The Food Doctor plan, which illustrates how eating the right foods at certain times can help you avoid the lows that might otherwise occur, and keep your energy level constant.

This breakfast of natural yoghurt, seeds and pear tops up your energy levels after a night's sleep.

A snack of cold vegetable omelette left over from last night's supper keeps you going through the morning

THE FOOD DOCTOR PLAN

AVERAGE DIET

Processed cereal for breakfast sends your blood-glucose levels soaring, then soon leaves you hungry again.

A piece of fruit such as a watermelon is high in sugar and low in fibre, and so makes an insubstantial snack.

08:00   09:00   10:00   11:00   12:00

steady supply of glucose enters the bloodstream to be converted into energy. Together, these two factors create a potent mix of the right food at the right time, leading to effective weight loss and stable energy levels.

How it works in practice

Within two hours of eating breakfast your blood-glucose levels begin to drop. These levels continue to diminish until they reach a low point that the body interprets as hunger. There is an optimal period of time just before you begin to feel the pangs of hunger, and it is during this time that eating something satisfying and healthy will make all the difference to your energy levels. This may mean that you have to teach yourself to recognize the first signs of hunger, which can take a number of forms ranging from loss of concentration to feeling slightly shaky. If you have dieted previously, you

will be familiar with the big mid-morning dip depicted in the diagram below. If, however, you follow The Food Doctor plan and choose to eat an appropriate snack *(see pp.210–211)* mid-way through the morning, you will be able to combat a slight dip in energy levels and any associated symptoms of hunger.

Ideally, you should eat approximately every two or three hours through the day. So you need to eat a proper lunch and another healthy snack in the middle of the afternoon before your evening meal.

Think of this principle as the equivalent of filling up your car with just enough premium grade fuel to last you to the next filling station, and then doing the same again and again throughout the day. In this way you can combat hunger pangs and bad food choices, minimize insulin production, maximize your energy levels and lose weight, all at the same time.

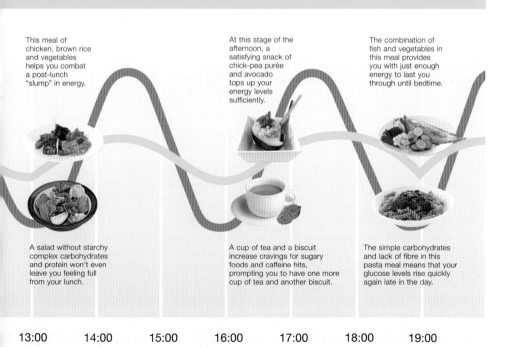

This meal of chicken, brown rice and vegetables helps you combat a post-lunch "slump" in energy.

At this stage of the afternoon, a satisfying snack of chick-pea purée and avocado tops up your energy levels sufficiently.

The combination of fish and vegetables in this meal provides you with just enough energy to last you through until bedtime.

A salad without starchy complex carbohydrates and protein won't even leave you feeling full from your lunch.

A cup of tea and a biscuit increase cravings for sugary foods and caffeine hits, prompting you to have one more cup of tea and another biscuit.

The simple carbohydrates and lack of fibre in this pasta meal means that your glucose levels rise quickly again late in the day.

| 13:00 | 14:00 | 15:00 | 16:00 | 17:00 | 18:00 | 19:00 |

Principle 5
Eat breakfast

Unlike many diets that leave you hungry and craving forbidden foods, this diet plan promotes eating little and often as the key to keeping your energy levels consistent and achieving successful weight loss. So it is essential that at the start of each day you eat a healthy breakfast.

Skipping any meal is one step to failure, and by far the worst meal to skip is breakfast. You may not have much of an appetite first thing and I appreciate that mornings can be stressful with kids to organize as well as getting yourself ready for work, but investing time in eating breakfast is fundamental to losing weight.

Time for a change

If you are the sort of person who has a cup of tea or coffee and a bowl of processed breakfast cereal to kick-start your day, then the time has come to make some changes to your diet.

Let's look at what this typical breakfast does to your body. The cereal almost certainly lacks protein. It is converted into glucose rapidly by the body, and so produces only short-term energy. Coupled with the caffeine, it may make you feel satisfied, but only for a short time. If you eat breakfast at 8am, by 10am it is likely that you will experience an energy slump, which is perceived as hunger. If you have another cup of coffee and a biscuit or two, the whole cycle starts again. As the Food Doctor plan is designed to help you feel energetic and reduce hunger pangs, your intake of caffeinated drinks and sugary foods should be kept to a minimum.

A better approach

Eating the right foods little and often is the key to increased energy and sustained weight loss. If you eat a healthy breakfast, such as muesli or natural yoghurt with fruit and seeds, you shouldn't feel hungry until 10.30–11am, which is the best time to eat a snack in order to sustain your energy levels. These types of breakfasts are easy to prepare and have the right

combination of food groups: the nuts, seeds and yoghurt provide your body with plenty of protein and the wholegrains are rich in complex carbohydrates. If you do not enjoy yoghurt or muesli, there are many other healthy options for breakfast, including eggs, toast, crackers, fruit and smoothies. See pages 204–205 for a range of suggestions to inspire you. Whatever you decide to eat, remember that taking a few minutes to eat a good breakfast is essential and sets the scene for the rest of the day.

CAN I HAVE COFFEE?

I love coffee and I feel that no morning is complete without it. As long as you have coffee with or after a meal or snack containing protein and fibre, you should be able to keep your energy levels high. However, do not have more than one or two cups a day because caffeine stimulates your adrenal glands to produce adrenaline. This is the same response your body has under stress, and is part of what is known as the "flight or fight" response – providing short-term energy, a heightened sense of sight and hearing and quickened responses. Once the "danger" has passed, adrenaline production stops, energy levels drop and you may experience fatigue and hunger, which in turn encourages you to make poor food choices. Try to limit yourself to one cup a day, and don't add sugar to your drink.

Is your breakfast balanced?

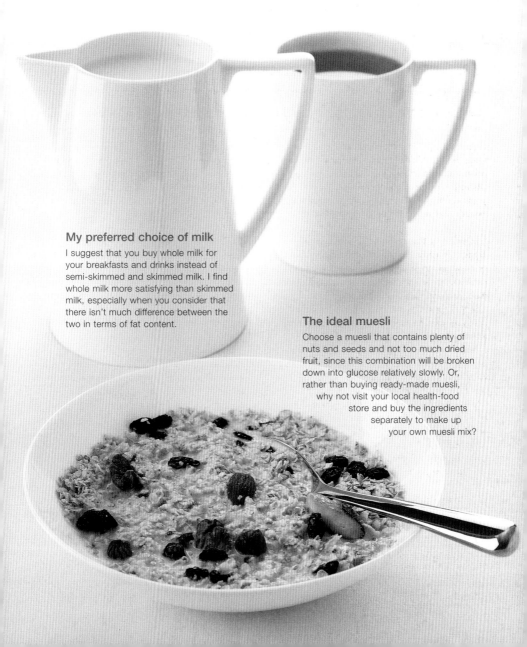

My preferred choice of milk

I suggest that you buy whole milk for your breakfasts and drinks instead of semi-skimmed and skimmed milk. I find whole milk more satisfying than skimmed milk, especially when you consider that there isn't much difference between the two in terms of fat content.

The ideal muesli

Choose a muesli that contains plenty of nuts and seeds and not too much dried fruit, since this combination will be broken down into glucose relatively slowly. Or, rather than buying ready-made muesli, why not visit your local health-food store and buy the ingredients separately to make up your own muesli mix?

Principle 6
Avoid sugar

I believe that sugar is just as much to blame for weight gain as is fat. You will benefit enormously by cutting down on the amount of sugar in your diet and, as The Food Doctor plan is designed to help you achieve good digestive health, avoiding sugar takes on added importance.

It is worth explaining exactly what I mean by the word "sugar". There are many variations on the white or brown granules that you buy in packets, such as sorbitol, malt and even honey (*see box, below*). With so many different names for sugar, it's no wonder that most people have little idea just how much of it may be present in their diet.

The aim of limiting your sugar intake is to reduce the amount and frequency of insulin secretion in the body. Sugar in all its forms is broken down by the digestive system into glucose extremely quickly. As the blood-glucose levels suddenly rise high in response, they trigger the production of insulin, which in turn forces the glucose levels down again by converting the glucose into fat through a series of biochemical changes. This is the reason why we need to minimize insulin production if we want to lose weight. Foods that are converted into glucose rapidly should be avoided or, at the very least, combined with those that are broken down at a slower rate.

The fat-free myth
Sugars of one kind or another are almost always added to processed and ready-made foods, and it's not uncommon for a product to contain several different types of sugar. The more sugar there is in a product, the less fat it contains, which allows manufacturers to claim that it is low in fat or that it contains less than a certain percentage of fat. In reality, this means that in your desire to lose weight you buy, for example, a product that is labelled 95 per cent fat-free. You have probably done so for years. So why don't you become the thin person you want to be when all you eat is this type of food? The answer is that the sugars in these products are always higher when the fat content has been decreased.

How the theory works
Let's see how this theory works in practice. You choose a low-fat muffin for breakfast or a snack (*see right*). As its sugar content is higher than that of a regular muffin your blood-glucose levels rise sharply and fall quickly, leaving you hungry again all too soon. You battle with your food cravings, give in and eat another low-fat snack.

If you eat a meal or snack containing complete protein and complex carbohydrates (*see pp.14–21*), the insulin produced is minimal by comparison. Your prolonged energy levels and reduced hunger pangs even enable you to make sensible choices about what to eat next.

ALTERNATIVE NAMES FOR SUGAR

Although these substances are derived from a variety of sources, they are all classed as sugars.

- Sucrose
- Mannitol
- Glucose
- Honey
- Lactose
- Fructose
- Sorbitol
- Corn syrup
- Malt
- Malt extract
- Maltose
- Rice syrup
- Rice extract
- Molasses
- Golden syrup
- Invert sugar

Can I use artificial sweeteners instead?

Sweeteners are usually added to so-called diet drinks and processed foods. In The Food Doctor plan you won't be eating any of these foods, so the issue of sweeteners shouldn't come up. If you add sweeteners to your tea and coffee, I suggest that you try to stop. Sweeteners have no nutritional value and can affect the overall benefits of the plan by perpetuating any cravings you might have for sweet foods.

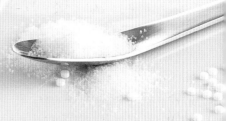

Which is the best option?

If you choose to eat a low-fat muffin, its calorie count may be low but check its sugar content against a regular muffin. The low-fat muffin almost certainly contains a higher percentage of sugars, and thus it is classed as a simple carbohydrate. The body can convert it from food to glucose with ease. As a result, blood-glucose levels rise and insulin is released, which in turn increases fat stores in the body.

Full-fat cranberry muffin

A full-fat muffin is typically made of white flour, sugar and fat. Any fruit, such as cranberries, or fibre, such as bran, supplies a small amount of complex carbohydrates.

simple carbohydrates 80%
of which sugar 40%, white flour 40%

vegetable fat 15%

complex carbohydrates 5%

Low-fat cranberry muffin

This low-fat muffin may now contain less saturated fat, but to compensate far more sugar has been added during the manufacturing process.

simple carbohydrates 90%
of which sugar 60%, white flour 40%

vegetable fat 5%

complex carbohydrates 5%

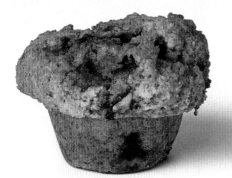

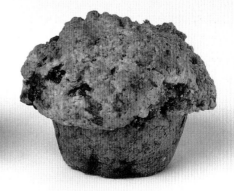

Principle 7
Exercise is essential

A weight-loss programme will not prove to be very successful if you don't exercise, just as exercising frequently while eating the wrong foods isn't likely to result in a healthier lifestyle either. Even with the busiest schedule there is time to do more if you want to, so make exercise a priority.

My expertise is in food, not in exercise, but I do know that the benefits of exercising are far-reaching, and not just in the area of weight-loss. A regular exercise programme can help reduce the risk of cardiovascular disease, osteoporosis and Type 2 diabetes. Exercise can even help you cope with stress more effectively.

Adjusting your metabolic rate

Exercise increases your metabolic rate, that is, the speed at which your body uses up food as energy. Likewise, the aim of exercise in the context of The Food Doctor plan is to increase the rate at which the food you eat, and any stores of fat, are utilized for energy.

Remember that this eating plan relies on supplying premium-grade fuel in the form of whole foods to the body, where it is converted into glucose and circulated in the bloodstream to cells to be used as fuel for energy production. On my plan the rate of glucose entering the cells is steady enough to keep energy levels consistent and avoid lows (which we interpret as hunger).

However, it is possible to influence how that glucose, or fuel, is managed at cellular level. In each cell there is a tiny power plant, called a mitochondria, which effectively converts the glucose into energy. Cells are amazingly advanced structures that respond to requirement, so if you increase your energy output, the cells respond accordingly by creating more of these tiny mitochondria in each cell to make yet more energy. Thus you can affect how much glucose is used up as energy. Exercising encourages this smooth conversion of glucose into energy because consistent and increased energy helps your body burn off that unwanted fat.

What sort of exercise is best?

I am a firm believer that you should always consult an appropriate professional if you need advice about what sort of exercise to undertake. I wouldn't suggest taking nutritional advice from instructors else unless they are fully qualified, and since I am not an expert in exercise I only make suggestions as to what might suit you.

If you decide to join a gym, ask a trained instructor to help you devise a simple routine that you can stick to and enjoy, since I have found that, even with the best intentions, the gym can sometimes become boring after a while. Try to vary your exercise routine, or exercise with a friend who has similar goals to your own. This makes it more fun, and you can chat as you exercise.

Depending on your current level of fitness, you could also try jogging, aerobic classes, swimming, walking the dog or playing football, tennis or squash. The list is endless.

If the thought of exercising is abhorrent to you, then start off gently. Try walking to your local shops every other day instead of taking the car, or getting off the bus or train a stop early on the way to work and walking briskly the rest of the way. As long as you exercise for a minimum of 30 minutes, three times a week, the exercise you choose isn't that important. You needn't punish yourself in the gym. Instead you must raise your heartbeat to a level at which you break out in a sweat at some point over the half hour, but while still being able to continue a conversation.

So, be creative with your choice of exercise because the benefits are many and because your progress with The Food Doctor plan will be greatly enhanced.

What to eat after exercise?

You may well find that you feel hungrier if you are exercising regularly. I suggest that you increase your portion sizes a little at mealtimes to match this, but by no more than ten per cent. You should also ensure that you have appropriate snacks to eat immediately after you have exercised: it is especially important to replenish spent glucose levels after any exercise, so eat something that contains complex carbohydrates as well as protein, such as a cereal bar that contains oats, fruit, nuts and seeds

Which type of exercise?

The bottom line is that you must be physically active, be it swimming, jogging, playing tennis, football, squash, going to the gym or simply walking. You should aim to complete at least 30 minutes of any form of exercise three times a week or more. This will help to raise your metabolic rate and improve your overall digestion, helping you to get rid of any fat stores that you have accumulated.

Principle 8
Follow the 80:20 rule

Perhaps you have followed diets in the past that revolve around sticking to the prescribed plan 100 per cent of the time. The problem is that it's in our nature to veer off course after a while – usually out of frustration or boredom – hence the all-important 80:20 rule.

The Food Doctor plan encourages you to eat little and often so that your hunger pangs are minimized and you are unlikely to suffer from food cravings.

However, life just isn't that easy, as we all know, and from time to time you will eat out of line with the plan. I know that however many practical suggestions for coping with special occasions, interesting recipes or sound advice this book contains, there will be times when nothing will work for you apart from your chosen treat, be it chocolate cake, sweets or ice cream. The good news is that this is entirely possible, within reason.

Putting the rule into practice

So what constitutes the 80:20 rule? If you follow the Plan for Life principles – such as combining the right food groups and avoiding refined carbohydrates and sugars – as closely as possible, then I believe that your food will satisfy you and your success rate will be high.

By eating regularly to keep blood-glucose levels more even, you won't want to eat the sort of foods you probably see as treats now. Yet the experience of eating goes further than just supplying energy. Follow the plan for 80 per cent of the time and you will still achieve success, albeit more slowly. For example, if you eat healthily through the day, you can save your remaining 20 per cent for when you are out to dinner or at a party. There is more information about this in special situations *(see pp.224–227)*.

Try not to veer from The Food Doctor plan every day as this could create a habit in which you crave the wrong types of food. As a consequence, eating in line with the Plan for Life will become harder to do and the possibility of slipping back into old habits increases. On average, use the 80:20 rule to treat yourself two or three times a week, perhaps taking into account any situations you may have coming up that mean you can't eat what you would ideally like.

EATING OUT

When you have a choice about where to eat, stick to a restaurant or café that you know will enable you to eat in line with the Plan for Life principles. It's possible to eat well nearly everywhere as long as you keep food proportions in your mind when ordering. For example, have a vegetable-based starter without pastry and a complete protein for your main course. If you have no choice as to the venue, then hopefully you can allocate your 20 per cent quota to this meal. If not, then eat as carefully as you can and make up for it later.

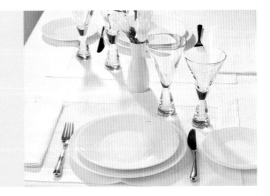

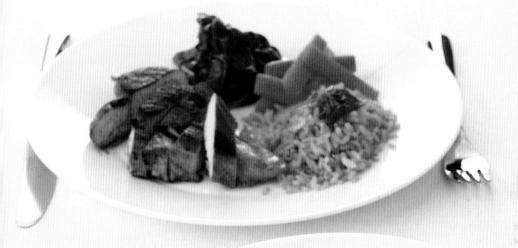

What can I do about chocolate?

Chocolate tends to be by far the one food that is craved more than any other, and it can be the downfall of so many dieters. Here are some guidelines to follow:

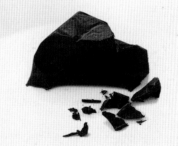

- The pleasure in eating chocolate should come from the flavour of the bean, not from the fats and sugar that make up around 80 per cent of many popular brands.

- If you crave chocolate, eat a couple of squares of the richest, darkest variety you can find – preferably one that contains more than 70 per cent cocoa. The higher the bean content, the lower the sugar and fat content. Two squares of dark chocolate are far more satisfying than lesser varieties.

- If you are the sort of person who can't eat just two squares of chocolate, try buying mini bars or breaking off two chunks and putting the rest out of sight and reach.

Principle 9
Make time to eat

Eating is an essential yet pleasurable social ritual, and one that I feel has become devalued in our society. Fast food, ready-made meals and the pressure we all impose on ourselves to save time have eliminated the importance of sitting down to enjoy a meal. So make time to eat.

I have had consultations with many clients who, while they are accountable in other areas of their lives as parents or employees, for example, seem to take no interest in or responsibility for what they eat. Ironically, some of these clients will change their eating habits if they find that they are pregnant, or planning pregnancy, only to change back again after their baby is born. This is often in spite of feeling much better on the healthier eating plan while pregnant.

I have also worked with many families who rush through dinner, both cooking and eating their meal, simply so that they can spend the rest of the evening in front of the television watching cookery programmes!

Modern life appears to have taken the pleasure out of cooking and eating food. It seems to be something that is not worth fussing over and it wastes valuable time: let the food manufacturers do your work for you so that you can do something else more important instead. If this lifestyle sounds familiar to you, then ask yourself how ready-made meals and processed foods have contributed to your weight problems. If you learn to value and respect good food, making time to eat will become normal practice for you and your family. Try to sit down and eat at least one meal a day together. Take your time eating, and you may even find that you linger at the table chatting after your meal is over.

Eating at work

If your job is stressful and you never get a chance to eat a proper meal, you will probably snack when you can and rush through a sandwich at lunchtime. However, on The Food Doctor plan I want you to eat little and often, and this means eating mid-morning and mid-afternoon snacks that may require you to leave your desk and take a few minutes to prepare and eat them (see pp.210–211). You may need to plan ahead in the early stages until you become used to the plan, but your snack doesn't have to be complicated or take more than a minute to prepare. More importantly, taking the time to eat properly and chew well will ensure that you supply yourself with enough energy to see you through until your next meal.

If you really cannot leave your desk, keep a bag of raw, unsalted nuts in your drawer and measure a palmful of them in your hand to eat with an apple. If you have appointments or meetings throughout the day, try to leave a gap of a few minutes between them so that you can eat. If you don't, you are more likely to rely on coffee and biscuits and then make a poor food choice at lunchtime because your energy levels will be low and need to be replenished quickly.

THE BENEFITS OF TAKING TIME TO EAT

- Your stress levels are reduced.

- Chewing slowly and thoroughly enables you to digest your food properly and maintain good digestive health.

- Your body can absorb the nutrients from your food more effectively.

- A feeling of satisfaction that you have eaten a tasty, filling meal.

Why should I stop to eat at work?

Try to view eating your lunch or snack at work as a separate
activity that you should concentrate on – don't treat
it as an adjunct or an afterthought. You must
take the time to eat slowly and digest your
food properly, so stop working
or close down your computer
while you eat.

Principle 10
Eat fat to lose fat

If you come from a background of calorie-counting, you probably see fat as the enemy. Yet although the fat accumulated in our bodies and the fats in food are, in theory, similar, they are actually quite different: the essential fats present in a variety of foods are crucial for the body to function properly.

Fat contains nine calories per gram, the highest calorie count of any food there is, and this is why many diet plans advocate limiting your intake of fatty foods. However, I believe that it is saturated fats, not the all-important essential fats, that should be avoided.

What's the difference?

There are many types of fats that the body uses in a variety of different ways. Some fats are termed "essential" as they must come from the food we eat (*see right*). The conversion of these essential fats into substances that can be used internally is dependent upon several enzymes, which themselves require specific nutrients in order to work efficiently. Even those fats that are deemed non-essential to the body have a role to play, although saturated fats are not required in any great amount. Furthermore, fat adds to the satisfaction of eating – known in the food industry as "mouth feel" – and is considered a vital part of the eating experience. When we eat fat a substance called galanin, which actually increases our desire to eat more fat, is released into the body. This is why we often crave fatty foods, and why they are so pleasurable to eat. Luckily, this same feeling is experienced when we eat essential fats, which should form the bulk of our fat intake.

How much is too much?

Research has shown that a diet supplying not more than 30 per cent of energy from fat is the best way to lose weight. So you will find that by including 20 per cent of fat in the form of essential fats in your diet you will still enjoy the satisfaction of eating, yet the rate at which your food is converted into glucose is slowed down, thus fitting in perfectly with the Plan for Life principles.

LOW-FAT FOOD LABELS

If you buy, for example, a packet of crisps that claims to be low in fat, you may see something like "33 per cent less fat" advertised on the packet. The food label (*see top right*) lists the product as containing just over five grams of fat, but this figure does not take into account the number of calories you will eat. Bear in mind that fat contains nine calories per gram, and the total calorie count of this product is

	Per 24g bag
Energy	113 calories
Protein	1.8 g
Carbohydrates	14.4 g
of which sugars	0.1g
Fats	5.3g

	Per 24g bag
Energy	113 calories
Fats	45 calories
Calories from fat	42%

113 calories. When you eat the crisps, you must multiply five grams by nine calories to determine how much energy this food supplies – in this case it is 45 calories. That's how many calories are provided by fat alone in this product, which is what the label should really say (*see bottom left*). So although the fat, by weight, is about three grams less than a regular bag of crisps, the percentage of calories from fat is still high: 42 per cent of the total calorie count. You are only eating five grams of fat by weight, but 42 per cent of all the calories in the product comes from fat.

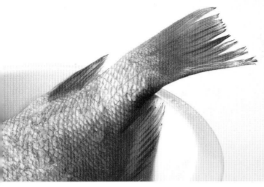

Which fats are good?

Foods that contain essential fats

Overall, the fats that are naturally found in fish (such as salmon, mackerel, tuna, trout, eel and sardines), raw nuts, seeds and olives are those that are most beneficial to your diet. However, don't go overboard with these foods: keep an eye on how much you are eating, and aim to eat no more than a palmful of nuts daily and fish four or five times a week.

The good oils

All of the foods illustrated below are good sources of valuable essential fats in their most natural form. In addition, the oils derived from these foods are beneficial in small quantities. Choose cold-pressed, good-quality oils as the basis for salad dressings and marinades, and avoid cooking with these oils at high temperatures as this causes them to lose their nutritional value.

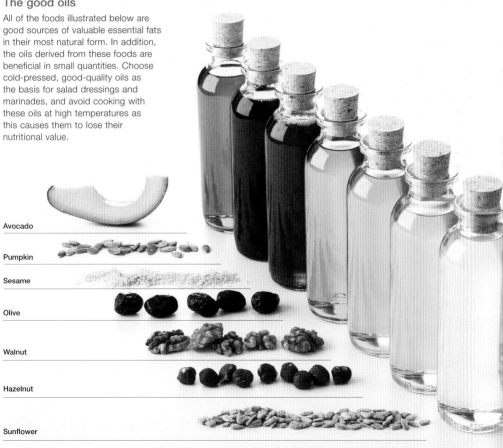

Avocado

Pumpkin

Sesame

Olive

Walnut

Hazelnut

Sunflower

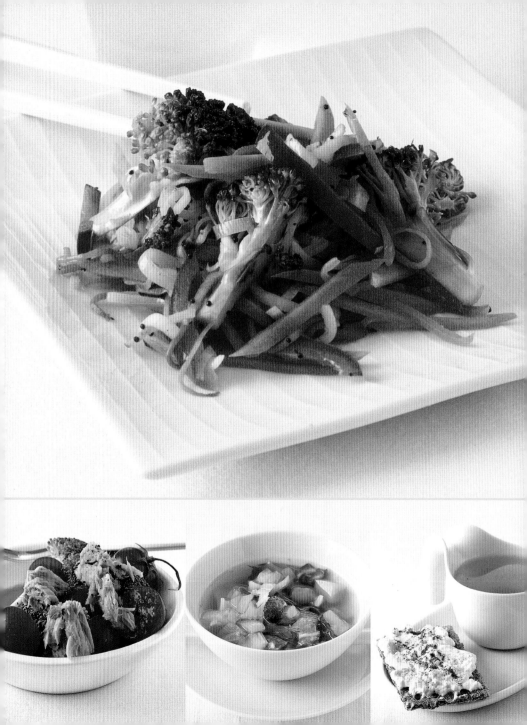

Seven-day Diet

This diet encourages good digestive health by reducing the amount of sugars and saturated fats you eat. Seven days is sufficient for you to adapt to, and benefit from, the changes in your diet, and still achieve realistic goals. You will eat frequently, so you shouldn't feel especially hungry. Try to stick to the suggested meals as this balanced plan is designed to promote health and well-being, but if there are foods that you would prefer not to eat, substitute one recipe for another recommended at a similar time of day. Before you start, see the Note at the front of the book.

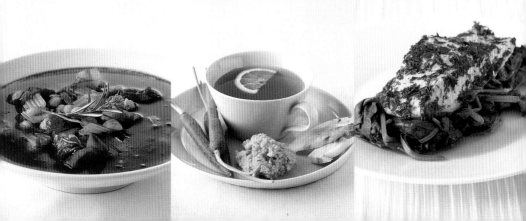

Preparing for the seven-day diet

Before you begin the Seven-day Diet, keep a food diary of what you eat and drink over three days. This will help you to identify which foods presently make up the bulk of your usual diet, and to clarify the current state of your health (*see pp.48–49*). During this time you can shop for the ingredients you will need for the week.

Three-day diary

Before you begin the diet, the most important step is to keep a food diary. Photocopy this blank diary plan and fill it in as diligently as you can. I suggest that you write down a list of everything you eat and drink, and at what time, over three consecutive days. There is also space to write down how you feel. This could include physical symptoms – for example, whether you feel lethargic or bloated – and even, perhaps, how you feel emotionally.

The changes in your eating habits over the next week may take some getting used to, so this food diary will serve to remind you of the meals and treats you currently eat, the impact such foods have had on the state of your health and how positive the Seven-day Diet will be for your future well-being. Write yourself notes and post them in places where you keep food (the larder, fridge, your desk drawer) so that you will remember to stay resolute and not waver while you are on the diet.

DAY ONE

Time	All meals, snacks, treats and drinks

How do I feel?

DAY TWO

Time   All meals, snacks, treats and drinks

How do I feel?

DAY THREE

Time   All meals, snacks, treats and drinks

How do I feel?

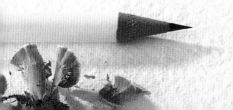

Shopping list for the seven-day diet

Once you decide which day you'll begin the Seven-day Diet (*see box, below*), you can shop for most of the food you'll require before you start, leaving yourself just a few vegetables and some fresh fish to buy during the week. If you are well-stocked with all the right ingredients for the recipes, the Seven-day Diet will be much easier to follow and you will also have no excuses for straying into shops and buying unsuitable alternatives at the last minute. Photocopy the lists on these pages and tick off the ingredients as you shop for them. Buy organic food if you prefer, although the success of this diet does not depend on it.

Don't start on a Monday

How many times have you overdone things or veered from your eating plan at the weekend and then justified your actions by promising to start again on Monday? I know from experience that starting the Seven-day Diet on a Monday makes the weekend feel a long way away. I recommend starting the diet on a Wednesday or Thursday so that if you feel you need more sleep, or if you experience any of the symptoms on pages 48–49, then the weekend is just around the corner, allowing you to take things easy. By the time Monday comes around, you should be feeling good, making it easier to tackle whatever the following week holds.

Dried foods

☐ 450g (1lb) porridge oats
☐ 450g (1lb) quinoa

☐ 1 packet unsalted rice cakes
☐ 1 packet olive oil oatcakes
☐ 1 packet rye crispbreads

☐ 1 small packet pumpkin seeds
☐ 1 small packet sesame seeds
☐ 1 small packet sunflower seeds
☐ 1 small packet linseeds
☐ 1 small packet pine nuts
☐ 1 small packet cashew nuts

☐ 250g (9oz) raisins
☐ 2 small packets mixed nuts, including cashew nuts, Brazil nuts, almonds, walnuts and hazelnuts

For the muesli mix

To make the Seven-day Diet muesli mix, buy a small packet of each of any **four** of the following grains:

☐ Barley flakes
☐ Rye flakes
☐ Oat flakes
☐ Millet flakes*
☐ Rice flakes*
☐ Quinoa flakes*
☐ Buckwheat flakes*

Spices, flavourings and oils

☐ Cold-pressed olive oil
☐ Cold-pressed sesame seed oil
☐ Yeast-free vegetable bouillon

*Choose these grains if you require a gluten-free diet.

☐ Mango powder, available from spice shops or Indian food shops (or substitute with fresh lemon juice)

☐ 1 whole nutmeg
☐ 1 small jar ground cinnamon powder
☐ 1 small jar cardamom pods
☐ 1 small jar caraway seeds
☐ 1 small jar cumin seeds
☐ 1 small jar coriander seeds
☐ 1 small jar garam masala
☐ 1 small jar black peppercorns
☐ 1 small jar cayenne pepper
☐ 1 small jar tahini paste
☐ 1 small jar tumeric
☐ 1 small jar paprika

Canned foods
☐ 1 can mixed beans†
☐ 1 can lentils†
☐ 2 cans chick-peas†
☐ 2 cans chopped tomatoes†
☐ 2 cans tuna in spring water, unless you prefer fresh tuna

Fresh vegetables
☐ 4 medium onions
☐ 1 small red onion
☐ 1 pumpkin
☐ 10 carrots
☐ 250g (9oz) leaf spinach
☐ 1 small bulb Florence fennel
☐ 2 small or 1 large head celery
☐ 2 medium leeks

†I list canned food for simplicity. If you use dried legumes or fresh tomatoes, allow for extra soaking and cooking time. Ensure that cans contain no sugar or salt.

The Seven-day Diet recipes are all simple assemblies of ingredients that require minimal preparation and cooking time.

☐ 2 heads pak choi
☐ 4 small heads broccoli
☐ 1 small green cabbage

☐ 5cm (2in) root ginger
☐ 6 lemons
☐ 2 bulbs garlic

Salad vegetables
☐ 12 baby/cherry tomatoes
☐ 4 medium tomatoes, if not using tinned
☐ 1 bag mixed leaf salad
☐ 1 avocado
☐ 1 cucumber
☐ 3 peppers, yellow, red or orange
☐ 1 bunch watercress

Frozen foods
☐ 50g (2oz) peas
☐ 50g (2oz) frozen prawns, if not using fresh

Chilled foods
☐ 1 tub cottage cheese
☐ 150g (6oz) tofu
☐ 1 tub live natural yoghurt

☐ 1 tub houmous, or make your own fresh (see recipe, p.54)
☐ 50g (2oz) prawns if not using frozen
☐ 100g (4oz) white fish

☐ 6 free-range eggs

Fresh herbs
☐ Basil
☐ Mint
☐ Parsley
☐ Coriander
☐ Dill
☐ Rosemary
☐ Bay leaves
☐ Thyme

Food to buy during the week
☐ 6 medium tomatoes for day six if not using tinned tomatoes
☐ 300g (10oz) salmon fillet if you choose this option for dinner on day five and lunch on day six

Changes that may take place

The Seven-day Diet is designed to encourage better overall digestion by excluding the three "S"s – simple carbohydrates, stimulants and saturated fats. Since your usual diet may include some or all of these elements, it's important that you are aware of what is happening to your body during the seven days, and what these changes to your health mean.

IMPORTANT PRECAUTIONS

I do not recommend that children follow any diet unless it's absolutely necessary, and then only under the supervision of an appropriate healthcare professional. No one under the age of 16 should undertake this diet plan. Likewise, do not follow this diet if you are pregnant. If you have a diagnosed medical condition, such as diabetes, please consult your doctor first.

The state of your health

Some people feel energized while they are on the Seven-day Diet, finding that they sleep well and have a clear mind. However, even if you don't feel especially good, rest assured that this programme is an important first step in achieving your goal of feeling well and eating healthily. I believe that the more of the three Ss you normally eat, the more likely you are to experience any one of the following symptoms while on the diet:

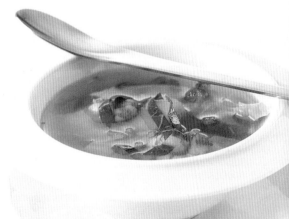

- Fatigue
- Food cravings
- Bad breath
- Mild diarrhoea
- Increased need for sleep
- Skin breakouts

Not everyone experiences unpleasant symptoms, so don't be put off by the possibility that these conditions might affect you. They are all really positive signs that things are changing for the better.

The Seven-day Diet is a short and simple programme that will help cleanse your body of the detrimental effects of the three Ss.

Signs of change

These are some of the common symptoms that you may experience during the initial stages of the Seven-day Diet, depending on how much you have previously indulged in the three Ss.

Do you feel more tired than usual?

If you have previously relied on caffeine and simple carbohydrates to give you short-term energy, then removing these substances from your diet will help to normalize the way your adrenal glands behave. Instead of triggering adrenaline repeatedly through the day, the adrenal glands should start to respond less often, which will keep the levels of glucose in your blood more even and help you to avoid "highs" and "lows". As this process takes place you may feel more tired than usual but don't worry, this feeling will soon pass.

Have you an increased need for sleep?

One key requirement of the Seven-day Diet is to rest, and you may notice that you have an increased need for sleep. For this reason I suggest that you don't make any plans for the week and that you stay at home whenever possible. Many people find that they sleep really deeply during the Seven-day Diet, and perhaps need more sleep than usual, so plan some early nights.

Are you craving sugary foods?

You will probably find that if you have eaten simple carbohydrates for energy in the past, you are now craving sugar and sweet foods. Such foods have encouraged the unfriendly bacteria and yeasts in your gut to proliferate, and since you are removing the simple sugars they feed on by following this diet – in effect, starving them – they can become a little demanding! If you do experience any food cravings, these should pass quickly.

Does your breath smell?

Rather than being hindered by the three Ss and processed foods, your digestive system is being encouraged to function more efficiently. As a result, you may find that you develop a green or white coating on your tongue. This may be accompanied by bad breath. There is no need to worry as this is only a temporary symptom. Chewing parsley can help alleviate bad breath, as can cleaning your teeth and gargling with a sugar-free mouthwash.

Are you experiencing mild diarrhoea?

The increase in liquids (including water and soups) and fibre that this diet provides can stimulate bowel movements and soften the stools. This is a healthy sign, showing that the Seven-day Diet is working. Conversely, some people get slightly constipated for the first day or two but this, too, is likely to be temporary.

Have you broken out in spots?

It is possible that you may get some spots, especially around the chin area. This suggests that your digestive system is undergoing a mild cleansing. As this is a good sign that things are changing, you may have to just bear with it, and they shouldn't last long.

Seven-day diet soups

These soups are an integral part of the Seven-day Diet for several reasons. The clear soup is a highly concentrated, cleansing drink rich in minerals. It is designed to help improve the workings of the digestive system as quickly as possible, and will also be used throughout the week to increase your fluid intake.

The other two vegetable-based soups provide your body with a high degree of easily absorbed nutrients, together with vital fibre and liquid. They will also help to promote better digestive health, which is the main aim of The Food Doctor diet.

The soups are all easy to prepare by even the most inexperienced cook, and can be stored in the fridge for up to a week, or in the freezer. Try to make these soups one day ahead of beginning the Seven-day Diet. If you work, you may like to invest in a thermos to enable you to drink these soups during the day.

Clear soup
for the 14 snacks in the Seven-day Diet

3.5 litres (6 pints) water
4 carrots, roughly chopped
½ head celery, roughly chopped
1 medium onion, quartered
2 cloves garlic, crushed
2 bay leaves
4 sprigs fresh thyme (or 1 teaspoon dried thyme)
4 whole cloves
6 black peppercorns
6 sprigs of parsley
Large handful fresh leaf spinach, coarsely shredded
Juice of 1 lemon
1 teaspoon Dijon mustard
Freshly ground black pepper, to taste
2 lemon and ginger tea bags (optional)

Put all of the ingredients, except the lemon juice, mustard, black pepper and tea bags, in a large saucepan, bring to the boil and simmer gently for 30 minutes.

Strain the liquid into a jug and throw the vegetables away. Return the broth to the pan and stir in the remaining ingredients. If using the tea bags, leave them to brew for about a minute, then lift out and discard. Store the soup in the fridge for the duration of the Seven-day Diet. The tea bags are optional but do add a freshness to the taste, and ginger is good for the digestive system.

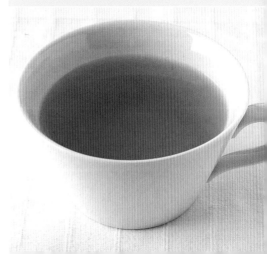

Tomato and rosemary soup
for three meals on days one, two and three

1 medium onion, diced

2 stalks celery, sliced

1 carrot, diced

1 large clove garlic, crushed

1 400g (14oz) can plum tomatoes, chopped

1 sprig fresh rosemary

1 flat teaspoon mango powder, or the juice of ½ lemon

1 litre (1¾ pints) fresh chicken or vegetable stock, or add 1 tablespoon yeast-free bouillon powder to 1 litre (1¾ pints) water

50g (2oz) shredded spinach

1 medium head pak choi, shredded

Heat two tablespoons of olive oil in a large saucepan. Add the onion, celery, carrot and garlic and cook gently over a low heat until the vegetables begin to soften. Stir in the tomatoes and add the rosemary and mango powder or lemon juice. Simmer for five minutes, then add the stock and simmer for 15 minutes or so until the vegetables are cooked but not soggy.

Stir in the spinach and pak choi and cook for two or three minutes more until they wilt. Remove the rosemary and season with freshly ground black pepper. Divide the soup into three individual portions and store in the fridge.

Chunky vegetable soup
for three meals on days four, six and seven

1 teaspoon each of caraway and cumin seeds

1 medium onion, diced

1 clove garlic, crushed

200g (7oz) pumpkin, peeled and cut into small cubes

½ small green cabbage, shredded

1 small head broccoli, broken into florets

1 stick celery, sliced

1 small carrot, diced

½ medium leek, finely sliced

1.5 litres (2½ pints) fresh chicken or vegetable stock, or add 1½ tablespoons yeast-free bouillon powder to 1.5 litres (2½ pints) water

1 bay leaf

Put the seeds in a small, heavy-based pan and toast over a medium heat for a few minutes until lightly browned.

Gently heat two tablespoons of olive oil in a large pan and soften the onion and garlic for five minutes. Add the rest of the vegetables and the seeds. Heat them together in the oil for another five minutes or so, then add just enough stock to cover the vegetables and simmer for ten minutes. Add the remaining stock and bay leaf, season with black pepper and simmer for about 20 minutes until all the vegetables are cooked. Divide the soup into three portions and store in the fridge or freezer.

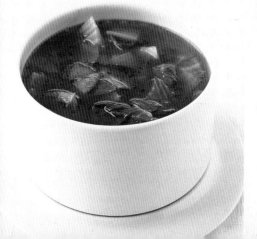

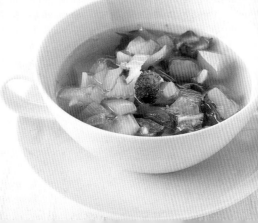

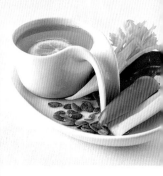

Day

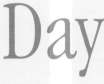

7-DAY DIET

You are probably full of good intentions as this is day one. This first day shouldn't prove too difficult as your food choices are tasty and varied and you won't begin to feel the effects of your change in eating habits until tonight or tomorrow morning.

Remember to drink plenty of water and herbal teas in between meals, and try to take things easy in the evening. All menus serve one.

Breakfast

This meal provides the right mix of ingredients to give your body sufficient energy and to enable you to have the best start to the day.

Glass of hot water with juice of ½ lemon

Cinnamon porridge

RECIPES

2 tablespoons porridge oats
50ml (2fl oz) water
2 tablespoons live natural yoghurt
A pinch of ground cinnamon

Combine the oats and water in a small saucepan, bring to the boil and simmer for one minute until the oats are soft.

Let the mixture stand off the heat for another minute before serving. Top with the yoghurt and a sprinkle of cinnamon.

Mid-morning snack

Your breakfast should have lasted you well into the morning but by 10.30am or so you will probably be feeling hungry enough to need this snack.

200ml (7fl oz) clear soup

2 strips each of red and orange pepper, 1 stick of celery and 1 tablespoon of pumpkin seeds

MANAGING YOUR TIME

This diet is based upon fresh, homemade meals, so you may need to allow yourself a little more time before each meal to prepare the ingredients and cook your food.

In practice, this really means getting up ten minutes earlier or so each morning to give yourself extra time to prepare your food and eat breakfast. You may even enjoy the chance to slow your pace and switch off in the evening as you prepare dinner.

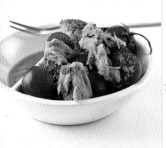

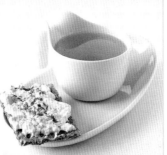

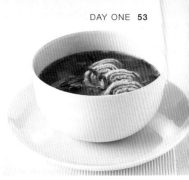

Lunch

Assuming that you ate your mid-morning snack about 10.30am, you should eat lunch around 1pm so that your energy levels stay constant.

Broccoli and tomato salad with tofu or tuna

Juice of ½ lemon
25g (1oz) tofu or 50g (2oz) canned tuna
50g (2oz) broccoli florets
4 cherry tomatoes, halved

Mix up a marinade of lemon juice in a small bowl and season with freshly ground black pepper.

If you are using tofu*, cut it into cubes and add it to the marinade.

If you are using tuna*, separate the flakes loosely with a fork and add them to the marinade.

Place the broccoli and tomatoes in a bowl, scatter the tofu or tuna over the top, drizzle with olive oil and serve.

*Store the remaining tofu or tuna in the fridge for lunch on day four.

Mid-afternoon snack

Eating in the afternoon is really important since the gap between lunch and dinner can be a long one. Aim to eat this snack around 4pm.

200ml (7fl oz) clear soup

Plain cottage cheese spread on 1 rye crispbread and topped with a pinch of garam masala

MEALS TO GO

If you work in an office or are out and about most days, you may be wondering how you will manage to stick to the diet. Why not prepare your snacks and lunch the previous evening, or first thing in the morning, and store them in tupperware boxes? You can also heat your soup in the morning and bring it into work in a thermos flask.

Try to ensure that you take a break from work to eat so that the stress of the day doesn't impair your digestive process.

Dinner

This meal is quick and convenient if you made your soups in advance, or cook a batch of soup now *(see p.51)* and store the remainder in the fridge.

Tomato and rosemary soup with mixed beans or shredded omelette

350ml (12½fl oz) tomato and rosemary soup
2 tablespoons mixed beans, canned or soaked and cooked, or 1 egg
A pinch of turmeric powder

If you are using mixed beans, ladle the soup into a saucepan and add the beans. Warm through over a low heat and serve.

If you are using an egg, beat it with a tablespoon of water and season with freshly ground pepper and turmeric. Lightly oil an omelette pan using a little olive oil. Pour in the egg mix and cook over a gentle heat until it sets. Flip the egg over and cook until golden. Turn it onto a wooden board, and when cool roll it up and cut into fine shreds.

Heat the soup through, stir in the shredded omelette and serve.

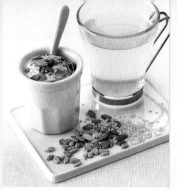

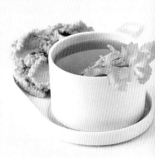

Day

7-DAY DIET

Don't give in to temptation today, since the cleansing effects of this diet are now under way, improving your digestion. Once again, ensure that you drink plenty of water, perhaps flavoured with some sliced cucumber or a squeeze of fresh lime if you need some added taste.

If this is a work day, prepare your snacks and lunch to take in with you so that you can stick to the plan.

Breakfast

Ideally, you should eat within an hour of waking to replenish energy levels that have become depleted overnight. Today's breakfast is quick and easy.

Glass of hot water with juice of ½ lemon

Three-seed yoghurt

RECIPES

3 tablespoons live natural yoghurt
1 tablespoon pumpkin seeds
1 tablespoon sunflower seeds
1 heaped teaspoon sesame seeds
A pinch of ground cinnamon

Spoon three generous tablespoons of yoghurt into a bowl. Sprinkle the pumpkin, sunflower and sesame seeds over the top. Flavour with a pinch of cinnamon and serve.

Mid-morning snack

A mid-morning snack is essential to ensure that you don't feel too hungry by lunchtime. This combination will sustain you until your next meal.

200ml (7fl oz) clear soup

Houmous spread on 1 rice cake

1 420g (15oz) can chick-peas*
2 tablespoons tahini paste
2 tablespoons lemon juice
1 clove garlic, crushed
Olive oil and cayenne pepper to garnish

Blend the chick-peas, tahini, lemon juice, garlic and some freshly ground black pepper into a smooth paste in a food processor. Scrape into a small bowl, drizzle with a little olive oil and sprinkle with cayenne pepper. Cover and keep refrigerated.

Spread a rice cake with one tablespoon of the houmous for your snack.

*Save two tablespoons of chick-peas for dinner tonight if you want to add them to your soup.

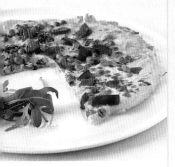
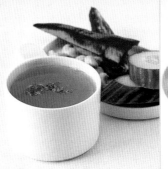
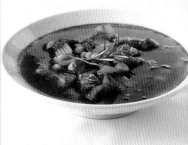

Lunch

If you made your omelette first thing this morning before going out for the day, eat it cold or reheat it if you can. Take time to chew each mouthful.

Vegetable omelette*

Mid-afternoon snack

Like your mid-morning snack, this combination of nuts and raw vegetables should help you to feel satisfied until dinner.

200ml (7fl oz) clear soup

10 cashew nuts, 2 thick slices of cucumber, 2 strips of pepper

Dinner

All evening meals consist of protein and vegetables. You don't need to eat carbohydrates this late in the day as you will not use the energy they give.

Tomato and rosemary soup with chick-peas or flaked fish

---

1 small red onion, finely chopped
1 clove garlic, crushed
2 eggs
1 tablespoon live natural yoghurt
½ teaspoon paprika
1 tablespoon chopped parsley
½ teaspoon chopped thyme
2 tablespoons peas
1 medium-ripe tomato, chopped

In a small frying pan, heat a tablespoon of olive oil over a low heat. Gently soften the onion and garlic. Beat the eggs with the yoghurt and paprika, add the herbs, season with black pepper and pour into the pan. Scatter the peas and tomato on top, cook gently until the egg sets, then turn out onto a plate and serve.

*Leave a small serving for your mid-afternoon snack tomorrow.

WHAT CAN I DRINK?

This diet, though very short, depends on you adhering to some basic rules that will make the difference between feeling great at the end or not noticing much change at all. One important rule is to avoid alcohol, tea and coffee. This may sound like an impossible task but try it and see: you will probably find that you sleep better, wake up feeling refreshed, and experience fewer energy slumps. You should aim to drink at least eight generously sized glasses of water through the day to stay hydrated.

350ml (12fl oz) tomato and rosemary soup
2 tablespoons chick-peas
or 100g (4oz) white fish fillet, cut into bite-sized pieces
Juice of ½ lemon
1 teaspoon ground coriander

If you are using chick-peas, add two tablespoons of cooked chick-peas to the soup before heating it thoroughly in a saucepan over a low heat.

If you are using fish, let it marinate in the lemon juice, ground coriander and a seasoning of freshly ground black pepper while you ladle the soup into a saucepan and heat it thoroughly. Add the fish and simmer for five minutes or until just cooked, and serve.

Day 3

7-DAY DIET

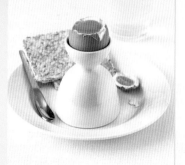

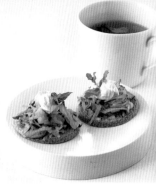

You are now nearing the halfway point of the diet, so you should be feeling a little lighter and hopefully less hungry too. Don't stray from the recommended foods, and take care to not overeat.

If you are going to be out and about today, take one portion of tomato and rosemary soup out of the fridge first thing in the morning and blend it until smooth in a processor.

Breakfast

Eggs are a great source of protein for breakfast. Boil your egg according to personal preference; the ideal time to cook a soft-boiled egg is four minutes.

Glass of hot water with juice of ½ lemon

1 boiled egg with 2 rice cakes

RECIPES

EXCLUSION ZONE

You may have noticed that the Seven-day Diet excludes any kind of meat. This is because I believe that the saturated fats in meat – and especially in red meat – promote the proliferation of unfriendly bacteria and potential yeasts in the gut (see p.18). These fats are detrimental to your overall digestive health in large quantities, so meat is not an option on the Seven-day Diet.

Mid-morning snack

If you work in an office, make this cucumber mint yoghurt in advance so that you can take it in to work with you and store it in a fridge.

200ml (7fl oz) clear soup

Cucumber mint yoghurt on 2 oatcakes

50g (2oz) cucumber, grated
2 tablespoons live natural yoghurt
A sprig or two of fresh mint, shredded

Mix the cucumber and yoghurt. Add the mint, season with freshly ground black pepper and mix well.

Spread on two oatcakes and serve with the soup.

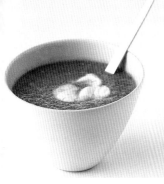
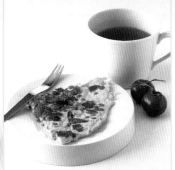
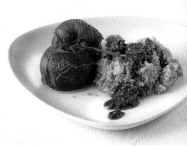

Lunch

This is the last portion of
the tomato and rosemary soup,
so blending it into a smooth
texture will help to make it
taste slightly different.

**Smooth tomato and rosemary
soup with yoghurt**

Mid-afternoon snack

For this instant afternoon snack,
take the slice of omelette left over
from yesterday lunchtime out of the
fridge and eat it cold.

200ml (7fl oz) clear soup

**1 small slice of omelette
with 2 cherry tomatoes**

Dinner

This meal is very nutritious and
will take you about 25 minutes
to cook. Remember to save a
spoonful of pesto for tomorrow
morning's snack.

**Quinoa with pesto
and roast tomatoes**

350ml (12fl oz) tomato and
rosemary soup
1 tablespoon live natural yoghurt

Blend the soup in a food
processor and then heat it
thoroughly in a small pan
over a low heat.

Pour the hot soup into a bowl
and swirl the yoghurt into it
just before serving.

FRUIT-FREE WEEK

Fruit is also off-limits on the
Seven-day Diet for the simple
reason that it contains a form of
sugar. The natural sugar in fruit,
known as fructose, can act like
other sugars in the way that it
encourages the growth of
unfriendly bacteria and yeasts
in the gut. The aim of this diet
is to make your digestive system
as healthy as possible, so fruit is
off the menu for the duration of
these seven days only.

2 medium tomatoes
2 sprigs fresh rosemary
For the pesto:
  1 large handful fresh basil
  100ml (3½fl oz) olive oil
  100g (4oz) pine nuts
  1 small clove garlic
50g (2oz) quinoa
100ml (3½fl oz) water with ½ teaspoon of
yeast-free bouillon powder added

Preheat oven to 200°C/400°F/Gas 6.

Put the tomatoes and rosemary in a
baking dish, drizzle with olive oil
and roast for 20 minutes. Blend the
pesto ingredients in a processor.
Simmer the quinoa and water in a
pan until soft, stir in three teaspoons
of pesto and serve with the tomatoes
(remove the rosemary sprigs first).

Day

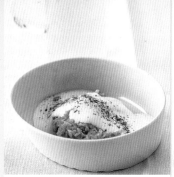

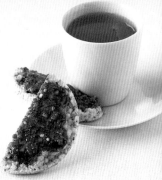

7-DAY DIET

Today you will continue to eat lightly, so try to make sure that you are busy doing something you enjoy in order to keep yourself occupied.

If you have already cooked and frozen the chunky vegetable soup, take a portion out of the freezer in the morning and let it defrost in the fridge during the day, ready for dinner. Try to rest in the evening and have an early night if you need to.

Breakfast

The oats in porridge aid the efficient functioning of your digestive system and provide much-needed energy to get you through the morning.

Glass of hot water with juice of ½ lemon

Nutmeg porridge

RECIPES

2 tablespoons porridge oats
50ml (2fl oz) water
2 tablespoons live natural yoghurt
Freshly grated nutmeg

Combine the oats and water in a small saucepan, bring to the boil and simmer for one minute until the oats are soft.

Let the mixture stand off the heat for another minute, then add the yoghurt and nutmeg and serve.

Mid-morning snack

Use the remaining pesto left over from last night's meal for this snack. Squeeze a little lemon juice over the top if you want to lift the flavours.

200ml (7fl oz) clear soup

Pesto spread on 1 rice cake

Spread a rice cake with a generous helping of pesto to eat with your soup.

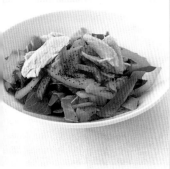

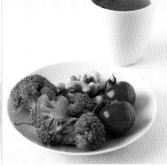

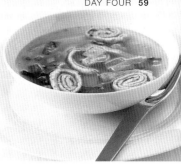

Lunch

Try to take time to sit down and eat your lunch slowly without any stress. Chewing thoroughly will also enable you to digest your food properly.

Pepper and pak choi salad with tuna or tofu

Mid-afternoon snack

This energizing snack will help you to avoid the mid-afternoon slump in energy that often follows after lunch or a busy morning's work.

200ml (7fl oz) clear soup

10 cashew nuts, 5 small florets of broccoli and 2 cherry tomatoes

Dinner

Try not to eat dinner too late in the evening. You should allow for a minimum of at least two hours in between eating and going to bed.

Chunky vegetable soup with mixed beans or shredded omelette

Juice of ½ lemon

A pinch of garam masala

25g (1oz) tofu, cut into bite-sized pieces, or 50g (2oz) canned tuna from day one

½ red or yellow pepper, cut into strips

1 small head pak choi, shredded

1 tablespoon grated carrot

Combine the lemon juice and garam masala in a small bowl and season with freshly ground black pepper. Add the tofu or tuna to this marinade and leave to one side for a few minutes.

Put the pepper and pak choi in a salad bowl and toss in a dressing of olive oil and freshly ground black pepper. Top with the carrot, spoon over the tuna or tofu with its marinade and then serve.

SHOP FOR THE NEXT FEW MEALS

Look ahead now to tomorrow's menu to make sure that you have all the ingredients you will require.

You'll need to buy some fresh salmon today or tomorrow if you intend to have this option for your evening meal on day five. You may also need to buy a few extra vegetables and some more live natural yoghurt if you have used up these ingredients.

350ml (12½fl oz) tomato and rosemary soup

2 tablespoons mixed beans, canned or soaked and cooked, or 1 egg

A pinch of turmeric powder

If you are using mixed beans, ladle the soup into a saucepan and add the beans. Warm through over a low heat and serve.

If you are using an egg, beat it with a tablespoon of water and season with freshly ground pepper and turmeric. Lightly oil an omelette pan using a little olive oil. Pour in the egg mix and cook over a gentle heat until it sets. Flip the egg over and cook until golden. Turn it onto a wooden board, and when cool roll it up and cut into fine shreds.

Heat the soup through, stir in the shredded omelette and serve.

Day

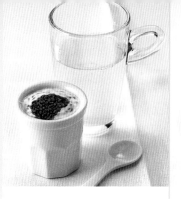
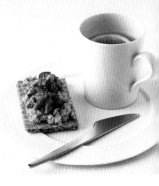

7-DAY DIET

You are now over the halfway point, and your body is responding to the different elements in your diet. You may also notice some of the physical changes that are described on pages 48–49.

There are only three days to go, so resist giving in to any temptation at this stage. If it is the weekend, keep yourself busy and concentrate on the sense of well-being you might now be feeling.

Breakfast

Linseeds encourage regular bowel movements and provide essential nutrients. You will need to chew the linseeds well to break them up.

Glass of hot water with juice of ½ lemon

Soaked linseeds with natural yoghurt

RECIPES

1 tablespoon linseeds
3 tablespoons live natural yoghurt
A pinch of ground cinnamon

Soak the linseeds overnight in enough water to just cover them.

In the morning drain the water away and combine the seeds with the yoghurt. Serve with a sprinkle of cinnamon on top.

Mid-morning snack

If you need to make this snack in advance, squeeze plenty of lemon juice over the avocado to prevent it going brown and store it in the fridge.

200ml (7fl oz) clear soup

Avocado spread on 1 rye crispbread with chopped tomato

½ small avocado
A good squeeze of lemon juice
1 cherry tomato, chopped

Combine the avocado, lemon juice and a seasoning of freshly ground black pepper in a bowl and mash together with a fork.

Spread the mixture on the rye crispbread, scatter the chopped tomato over the top and serve with the soup.

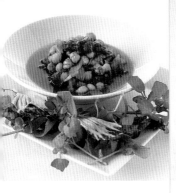
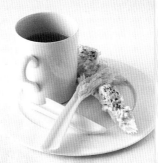
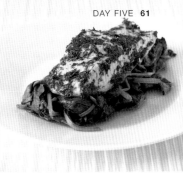

Lunch

Don't increase the portion size of this recipe according to how hungry you think you might be. The serving listed here is designed to satisfy you.

Quick chick-pea stew

Mid-afternoon snack

Eating this snack at about the same time each day enables your energy levels to stay even so that you don't feel tempted to stray from the diet.

200ml (7fl oz) clear soup

Tuna dip with celery or carrot sticks

Dinner

Don't forget to save a spoonful of spinach and a small portion of salmon for tomorrow. Alternatively, you may prefer a poached egg with the spinach.

Spinach with herb salmon or a poached egg

½ teaspoon cumin seeds

2 cardamom pods

1 medium onion, chopped

2 cloves garlic, crushed

400g (14oz) ripe or canned tomatoes, chopped

1 420g (15oz) can chick-peas

475ml (17fl oz) water

Gently heat a tablespoon of olive oil in a medium-sized saucepan, add the spices and cook for one minute. Add the onion and garlic, soften for five minutes, then stir in the tomatoes and chick-peas. Pour in the water and simmer for 10–15 minutes, stirring occasionally, until the sauce thickens.

Serve two tablespoons of stew with a salad. Refrigerate the remaining stew.

20g (1oz) canned tuna

2 tablespoons live natural yoghurt

A few sprigs of fresh parsley, chopped

A pinch of cayenne pepper

Mash the tuna with the yoghurt, season with freshly ground black pepper and stir in the chopped parsley.

Scoop up the dip with celery, chopped carrot sticks or Florence fennel and sprinkle a little cayenne pepper on top before serving with the soup.

300g (10oz) salmon fillet or 1 egg

A handful of chopped dill, coriander, parsley

Juice of ¼ lemon

1 clove of garlic, finely chopped

100g (4oz) fresh leaf spinach, washed

A pinch of garam masala

If you are using salmon, preheat the oven to 180°C/350°F/Gas 4. Coat the fish in the herbs, place on an oiled sheet of foil and season with lemon juice, black pepper and garlic. Fold the ends of the foil into a parcel. Cook for 20 minutes.

If you are using an egg, poach it in a frying pan of boiling water until set. Cook spinach in a medium saucepan over a gentle heat. Drain well. Drizzle with a little sesame seed oil, lemon juice and garam masala. Top with the salmon or egg and serve.

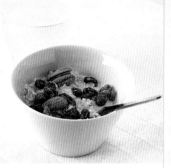

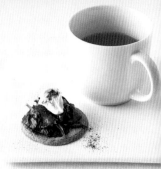

Day

7-DAY DIET

You are almost there, so persevere for these last two days and you will soon be reaping the benefits.

If you have frozen your home-made soup, then take the last two portions out of the freezer this morning and let them defrost in the fridge over the course of the day.

Take things easy if you are tired, although some people can feel energized by now.

Breakfast

If you are following a gluten-free diet, make sure you choose those grains marked with an asterisk* when you mix up your muesli.

Glass of hot water with juice of ½ lemon

Muesli with whole milk or natural yoghurt

RECIPES

Choose 1 tablespoon each from any **four** of the following grains:

   Barley flakes
   Rye flakes
   Oat flakes
   Millet flakes*
   Rice flakes*
   Quinoa flakes*
   Buckwheat flakes*

8–9 mixed nuts, including hazelnuts, Brazil nuts, cashew nuts, almonds, walnuts

1 teaspoon raisins

Combine the dried ingredients in a bowl, add one tablespoon of live natural yoghurt or your choice of milk (either whole cows', goats' or sheep's milk or an unsweetened substitute such as rice or soya milk) and serve.

Mid-morning snack

Use the extra spoonful of spinach from last night's meal for this snack. Squeeze over a little lemon juice if you want to lift the flavours slightly.

200ml (7fl oz) clear soup

Spinach and yoghurt on 1 oatcake

Chop the spinach and spread it on one oatcake. Top with a teaspoon of yoghurt and sprinkle over a little cayenne pepper before serving with the soup.

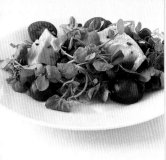
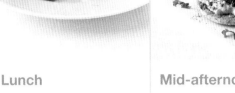
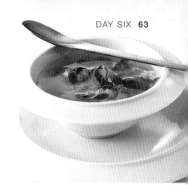

Lunch

If you had salmon for dinner last night, then use the remaining fish in this salad. If you had a poached egg, slice up an avocado instead.

Avocado or cold salmon with watercress salad

½ teaspoon of cumin seeds

A handful of fresh watercress, rocket, lambs lettuce or other green salad leaves

A squeeze of lemon juice

4 cherry tomatoes, halved

½ avocado, sliced, or cold salmon

Toast the cumin seeds gently in a small heavy-based saucepan for one minute, then remove from the heat.

Dress the salad leaves with the dry-roasted cumin seeds, lemon juice, a drizzle of olive oil and freshly ground black pepper. Add the tomatoes, mix well and serve with the salmon or avocado.

Mid-afternoon snack

Any cravings you may have had for sweet, sugary food will hopefully have passed by now, so you should enjoy this sustaining snack.

200ml (7fl oz) clear soup

Cottage cheese spread on 1 rice cake, topped with chopped fresh coriander

EXERCISE

It is fine to exercise while you are on the Seven-day Diet, although don't overdo things and make sure you can rest for a while afterwards. You may want to time your exercise to fit in before a snack or a meal so that you can refuel quickly and not feel overly hungry.

Don't attempt any unfamiliar sports or training sessions while on this diet, since this may exhaust you or prove to be too excessive.

Dinner

Add either a spoonful of yesterday's quick chick-pea stew to tonight's soup or include a few cooked prawns instead if you prefer.

Chunky vegetable soup with chick-peas or prawns

300ml (10fl oz) chunky vegetable soup

50g (2oz) cooked prawns

or 1 tablespoon quick chick-pea stew

Pour the soup into a saucepan and add the prawns or the chick-pea stew. Heat thoroughly over a low heat and serve.

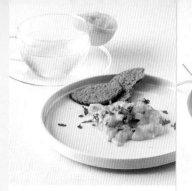

Day 7

7-DAY DIET

Well done, it's your last day. I hope that you didn't find the diet too difficult to follow and that by now you are feeling well, more energized and inspired to move on to the next stage, the Plan for Life. If you wish to continue with the daily eating plan, go straight to week two of the 30-day Diet Plan (p.108).

Breakfast

Try to continue the routine of preparing a nutritious, well-balanced breakfast of protein and carbohydrate such as this after you finish the diet.

Glass of hot water with juice of ½ lemon

Scrambled egg with 1 oatcake

RECIPES

1 egg
1 teaspoon live natural yoghurt
A pinch of turmeric powder
1 tablespoon fresh parsley, chopped
1 oatcake

Beat together the egg and the yoghurt, then season with freshly ground black pepper and add a pinch of ground turmeric powder.

Heat a little olive oil in a small saucepan, pour in the beaten egg and cook over a low heat until the egg forms soft curds. Once cooked, stir in the parsley and serve with one oatcake.

Mid-morning snack

If you made your own houmous on day two, you can use up the rest of it for this snack. Otherwise use some shop-bought houmous.

200ml (7fl oz) clear soup

1 tablespoon of houmous with raw vegetables

1 tablespoon houmous
A small selection of raw vegetables such as carrots, Florence fennel or celery, sliced

Serve the dip and crudités with the soup, using the vegetables to scoop up the houmous.

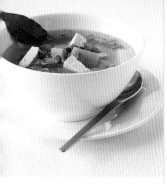
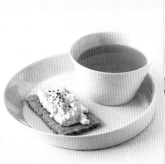
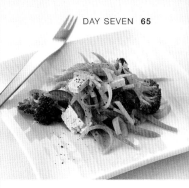

Lunch

Add a few pieces of tofu or some pumpkin seeds to this final serving of your homemade soup in order to vary the taste slightly.

Chunky vegetable soup with tofu or pumpkin seeds

Mid-afternoon snack

This is the last of the nutrient-rich clear soup that has helped to cleanse and improve your digestive system and kept your fluid intake high.

200ml (7fl oz) clear soup

Cottage cheese spread on 1 rye crispbread

Dinner

Use up the remaining vegetables in your fridge for this stir-fry and add some pumpkin seeds or the remaining tofu that you saved from lunchtime.

Stir-fried vegetables with marinated tofu or pumpkin seeds

350ml (12fl oz) chunky vegetable soup
50g (2oz) tofu*, finely cubed, or 1 heaped teaspoon pumpkin seeds

Pour the soup into a saucepan and warm it up gently over a low heat. Add the tofu or pumpkin seeds, transfer to a bowl and serve.

*Store the rest of the tofu in the fridge for tonight's supper.

THE BENEFITS OF THE SEVEN-DAY DIET

As you come to the end of the Seven-day Diet you should hopefully feel some or all of the following:

* Improved digestion, and therefore enhanced absorption of nutrients

* Sense of well-being

* More energy

* Reduced sugar cravings

* Reduced cravings for caffeine and alcohol.

Approx. 150g (5½oz) various vegetables such as carrot, pepper, leek, broccoli
2 tablespoons lemon juice
½ teaspoon fresh ginger, grated
2 cardamom seeds, ground (see p.129)
50g (2oz) tofu, finely cubed, or 1 heaped teaspoon pumpkin seeds

Slice the vegetables finely. Mix the lemon juice, ginger and cardamom seeds in a bowl and season with freshly ground black pepper. If using tofu, toss the vegetables and tofu in the marinade; leave for 15 minutes.

Heat a tablespoon of water in a wok, add the vegetables and cook them over a high heat until crisp. Drizzle with cold-pressed sesame seed oil. If using pumpkin seeds, sprinkle them over just before serving.

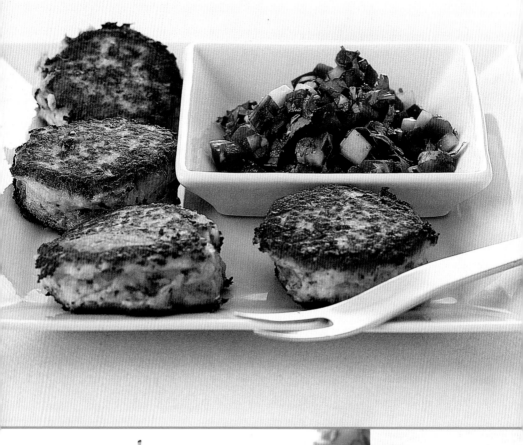

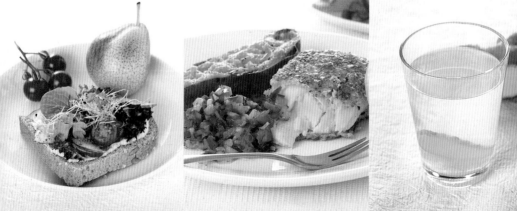

30-day
Diet plan

This plan is 30 days long: two days of preparation and four weeks of carefully structured menu plans and recipes. You'll avoid sugar, red meat and alcohol for the month, so don't be tempted to go to too many restaurants or parties if you want to ensure success. Preparation is all-important: read ahead, know what you're doing and shop for the necessary food beforehand. Preparation day 1 begins on a Tuesday, and weeks 1–4 start on successive Thursdays.

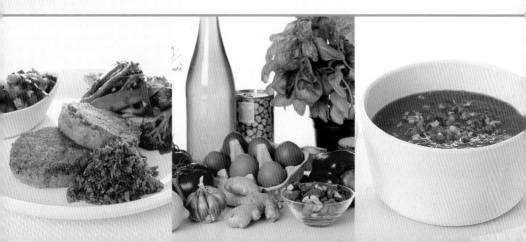

Pre-plan food diary

Before you begin The Food Doctor
30-day Diet plan, keep a food diary of what
you eat and drink over the next three days.
This will help you to identify which foods
presently make up the bulk of your usual
diet, and to clarify the current state of your
health. It will also be interesting for you to
look back after you finish the plan and see
how differently you ate.

Accurate accounts

To record an accurate diary, you should include
all drinks, snacks and meals, and the time you had
them. You should also make a note of how you feel
during, and at the end of, each day. Make sure you
don't leave anything out: although this is for your
reference only, it will help you to understand why
you feel like you do now when you compare
your results at the end of the plan.

FIRST DAY

Time	All meals, snacks, treats and drinks

SECOND DAY

Time   All meals, snacks, treats and drinks

THIRD DAY

Time   All meals, snacks, treats and drinks

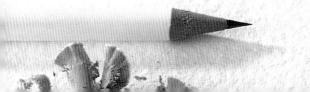

Shopping list for days 1 & 2 & soup recipes

Fruit

- [ ] Apples, 4
- [ ] Bananas, 1
- [ ] Lemons, 2
- [ ] Limes, 1
- [ ] Pears, 1

Vegetables

- [ ] Carrots, approx. 50g (2oz)
- [ ] Cherry tomatoes, 1 tub
- [ ] Cucumbers, small, 2
- [ ] Mixed raw vegetables, approx. 600g (1lb 3½oz)
- [ ] Mixed salad ingredients: enough for 2 portions
- [ ] Onions, medium, 1
- [ ] Onions, small, 2
- [ ] Peppers, green, 1
- [ ] Peppers, red, 1
- [ ] Red onion, small, 1
- [ ] Spring onions, 1 bunch
- [ ] Sweet potatoes, large, 1
- [ ] Tomatoes, medium, 2

Fresh herbs

- [ ] Basil, fresh, 1 packet
- [ ] Parsley, fresh, 1 bunch

Dairy

- [ ] Hen's eggs, 1
- [ ] Live natural low-fat yoghurt, 1 large pot
- [ ] Haloumi, 200g (7oz) (if making Oat-crumb haloumi, day 2)

- [ ] Orange or apple juice, 1 carton
- [ ] Peppermint tea, 1 packet
- [ ] Oatcakes, 1 packet

Meat & fish

- [ ] Beef mince, very lean, 200g (7oz) (if making Beef burgers, day 1)
- [ ] White fish fillet (cod, haddock etc.), 200g (7oz), (if making Oat-crumb fish, day 2)

Storecupboard foods

- [ ] *Chick-peas, 1x400g (13oz) can (if making Chick-pea burgers, day 1)
- [ ] Oat flakes, 1 packet
- [ ] Rice, Camargue (red) or brown, 1 packet
- [ ] Mixed seeds, 1 tub (or see p.93)
- [ ] Nuts, raw unsalted, 1 small packet

Spices & flavourings

- [ ] Chilli powder, 1 small jar
- [ ] Cumin powder, 1 small jar
- [ ] Herbes de Provence,1 pot
- [ ] Mustard, 1 small pot
- [ ] Olive oil, 1 bottle
- [ ] Soy sauce, 1 bottle
- [ ] Stock,vegetable, 150ml (¼ pint) or yeast-free bouillon powder, 1 tub

FOR THE WINTER SOUPS

(Carrot, leek & watercress soup, Tomato & mixed vegetable soup)

- [ ] Carrots, 500g (1lb 2oz)
- [ ] Celery, 1 bunch
- [ ] Garlic bulbs, 1
- [ ] Leeks, medium, 1
- [ ] Onions, medium, 1
- [ ] Onions, small, 1
- [ ] Red pepper, large, 1
- [ ] Watercress, fresh, 2 bunches
- [ ] *Cannellini beans, 1x400g (13oz) can
- [ ] *Chick-peas, 1x400g (13oz) can
- [ ] Plum tomatoes, chopped, 1x400g (13oz) can
- [ ] Basil (dried), 1 small jar
- [ ] Mango powder, 1 small jar
- [ ] Smoked paprika, 1 jar
- [ ] Vegetable stock, 2 litres (3½ pints) or yeast-free bouillon powder, 1 tub (if not bought for prep days)

FOR THE SUMMER SOUPS

(Light vegetable broth, Chilled summer soup)

- [ ] Lemons, 2
- [ ] Baby corn, 100g (3½oz)
- [ ] Carrots, 100g (3½oz)
- [ ] Cucumber, ½
- [ ] Baby leeks 100g (3½oz) or spring onions, 1 bunch

- [ ] Mangetout, 100g (3½oz)
- [ ] Pepper, 1 (any colour)
- [ ] Red onion, medium, 1
- [ ] Root ginger, fresh, 1 piece
- [ ] Fresh coriander, 1 bunch
- [ ] Apple juice, 1 carton
- [ ] Vegetable juice, 1 carton

- [ ] *Cannellini beans, 1x400g (13oz) can
- [ ] Plum tomatoes, chopped, 1x400g (13oz) can
- [ ] Miso paste, 1 packet
- [ ] Quinoa, 1 packet
- [ ] Tomato purée, 1 tube
- [ ] Tabasco, 1 bottle

- [ ] Vegetable stock (good quality) to make 1.6 litres (2¾ pints) or yeast-free bouillon powder, 1 tub (if not bought for prep days)

*All cans should be free from added salt and sugar

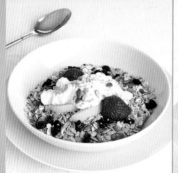

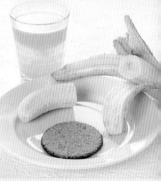

Preparing
for the
plan

days 1-2

30-DAY DIET

Breakfast

Have your usual cereal, but add 1 tablespoon of live natural low-fat yoghurt and some fresh fruit.

Dilute juice with water for a 50:50 mix. Avoid caffeine.

Morning snack

Diluted juice or herb tea with 12 mixed raw nuts or ½ banana and 1 oatcake.

If you usually eat biscuits around this time of day, eat 1 tablespoon of pumpkin seeds too.

DAY 2

Breakfast

50g (2oz) of your usual cereal with 1 tablespoon of pumpkin seeds, 1 chopped apple and 1 tablespoon live natural low-fat yoghurt.

Drink diluted juice or herb tea. Avoid caffeine.

Morning snack

Orange or apple juice diluted 50:50 with water, or a cup of peppermint tea.

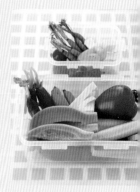

The Food Doctor

Tip for the day ...

When you shop, look out for varieties of flavoured seed mixes on sale, as they make a tasty alternative to plain seeds.

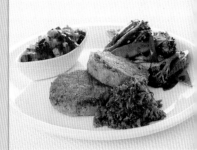

Lunch

Have 3–4 cherry tomatoes and an apple with your sandwiches or lunchtime meal.

Afternoon snack

Diluted juice or tea or coffee made weaker than you usually have it and without sugar.

If you normally eat sweet biscuits, have ½ banana and 1 tablespoon of pumpkin seeds instead.

Dinner

Home-made beef or chick-pea burgers with red rice & stir-fried vegetables *(p.74)*.

Lunch

Take away the top layer of your sandwiches and have it with 4 tomatoes. Eat either a pear or an apple with your lunch.

Afternoon snack

Diluted juice or herb tea with 2 oatcakes, ½ banana or 1 apple and 1 tablespoon of pumpkin seeds.

Dinner

Oat-crumbed fish fillet or haloumi with baked sweet potato & mixed salad *(p.75)*.

Foods to enjoy

Vegetables in as many different colours as possible, apples, pears, cherries, berries, lemons, limes, any other fruit in moderation, avocados, oats, quinoa, millet, rye, brown, red or wild rice, seeds, nuts in moderation, organic eggs, organic chicken, turkey, fish, tofu, unprocessed cheese such as goat's cheese, herb teas, herbs and spices. Make your own sprouted seeds now to enjoy while you are on the plan. See page 181 to find out how.

Foods to avoid

Tea, coffee, fizzy drinks, alcohol, undiluted fruit juice, salted snacks, crisps, sweet biscuits, cakes, confectionery, ice cream, white bread, white pasta, white rice, potatoes, most commercial cereals, processed cheese, flavoured yoghurts, fried foods, bacon, red meat, sausages, jams, marmalade and honey.

Burgers with stir-fried vegetables & red rice

DINNER DAY 1

It's easy to make home-made beef or chick-pea burgers. Prepare them while the rice is cooking, then cook the stir-fry. Serves two.

Beef burgers

| ready in **30** minutes |

200g (7oz) very lean beef mince
1 medium onion, finely chopped
A dash of soy sauce
A large pinch of chilli powder (optional)
1 tablespoon olive oil

Mix the ingredients in a bowl or a mixer. Blend into a paste. Season with freshly ground pepper. Form two 2.5cm (1in) thick burgers. Heat the oil in a pan and cook over a medium heat, turning once.

Stir-fry

300g (10oz) raw vegetables per person, chopped, or 1 packet ready-prepared vegetables

Cook the vegetables in a little water or lemon juice. If you wish, add a sauce after cooking *(p.171)*.

Red rice

½ small onion, finely chopped
½ tablespoon olive oil
50g (2oz) red rice
150ml (¼ pint) light vegetable stock

Soften the onion in the oil in a saucepan over a medium heat. Add the rice and stock and simmer for 25 minutes or until the rice is *al dente*.

Chick-pea burgers

1x400g (13oz) can chick-peas, drained and rinsed
1 small onion, chopped
50g (2oz) carrot, finely grated
2 tablespoons mixed seeds
1 tablespoon olive oil
½ teaspoon ground cumin
A dash of soy sauce

Mash the ingredients with a potato masher in a bowl, or put them in a mixer and blend into a paste. Form into four burgers. Heat the oil in a frying pan and cook over a medium heat until lightly browned on both sides. Serve with a red salsa *(p.195)*.

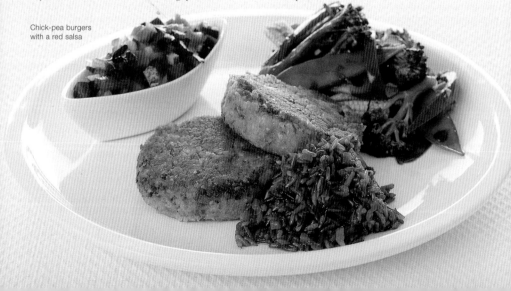

Chick-pea burgers with a red salsa

Oat-crumb fish or haloumi, sweet potato & salad

Preparing your own flavoured crumbs is cheap and simple. For this recipe, bake a large sweet potato and make the salad first. Serves two.

ready in 30 minutes

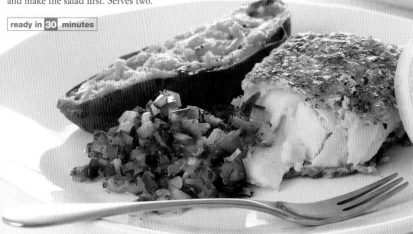

Oat-crumb fish fillets with half a baked sweet potato & a green salsa

Oat-crumb fish fillets

200g (7oz) white fish fillet (cod, haddock, etc.)
1 egg, beaten with 1 tablespoon mustard
4 heaped tablespoons oat flakes
1 tablespoon mixed dried herbs (Herbes de Provence)
1 tablespoon olive oil

Ask for the skin to be removed, or lie the fish skin-side down on a chopping board and use a sharp knife, blade horizontal and pointing away from you, to ease the flesh away from the skin.

Lightly beat the egg and mustard. Blitz the oat flakes in a blender for a few seconds to make a coarse powder. Mix it with the dried herbs. Put the egg and oat flakes on two separate flat plates.

Gently heat the oil in a frying pan. Coat the fish in the egg, then the oat flakes. Fry the fish on each side for 3 minutes or so. Serve with lemon wedges, a green salsa (p.195), a mixed salad and half the sweet potato each, drizzled with a little olive oil.

Oat-crumb haloumi

1 egg, beaten with 1 tablespoon mustard
4 heaped tablespoons oat flakes
1 tablespoon mixed dried herbs (Herbes de Provence)
1 tablespoon olive oil
200g (7oz) haloumi, cut into 6 slices approx ½cm (¼in) thick (cut the thin end to make long strips)

Lightly beat the egg and mustard. Zap the oat flakes in a blender for a few seconds to make a coarse powder. Mix it with the dried herbs. Put the egg and oat flakes on two separate flat plates.

Gently heat a tablespoon of olive oil in a frying pan. Coat the haloumi slices in the egg mix and then the oat flakes. Fry until the crumbs are brown, when the cheese will be soft and hot. Serve with lemon wedges, a green salsa (p.195), a mixed salad and half the sweet potato each, drizzled with a little olive oil.

Soup recipes

Make two soups: two are summer soups *(p.76)*, two winter *(p.77)*.
If you wish, make and freeze extra quantities in individual servings
to use later in the month. One serving is 250ml (8fl oz).

Light vegetable broth

| ready in **20** minutes |

100g (3½oz) carrots
100g (3½oz) baby corn
100g (3½oz) baby leeks (or
spring onions)
1.2 litres (2 pints) vegetable stock
100g (3½oz) mangetout
2.5cm (1in) cube fresh ginger root,
finely grated
1x400g (13oz) can cannellini beans,
rinsed and drained
2 tablespoons lemon juice
1 tablespoon dry apple juice
1 teaspoon soy sauce
1 teaspoon miso paste
Tabasco to taste
A small bunch fresh coriander, chopped

Slice the carrots into large
matchsticks. Cut the baby corn
in half lengthways and across.
Cut the leeks or spring onions
diagonally in fine slices.

Pour the hot stock into a saucepan,
add the carrots and cook for 2
minutes. Add the mangetout and
leeks and grated ginger. Simmer
together for about 10 minutes.
Add the cannellini beans and heat
for a couple of minutes. Stir in the
lemon juice, apple juice, soy sauce,
miso paste, Tabasco and fresh
coriander. Once the soup is cool,
freeze or refrigerate until needed.

Chilled summer soup

| ready in **20** minutes |

1 medium red onion, chopped
1 pepper, deseeded and chopped
½ cucumber, chopped
1x400g (13oz) can tomatoes
1 tablespoon lemon juice
1 tablespoon olive oil
1 tablespoon tomato purée
300ml (½ pint) vegetable juice
A good stem of parsley
and a couple of sprigs of basil
Finely chopped spring onion,
cucumber and tomato to garnish
200g (7oz) quinoa
400ml (¾ pint) light vegetable stock

Put all the ingredients except the
quinoa, stock, herbs and vegetable
garnish into a blender and blitz
until smooth. Stir in the garnish
and herbs. Simmer the quinoa
in the stock until cooked. Allow
to cool, then stir into the soup.
Freeze or refrigerate until needed.

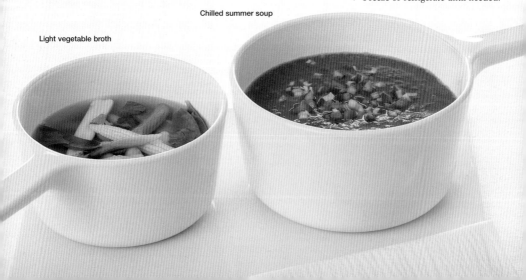

Chilled summer soup

Light vegetable broth

Tomato & mixed vegetable soup

ready in **30** minutes

2 tablespoons olive oil

1 medium onion, diced

2 sticks celery, finely sliced

1 fat clove garlic, crushed

1 large red pepper, deseeded and chopped

1x400g (13oz) can plum tomatoes, chopped

½ teaspoon paprika

1 teaspoon mango powder (or juice ½ lemon)

1 litre (1¾ pints) vegetable stock

1x400g (13oz) can cannellini beans, drained and rinsed

A few sprigs of fresh basil, shredded (or 1 teaspoon dried)

Heat the olive oil in a large saucepan. Add the onion, celery, garlic and pepper and cook gently until the vegetables begin to soften. Stir in the tomatoes, paprika and the mango powder (or lemon juice). Simmer for about 5 minutes. Add the stock and cook at a gentle simmer for about 20 minutes until the vegetables are cooked but not soggy. Stir in the cannellini beans and heat for 2–3 minutes. Add in the basil and season with freshly ground black pepper. Once cool, freeze or refrigerate until needed.

Carrot, leek & watercress soup

ready in **30** minutes

1 tablespoon olive oil

1 small onion, chopped

500g (1lb 2oz) carrots, chopped

1 medium leek, finely sliced

1x400g (13oz) can chick-peas, rinsed and drained

1 teaspoon ground cumin

1 litre (1¾ pints) vegetable stock

2 bunches watercress, chopped

Heat the oil in a saucepan and gently soften the onion. Add the carrots and leek and cook for 5 minutes. Add the chick-peas, cumin and stock. Simmer until the carrots are *al dente*. Tip into a blender, add the watercress and blend until smooth; add more stock if the mix is too thick. Add freshly ground black pepper to taste. Once cool, freeze or refrigerate until needed.

Carrot, leek & watercress soup

Tomato & mixed vegetable soup

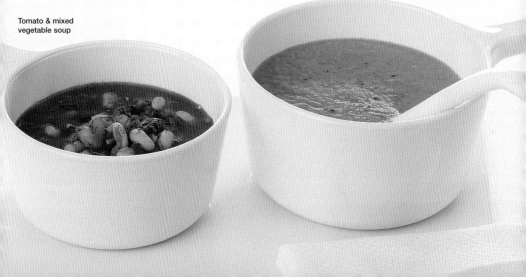

Shopping list for storecupboard foods

You may need to replace some of these items during the month.

- Barley flakes, 1 packet
- Buckwheat flour, 1 packet
- Quinoa flakes, 1 packet
- Quinoa seeds, 1 packet
- Rice, wholegrain puffed, 1 packet
- Oatcakes, approx. 4 packets
- Rye biscuits, approx. 2 packets
- Corn pasta shells, 1 packet
- Quinoa, 1 packet
- Lentils, dried puy, 1 packet
- Lentils, red, 1 packet
- Dried sea vegetables (optional) 1–2 packets

- Dried seaweed, 1 packet
- Mixed seeds, 1 tub (if not already bought for prep days) OR 1 packet each sunflower, sesame, pumpkin & linseeds to mix (see page 93)
- Sesame seeds, 1 small packet
- Sunflower seeds, 1 small packet
- Cashew nuts, raw unsalted, 1 small packet
- Mixed nuts, raw unsalted, 1 packet
- Herb teas, 1–2 packets (peppermint, rooibosch, lemon and camomile are best)
- Apricots, dried, 1 packet
- Raisins, 1 small packet
- Balsamic vinegar, 1 bottle
- Cider vinegar, 1 bottle
- Olive oil, 1 bottle (if not already bought for prep days and soups)

- Sesame oil, 1 bottle
- Soy sauce, 1 bottle (if not already bought for prep days and soups)
- *Butter beans, 1x400g (13oz) can

- ☐ *Cannellini beans, 1x400g (13oz) can
- ☐ *Chick-peas, approx. 5x400g (13oz) cans
- ☐ Coconut milk, 1x400g (13oz) can (or 50g/2oz creamed coconut)
- ☐ *Lentils, 1x400g (13oz) can
- ☐ *Mixed beans, 1x400g (13oz) can
- ☐ Passata, 1x500ml (17fl oz) carton
- ☐ *Puy lentils, 1x400g (13oz) can
- ☐ Plum tomatoes, approx. 2x400g (13oz) cans
- ☐ *Red kidney beans, 1x400g (13oz) can
- ☐ Black olives, 1 jar
- ☐ Dijon mustard, 1 pot

- ☐ Five-spice paste, 1 jar (also called Chinese five-spice paste)
- ☐ Five-spice powder, 1 jar (also called Chinese five-spice powder)
- ☐ Hot horseradish
- ☐ Mixed roast peppers, 1 jar
- ☐ Sun-dried tomatoes, 1 jar
- ☐ Tamarind paste, 1 jar
- ☐ Tabasco sauce (or cayenne pepper), 1 bottle
- ☐ Tapenade, 1 jar
- ☐ Thai fish sauce, 1 bottle
- ☐ Worcestershire sauce, 1 bottle
- ☐ Black peppercorns, 1 packet
- ☐ Black mustard seeds, 1 packet

- ☐ Caraway (or fennel) seeds, 1 packet
- ☐ Cardamom pods, 1 jar
- ☐ Cayenne pepper, 1 jar
- ☐ Celery seeds, 1 packet
- ☐ Cinnamon powder, 1 jar
- ☐ Cinnamon stick, 1
- ☐ Curry powder, 1 jar
- ☐ Dried dill, 1 jar
- ☐ Mixed dried herbs, 1 jar
- ☐ Nutmeg (fresh or dried)
- ☐ Turmeric powder, 1 jar
- ☐ Yeast-free bouillon powder, 1 tub (if not already bought for soups and prep days)

*All cans should be free from added salt and sugar

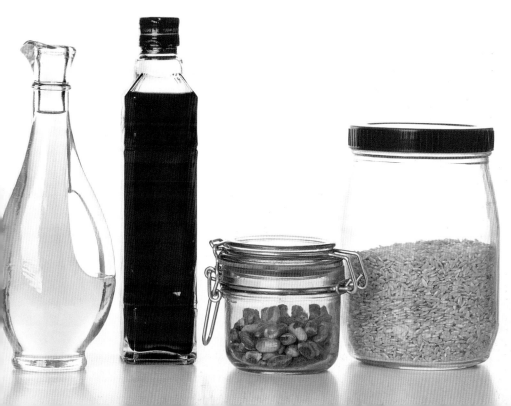

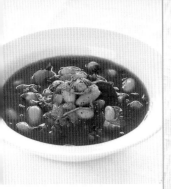
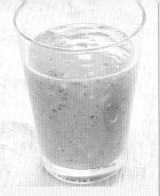
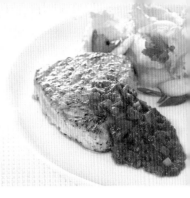

Lunch

Tomato & mixed vegetable soup, or Chilled summer soup, with 1 slice of rye bread

The recipes for all the soups are listed on pages 76–77.

Afternoon snack

250ml (8fl oz) Fruit smoothie

1 tablespoon mixed seeds, such as sesame, sunflower and pumpkin seeds *(or see p.93)*

To make the Fruit smoothie, see page 107. Either add the seeds to the smoothie mix as you blitz it in a blender, or eat them separately.

Dinner

Tuna or lentils in spicy tomato sauce *(p.101)*

Fresh tuna is an excellent source of essential fatty acids and protein, while cooked tomatoes are high in health-giving properties.

What to drink

Herb teas such as peppermint tea are an excellent choice of drink in addition to drinking plain water. These drinks can count towards your total daily fluid intake. Most fruit teas taste quite sweet, so check the ingredients and avoid any brands with added sugar. Good choices of herb or fruit teas include:

Juices diluted with water and Food Doctor soups can also count towards your daily intake of fluids. While you are following The Food Doctor 30-day diet plan, you should avoid all caffeinated tea and coffee, alcohol and soft fizzy drinks. During week 1 you should also avoid any decaffeinated drinks.

- [ ] Camomile tea
- [ ] Lemon tea
- [ ] Peppermint tea
- [ ] Rooibosch tea

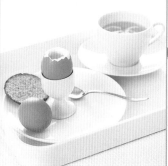
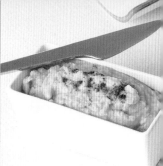

Week 1

day 5

30-DAY DIET

Breakfast

**Hot lemon & ginger drink
(p.84)**

Two boiled eggs with oatcakes
2 medium eggs
1 or 2 oatcakes, spread sparingly
with butter if you wish

Bring a small saucepan of water
to the boil and place the eggs in
the pan, one at a time, using
a tablespoon. Boil your eggs
according to your personal
preference; the ideal time to
cook a soft-boiled egg is four
minutes. Serve the eggs and
oatcakes with your morning
cup of hot lemon and ginger.

Morning snack

**250ml (8fl oz) Vitamin juice
(p.107)**

**1 oatcake generously spread
with houmous** *(below)*

Home-made houmous
1x400g (13oz) can chick-peas, rinsed
and drained
2 cloves garlic
3 tablespoons lemon juice
3 tablespoons olive oil
2 tablespoons sesame oil
2 teaspoons soy sauce

Put the ingredients in a food
processor. Blitz until smooth.
Season with freshly ground black
pepper. Add more soy sauce, or
lemon juice to taste. For an
interesting texture, stir in 1
tablespoon of toasted sesame
seeds. Cover and store in the
fridge for up to five days.

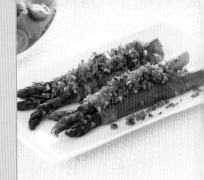

The Food Doctor

Tip for the day ...

If you tend to feel hungry again a couple of hours after eating dinner, save a small portion of your meal to eat as a late snack.

Lunch

**Roast vegetables
with feta cheese**

2 tablespoons roast vegetables
reserved from dinner, day 3

50g (2oz) feta cheese

1 oatcake

Crumble the feta cheese over the roast vegetables and serve with the oatcake.

Afternoon snack

250ml (8fl oz) Fruit smoothie

**1 tablespoon mixed seeds,
such as sesame, sunflower and
pumpkin seeds *(or see p.93)***

To make the Fruit smoothie, see page 107. Either add the seeds to the smoothie mix as you blitz it in a blender, or eat them separately.

Dinner

**Crumbed asparagus with ham
or haloumi & salad *(p.102)***

This recipe uses asparagus in a different way: roasted rather than steamed. Eating asparagus regularly can help maintain healthy bacteria in your digestive system.

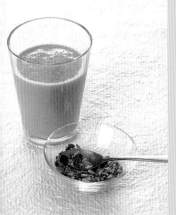

Alternative snacks

If you happen to forget to make your own vitamin juice or smoothie, or end up being on the go all day, try these substitutes – but only occasionally, as buying ready-made produce is not ideal.

For an alternative vitamin juice, buy a can of vegetable juice and have 250ml (8fl oz) with 1 tablespoon of mixed seeds and a couple of sprigs of watercress. If you have a blender to hand, blitz these ingredients together with a squeeze of lemon juice or a slice of fresh ginger.

To make a substitute smoothie, buy a fresh, ready-made fruit smoothie that contains no banana, yoghurt or added sugar. Mix the smoothie with 75ml (3fl oz) nut milk, 2 tablespoons of no-fat soft cheese and a squeeze of lemon. Measure 250ml (8fl oz) and have the smoothie with 1 tablespoon of mixed seeds.

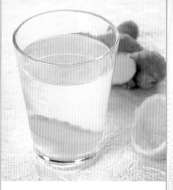

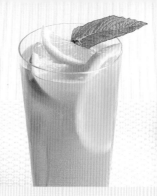

Week

day 6

30-DAY DIET

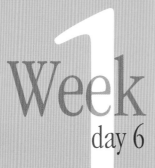

Breakfast

Hot lemon & ginger drink *(p.84)*

Apple & pear porridge with yoghurt

50g (2oz) oat flakes
150ml (¼ pint) water
25ml (1fl oz) dry apple juice
2 tablespoons live natural low-fat yoghurt
1 pear, cored and chopped

Gently simmer the oat flakes with the water and apple juice. Serve with the yoghurt and chopped pear on top.

Morning snack

250ml (8fl oz) Vitamin juice

1 tablespoon flavoured or plain no-fat soft cheese or houmous with crudités or 1 oatcake

To make the Vitamin juice, see page 107. Add fresh watercress if you are using a vitamin juice mix that you prepared previously.

If you are on the go today and need a more instant snack, have an apple or a pear with six or seven raw, unsalted nuts, such as almonds, walnuts and Brazil nuts.

The Food Doctor
Tip for the day

To give your meal tomorrow night a stronger flavour, marinate either the tofu or chicken tonight (*see p.104 for ingredients*).

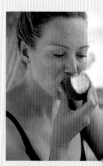

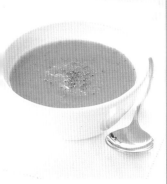
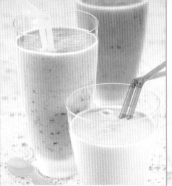
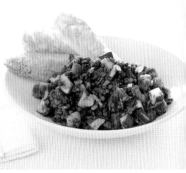

Lunch

Carrot, leek & watercress soup, or Light vegetable broth, with 1 slice of rye bread

All soup recipes are listed on pages 76–77.

Afternoon snack

250ml (8fl oz) Fruit smoothie

1 tablespoon mixed seeds, such as sesame, sunflower and pumpkin seeds *(or see p.93)*

To make the Fruit smoothie, see page 107. Either add the seeds to the smoothie mix as you blitz it in a blender, or eat them separately.

Dinner

Warm lentil salad *(p.103)*

Save a portion for lunch tomorrow

Lentils are a valuable source of vegetable protein, minerals and soluble fibre. Puy lentils taste wonderfully rich and meaty, which adds to the big flavours in this dish.

Make time to eat

Eating is obviously essential, but it's also meant to be pleasurable. Many of us lead such busy lives that we treat most of the meals we eat like fast food: we eat as quickly as possible in order to move onto the important tasks of the day.

If you stop what you're doing and make time to eat, the benefits are huge: you reduce your stress levels and gain a feeling of satisfaction that you've eaten a tasty, filling meal. Chew your food slowly and thoroughly so that you digest your food properly and maintain good digestive health. Your body can then absorb the nutrients effectively. Make time to eat is Principle 9 of The 10 Food Doctor principles *(pp.38–39)*.

Week 1

day 7

30-DAY DIET

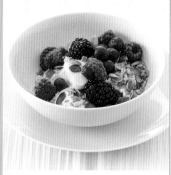

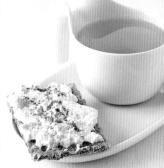

Breakfast

Hot lemon & ginger drink *(p.84)*

Yoghurt with toasted oat flakes or puffed rice, seeds & fruit

4 tablespoons live natural low-fat yoghurt

1 tablespoon toasted flakes or puffed rice *(see recipe, right)*

3 tablespoons mixed seeds

½ pomegranate or 2 tablespoons of mixed berries if in season

Put the yoghurt into a bowl and add the toasted cereal and seeds. Loosen the pomegranate seeds by gently squeezing the fruit and easing out the red seeds with a fork, avoiding the yellow pith. Spoon the pomegranate seeds or berries over the top and serve.

Morning snack

250ml (8fl oz) Vitamin juice

1 rye biscuit generously spread with flavoured or plain no-fat soft cheese *(p.84)*, houmous *(p.88)* or cottage cheese

To make the Vitamin juice, see page 107. Add fresh watercress if you are using a vitamin juice mix that you prepared previously.

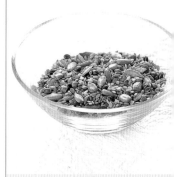

The Food Doctor

Tip for the day ...

To prolong the shelf life of your batches of toasted cereals and seeds, store the airtight jars in a cool, dark place.

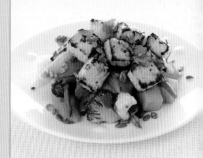

Lunch

Lentil salad

1 portion Lentil salad reserved
from dinner, day 6

Your choice of salad dressing
(pp.173, 175, 177)

A small side salad (optional)

Drizzle a little of the salad dressing over the lentil salad, add a few lettuce leaves if you wish and serve.

Afternoon snack

250ml (8fl oz) Fruit smoothie

1 tablespoon mixed seeds, such as sesame, sunflower and pumpkin seeds (or see p.93)

To make the Fruit smoothie, see page 107. Either add the seeds to the smoothie mix as you blitz it in a blender, or eat them separately.

Dinner

Spicy tofu or chicken with steamed rainbow vegetables (p.104)

Choose a colourful mix of seasonal vegetables for this meal. Brightly coloured fruit and vegetables provide high levels of beneficial nutrients, while soya and chicken are both ideal sources of lean protein.

Preparing a batch

Toasted flakes or rice

125–250g (4–8oz) oat flakes or wholegrain puffed rice, depending on how big a batch you want to make

Preheat the oven to 180°C/350°F/Gas mark 4. Spread the flakes or rice on a baking sheet. Cook for 20 minutes, turning occasionally. Once browned, leave to cool and store in an airtight jar.

Toasted cereal & Toasted seeds

For the cereal:

50g (2oz) quinoa seeds

50g (2oz) quinoa flakes

100g (3½oz) barley flakes

100g (3½oz) oat flakes

50g (2oz) raisins

For the seeds:

1 tablespoon each quinoa seeds, sesame seeds, pumpkin seeds, sunflower seeds, poppy seeds

Heat a heavy, dry pan until hot. Toast each seed or cereal for a few minutes until browned. Toss regularly. Leave to cool. When the cereal is cool, stir in the raisins. Store in airtight jars.

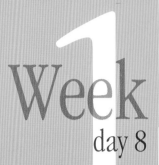

Week

day 8

30-DAY DIET

The Food Doctor

Tip for the day ...

Don't use lack of time as a reason not to exercise. Factor some activity into your day for the best possible results.

Breakfast

Hot lemon & ginger drink *(p.84)*

Spicy mixed flake porridge

1 star anise

100ml (3½fl oz) boiling water

30g (1oz) mixed flakes (use a mix of large and small flakes: oats, millet, quinoa, barley, rice, etc)

¼ teaspoon ground cinnamon

Juice ¼ lemon

1 tablespoon live natural low-fat yoghurt

1 apple, cored and grated

Rind ¼ orange

Sunflower seeds (optional)

Put the star anise into a jug and pour in the boiling water. Leave to stand for 5 minutes. Put the flakes in a pan, add the ground spice, lemon juice and water and stir well. Simmer gently for 3 minutes, or until the flakes are soft and the mix is a thick but soft consistency. Stir in the yoghurt. Serve topped with the apple, orange rind and seeds.

Morning snack

250ml (8fl oz) Vitamin juice

1 oatcake generously spread with houmous *(p.88)*, **flavoured or plain no-fat soft cheese or cottage cheese**

To make the Vitamin juice, see page 107. Add fresh watercress if you are using a vitamin juice mix that you prepared previously. If you don't have time to make your own houmous, try to buy organic houmous. The quality of olive oil used in organic products is usually better, which gives you some beneficial essential fats.

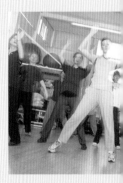

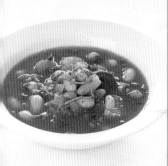
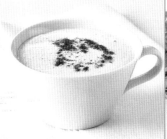
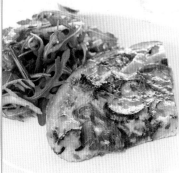

Lunch

Tomato & mixed vegetable soup, or Chilled summer soup, with 1 slice of rye bread

The recipes for both soups are listed on pages 76–77.

Afternoon snack

250ml (8fl oz) Fruit smoothie

1 tablespoon mixed seeds, such as sesame, sunflower and pumpkin seeds *(or see p.93)*

To make the Fruit smoothie, see page 107. Either add the seeds to the smoothie mix as you blitz it in a blender, or eat them separately.

Dinner

Frittata & green leaves *(p.105)*

Save a portion for lunch tomorrow if you wish

Egg dishes make a filling and satisfying fast meal, so it's always worth keeping some eggs in the fridge as an essential standby ingredient.

Exercise is essential

It's hard to find time to exercise if your week is busy, but fitting in a brisk walk every day, or a couple of workouts a week at the gym, will mean that your success rate on this diet will be much better than if you do nothing at all.

Any exercise that raises your heart rate consistently for a minimum of 20 minutes is ideal. And while exercise is essential, movement is even more crucial: take the stairs at work or walk to the next bus stop to keep physically active. But don't overdo things: if you over-exercise, your metabolic rate may actually slow down in time.

Have a small snack before and after you exercise to sustain your energy levels *(see also p.168)*. Exercise is essential is Principle 7 of The 10 Food Doctor principles *(pp.34–35)*.

Week
day 9

1
30-DAY DIET

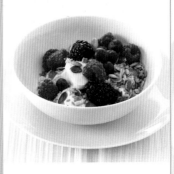

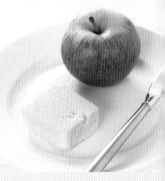

Breakfast

Hot lemon & ginger drink *(p.84)*

Your choice of cereal breakfast

Cereal recipes are listed on pages 84, 86, 90, 92 and 94.

Morning snack

250ml (8fl oz) Vitamin juice

1 apple with a small piece of feta cheese

To make the Vitamin juice, see page 107. Add fresh watercress if you use a juice mix you prepared previously. If you have to make a substitute juice, see page 89.

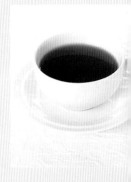

Tip for the day ...

You can buy ready-grown sprouted seeds in the shops, but if you want to grow your own sprouted seeds, see page 181.

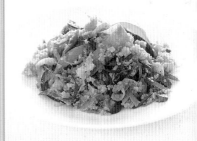

Lunch

Frittata or Chick-pea salad

1 portion reserved Frittata from dinner, day 8 with 2 tablespoons sprouted seeds, a dressing *(pp.173,175,177)* and 1 slice bread

OR

1 tablespoon canned chick-peas, 4 cherry tomatoes, 2 tablespoons sprouted seeds and a dressing, 1 tablespoon mixed seeds *(p.93)* and 1 slice bread

Drizzle the dressing over the frittata or salad and serve with the bread on the side.

Afternoon snack

250ml (8fl oz) Fruit smoothie

1 tablespoon mixed seeds, such as sesame, sunflower and pumpkin seeds *(or see p.93)*

To make the Fruit smoothie, see page 107. Either add the seeds to the smoothie mix as you blitz it in a blender, or eat them separately.

Dinner

Egg-fried quinoa

Either save a portion of egg-fried quinoa or reserve some raw vegetables for lunch tomorrow

If you'd prefer not to include egg in tonight's recipe, marinate 150g (5oz) tofu in soy sauce and lemon juice, cook it under the grill and add it to the dish.

Health check

This is the end of your first full week on the diet. You may be experiencing headaches, mild diarrhoea, spots or lethargy, but these symptoms should soon pass. If you have water retention, try drinking dandelion tea.

On the other hand, you may already be experiencing some positive benefits:

☐ Reduced cravings for caffeine, sugar and/or alcohol
☐ Improved digestion
☐ Enhanced absorption of ingredients
☐ More energy
☐ Improved sense of well-being

Don't worry if some or all of these beneficial effects don't apply to you yet – it's different for everyone.

Week 1 diary

During week 1, keep track of the foods
and recipes that you're enjoying, and
how you are feeling. Tick off each day
as you go, and make a daily record
of how you're coping and whether
you are becoming aware of any major
or minor changes to your health.

DAY 3

What I've enjoyed eating/How do I feel?

DAY 6

What I've enjoyed eating/How do I feel?

DAY 7

What I've enjoyed eating/How do I feel?

DAY 4
What I've enjoyed eating/How do I feel?

DAY 5
What I've enjoyed eating/How do I feel?

DAY 8
What I've enjoyed eating/How do I feel?

DAY 9
What I've enjoyed eating/How do I feel?

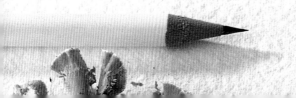

Roast vegetables & chick-peas with feta cheese

This meal is deliciously crunchy and filling. Butternut squash is a good alternative if you can't find acorn squash. Try using a vegetable peeler to take off the skin. Serves two.

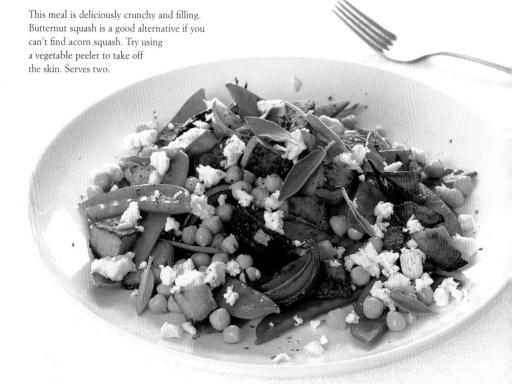

250g (8oz) red onion

250g (8oz) acorn (or other firm-fleshed) squash

1–2 tablespoons olive oil

2–3 sprigs fresh sage (or ½ teaspoon dried sage)

150g (5oz) mangetout, rinsed

1x400g (13oz) can chick-peas, rinsed and drained (reserve 1 tablespoon for day 8 dinner)

100g (3½oz) feta cheese, crumbled

Heat the oven to 180°C/350°F/Gas mark 4. Peel and slice the red onion coarsely from top to bottom. Peel and cut the squash into cubes.

Heat a tablespoon of olive oil in a roasting tin, add the onions and toss well. Cook for 10 minutes. Add the squash and the sage, mix well and cook for a further 15 minutes. Add the mangetout and chick-peas, mix well and add another tablespoon of olive oil if necessary. Cook for a further 5 minutes.

Remove 2 heaped tablespoons of the roast vegetables to save for lunch on Day 5. Divide the remainder onto two plates, top with the crumbled feta and a little chopped sage and serve.

Tuna or lentils in spicy tomato sauce

DINNER DAY 4

The tomato sauce for this dish is very spicy.
If you prefer a milder sauce, reduce the quantity
of chilli powder you use or leave it out altogether.
Serves two.

ready in **30** minutes

1 tablespoon olive oil, plus extra for brushing tuna

2 shallots, peeled and chopped

½ teaspoon smoked paprika

¼ teaspoon chilli powder (or to taste depending on the strength of the powder)

1x200g (7oz) can chopped tomatoes

1 teaspoon tomato purée

1 clove garlic, crushed

Juice ½ orange

1 teaspoon balsamic vinegar

2 tuna steaks (approx. 100g/3½oz each) or 150g (5oz) puy lentils and 400ml (¾ pint) light vegetable stock (if you make the stock too strong, the lentils taste salty)

To cook the tuna:

Cook the tomato sauce first, then brush
each steak with a tablespoon of olive oil
and cover with a good grinding of fresh
black pepper. Wrap each steak tightly
in foil. Heat a heavy-based pan until
very hot. Put the wrapped tuna in
the pan and press down hard to
cook it. Turn over and repeat.
Cook for approximately 5 minutes
on each side. Unwrap and serve with
the sauce and a large green salad.

To cook the lentils:

Cook the lentils first, then the sauce. Simmer
the lentils in the stock in a medium-sized
saucepan, uncovered, for about 25 minutes, or until
all the fluid has been absorbed. Stir the tomato sauce
into the lentils and serve with a large green salad.

To make the spicy tomato sauce:

Heat a tablespoon of olive oil in a small saucepan over
a medium heat. Add the shallots and let them soften for
a few minutes. Turn the heat down a little if they brown
too quickly. Add the paprika and chilli powder and stir
quickly. Add the tomatoes, tomato purée and garlic, stir
well and bring the sauce to simmering point. Stir in
the orange juice and vinegar and simmer gently for
5 minutes to allow the flavours to blend well.

Tuna in spicy
tomato sauce

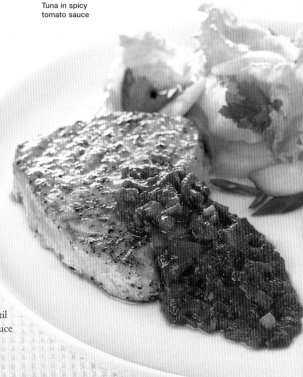

Crumbed asparagus with ham or haloumi & salad

If asparagus is not in season, try baking two heads of chicory until tender in a shallow dish half-filled with vegetable stock. Serves two.

ready in 25 minutes

12 spears fresh asparagus, tough ends snapped off
1–2 teaspoons olive oil
4 thin slices of Parma ham (or a good-quality cooked ham) or 4 thin slices haloumi

For the topping:
1 clove garlic, chopped or crushed
1 thick slice rye bread
1 teaspoon mixed toasted seeds (p.93)
Grated zest ½ orange
1 teaspoon olive oil

Preheat the oven to 200°C/400°F/Gas mark 6. Wash the asparagus spears thoroughly, put them in a baking tray, add a teaspoon or so of olive oil and lightly coat each spear in the oil. Roast for 10–12 minutes until just tender.

While the asparagus cooks, make the topping: either blitz all the ingredients in a small chopper, or grate the breadcrumbs, crush the seeds in a pestle and mortar and add the other ingredients.

Group the roasted spears in four bundles of three spears each. If using ham, wrap each bundle in one slice of ham. Top each parcel with some crumb mixture and brown gently under the grill for 5 minutes or so. Serve with a mixed salad.

If using haloumi, cover each bundle with one slice of haloumi. Top each parcel with some crumb mixture and brown gently under the grill for about 5 minutes. Serve with a mixed salad.

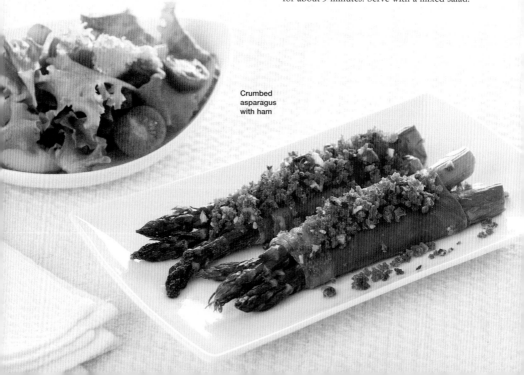

Crumbed
asparagus
with ham

Warm lentil salad

If time is short in the evening, you can use a can of lentils, and chop the pepper, onion and courgette in advance. Reserve a portion for lunch tomorrow. Serves two.

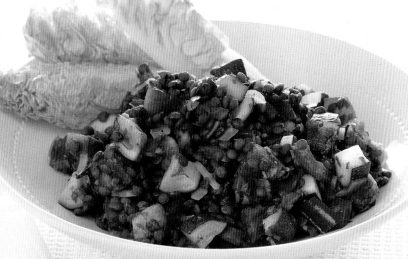

150g (5oz) dried puy lentils
(or 1x400g/13oz can puy lentils)

400ml (¾ pint) very light vegetable stock (if cooking dried puy lentils) with 1 thick slice lemon added

1 tablespoon olive oil

1 small onion, chopped

1 clove garlic, peeled

1 medium courgette, cubed

1 red pepper (such as Romano), chopped

3 good-sized, ripe tomatoes, skinned and chopped
(or in winter use 1x200g/7oz can chopped tomatoes)

1 teaspoon balsamic vinegar

2.5cm (1in) fresh ginger, grated (optional)

A small bunch fresh basil or coriander, chopped

1 tablespoon mixed seeds (*p.93*)

Simmer the dried lentils in the stock and lemon for 25–30 minutes until the stock is absorbed. Top wup with water if the stock boils away too fast. Discard the lemon slice.

Heat the oil in a frying pan or wok. Gently soften the onion, then add the garlic, courgette and pepper. Stir over a medium heat for a few minutes until they begin to soften, but still have a bite. Add the tomatoes, vinegar and ginger, and season with freshly ground black pepper. Cook until all the vegetables are piping hot.

Combine with the lentils, stir in the fresh herbs, add a spoonful of seeds and serve with a fresh green salad on the side.

If you would prefer to have this with extra protein, serve it with some grilled haloumi.

Spicy chicken or tofu with rainbow vegetables

If you can marinate the tofu or chicken overnight, the flavours will be more intense. Otherwise, marinate the ingredients for a minimum of 15 minutes. Serves two.

ready in 30 minutes

2 chicken joints (leg and thigh), skinned, with the flesh scored a couple of times, or 200g (7oz) tofu, cut into cubes
3–4 good sprigs fresh coriander, chopped
A few mixed seeds

For the marinade:
½ onion or 2 large shallots
2 cloves garlic, peeled
2.5cm (1in) fresh ginger, peeled and chopped
½ teaspoon ground cumin powder
Juice and grated zest ½ lemon
4 tablespoons live natural low-fat yoghurt

For the vegetables:
300g (10oz) mix of vegetables per person, cut into small chunks or 1 packet ready-prepared vegetables

Blitz the onion or shallot, garlic, ginger and cumin in a blender (or grate the onion and ginger and crush the garlic). Add the lemon and yoghurt and stir. Season with freshly ground black pepper Add the tofu or rub the marinade into the chicken joints and leave to marinate.

If using chicken, preheat the oven to 180°C/350°F/Gas mark 4. Place the chicken into a baking dish, cover with foil and cook for about 30 minutes until the juices run clear, but the chicken isn't dried out.

Put the vegetables in a steamer and steam for 10–15 minutes until they are just cooked, but not soft.

If using tofu, set the grill at medium hot and grill the pieces of tofu for a few minutes on each side until golden brown.

Divide the vegetables between two plates and pile on the chicken or tofu. Heat the remaining marinade, drizzle over each plate and serve with chopped coriander and seeds scattered on top.

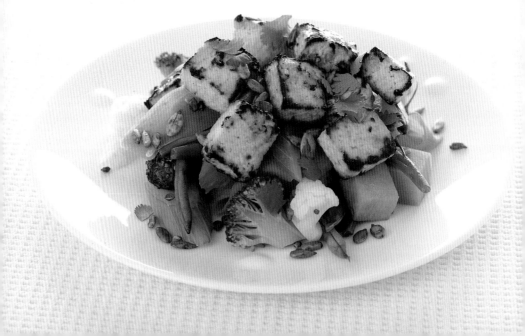

Frittata & green leaves

Buy a jar each of sun-dried tomatoes and peppers and use some frozen peas if you don't have time to roast vegetables tonight. Save a portion for lunch tomorrow. Serves two.

ready in 30 minutes

250g (8oz) mix of vegetables, chopped
1 tablespoon olive oil, plus a little extra to cook the onion
1 small onion, sliced
6 medium hen's eggs
1 tablespoon live natural low-fat yoghurt
1 tablespoon canned chick-peas, rinsed and drained
A handful fresh parsley or coriander, chopped

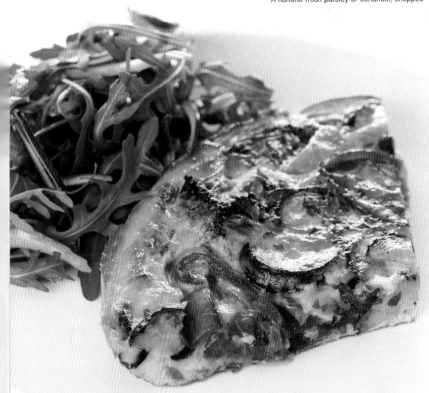

Preheat the oven to 180°C/350°/Gas mark 4. Use a small roasting tin to toss the mixed vegetables in a tablespoon of olive oil and roast for about 20 minutes until cooked. Cook the onion in a large omelette pan in a little olive oil until soft. Whisk the eggs and yoghurt, add the chick-peas and pour onto the onions. Stir in the roasted vegetables. Season with freshly ground black pepper, add chopped parsley or coriander and stir. Allow to cook gently until the bottom is set, then slip the pan under a medium grill to brown the top. Serve with a salad of green leaves.

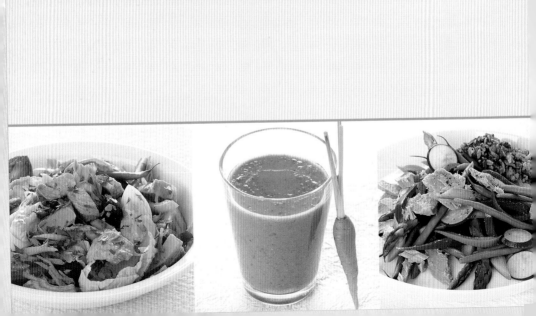

Weeks 2 & 3: readjusting

The following two weeks show how adaptable my plan is, as there are more choices for meals and snacks. Any side-effects experienced in the first week should now be a thing of the past, and you will really begin to see my principles in action.

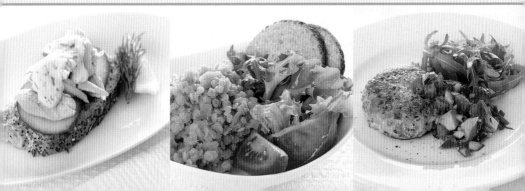

Readjusting: Ian's advice

Congratulations on getting through the first week. If you found week 1 challenging, you'll be pleased to hear that weeks 2 and 3 are more easy going, allowing you a little more freedom in what you can eat.

A good diet has innumerable benefits, so investing some time and thought into what you eat has to be a worthwhile exercise. If you found the first week especially tough then I am delighted you have got this far. The harder you found it, the more it suggests that your diet really needed some attention. The discipline that the first week demands is a useful exercise in understanding the level of priority that food has been for you in the past. Many clients report that after the first couple of days of being on my Food Doctor Diet plan, they find they get into the habit of preparing and planning food a little way in advance. They are often shocked to realize how little time they had previously spent on organizing and eating their food.

The **good news** is that **things get easier** from here on

Dealing with choice

The good news is that things get easier from here on. You will be able to mix and match to suit your tastes. If you flick through the next few pages, you will see that I'd still like you to start the day with the hot lemon and ginger drink, but that the breakfasts are more varied. You'll also be continuing with the mid-morning and mid-afternoon snacks, although it's up to you to

Ask yourself, "**Where's my protein?**" every time you **decide** what to **eat**

choose what you want to eat from the selection of juice, smoothie and snack recipes provided.

Some clients find that the prescriptive nature of the first week suits them really well, and they can be somewhat daunted by the choice that this next stage affords. If you find yourself feeling a little anxious about what's in store over the next two weeks, my advice is simple. Now that you have some flexibility in your routine, it's worthwhile reminding yourself often that you should be asking, "Where's my protein?" every time you make a decision about what to eat. If you keep this simple mantra in mind, you will find it much easier to stay within the guidelines of the plan and reap the benefits.

All in all, this gradual process of readjusting to a better way of eating should enable you to become accustomed to the extra effort of choosing the right types of food for yourself. There has been some really encouraging feedback from clients of their experiences in weeks 2 and 3, with

You should feel a **growing** sense of **confidence** when making **food** decisions

Sharing **thoughts** and **experiences** is a **great** means of moral **support**

comments ranging from "shopping for food is now more fun and stimulating", to "my awareness of foods around me is improving". In weeks 2 and 3 you should hopefully feel a sense of growing confidence when it comes to making great food decisions and planning ahead for meals.

Coping with difficult situations

For those of you who do shift work, I can appreciate that ensuring that you eat every two and a half to three hours can be a problem. Bear in mind that half an apple and a palmful of mixed seeds or nuts will do as a snack, and they are foods that can easily be slipped into your pocket or bag. This may not make for an exciting snack, but as we all have to adapt the food we can eat around our work and family commitments, this is probably the best solution.

I also know that weekend afternoons can be a problem when you have less to occupy yourself

with than usual. You might want to think back to what you had for brunch or lunch and check that it was correctly balanced with the right food types to ensure a slow and consistent level of blood glucose. If you truly are hungry, you may need to tweak your lunchtime accordingly or, if you had brunch,

I suggest that you have a small extra snack, such as sliced fruit with some sort of protein. If you find that you are eating or wanting to eat out of boredom, then please find something to do. It's an easy answer, but distracting yourself may really be the best way. If you have kids and are tempted to eat their tea, I recommend that you cook them food that you can also eat as a snack without veering away from the plan.

Late evenings can be a problem too, and in many ways this highlights the fact that in the past you may have been eating out of boredom rather than hunger. If you are hungry, then a little leftover dinner as a small snack should suffice, even if it's just a couple of mouthfuls. Some clients find that making themselves a cup of herbal tea satisfies their need to get something from the kitchen, so consider that option too.

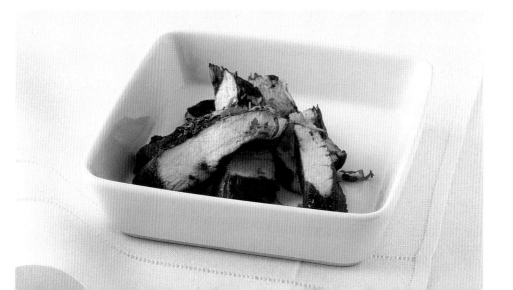

Shopping list for weeks 2 & 3, days 10–23

This shopping list includes approximate quantities for all the supper recipes and weekday lunches. It does not include ingredients for your choice of breakfasts, snacks, or weekend brunches or lunches.

FRESH FOOD FOR WEEK 2, DAYS 10–16

- [ ] Lemons, 2
- [ ] Limes, 1
- [ ] Oranges, 2
- [ ] Asparagus, 100g (3½oz)
- [ ] Avocado, 1
- [ ] Beetroot, raw or ready-cooked, 150g (5oz)
- [ ] Carrots, medium, 2
- [ ] Cherry tomatoes, 1 large tub
- [ ] Chicory, medium, 2 (or gem lettuce)
- [ ] Courgettes, medium, 1
- [ ] Fennel, medium, 1
- [ ] Mixed green vegetables, approx. 600g (1lb 3½oz)
- [ ] Mixed raw vegetables (eg, French beans, runner beans, mangetout, asparagus) approx. 450g (15oz)
- [ ] Mixed salad ingredients: enough for 9 portions
- [ ] Mushrooms, small, 150g (5oz), plus 8 mushrooms (if making Vegetable brochettes, day 12)
- [ ] Onions, small, 4
- [ ] Onions, medium, 2
- [ ] Peppers, red, 3
- [ ] Peppers, yellow, 2
- [ ] Root ginger, fresh, 1 large piece
- [ ] Spinach (fresh or frozen) or kale, 100g (3½oz)

- [ ] Sprouted seeds (if not growing your own), 1 tub
- [ ] Coriander, fresh, 1 bunch
- [ ] Parsley, fresh, 1 bunch
- [ ] Feta cheese, 150g (5oz)
- [ ] Haloumi, 200g (7oz) (if making Grilled haloumi, day 10)
- [ ] Hen's eggs, 3
- [ ] Reduced-fat fromage frais, 1 tub
- [ ] Tofu, 200–250g (7–8oz) (if making Smoked tofu salad, day 14)
- [ ] Dry apple juice, 1 carton
- [ ] Chicken thigh fillets, 250–300g (8–11oz) (if making Chicken brochettes, day 12)
- [ ] Duck breasts, 2, approx. 200g (7oz) each (if making Duck breast salad, day 14)
- [ ] Trout, 2, approx. 200g (7oz) after removing the head and tail (if making Baked trout, day 10)
- [ ] Tuna, 1 small can for lunch, day 10, and 1 large can (if you have run out) for lunch day 16

DAY 13 DINNER OPTIONS

Quick country soup

- [ ] Lemons, 1
- [ ] Mushrooms, button, 400g (13oz)
- [ ] Onions, medium, 1

- [ ] Dried sea vegetables, 1 small packet, or spinach, 50g (2oz)
- [ ] Vegetable stock, 500ml (17fl oz)

Four bean salad

- [ ] Lemons, 1
- [ ] Broad beans, 100g (3½oz)
- [ ] Green beans, 100g (3½oz)
- [ ] Mangetout or petit pois, 100g (3½oz)
- [ ] Pepper, 1 (red or orange)
- [ ] Spring onions, 1 bunch
- [ ] Fresh herbs of your choice, 1 bunch
- [ ] Feta cheese, 50g (optional)
- [ ] *Cannellini beans, 1x400g (13oz) can (if you have run out)

FRESH FOOD FOR WEEK 3, DAYS 17–23

- [ ] Lemons, approx. 4
- [ ] Limes, 2
- [ ] Aubergines, 1 (approx. 200g/7oz)
- [ ] Beefsteak tomatoes, 2
- [ ] Carrots, small, 2 (if making Vegetarian burgers, day 23)
- [ ] Cherry tomatoes, 1 tub
- [ ] Courgettes, 500g (1lb)
- [ ] Mixed raw vegetables, approx. 250g (8oz) or

- [ ] equivalent weight of ready-prepared vegetables in packets
- [ ] Mixed salad ingredients: enough for 9 portions
- [ ] Mushrooms, large, 4
- [ ] Onions, medium, 1
- [ ] Shiitake mushrooms, 4 (if making Vegetarian burgers, day 23)
- [ ] Spring onions, 1 bunch)
- [ ] Sprouted seeds, 1 tub (if you are not growing your own)
- [ ] Sweet potatoes, medium, 1
- [ ] Tomatoes, large, 5
- [ ] Coriander, fresh, 1 packet
- [ ] Parsley, fresh, 1 bunch
- [ ] Root ginger, fresh, 1 large piece (if you have run out)
- [ ] Cottage cheese, 1 tub
- [ ] Feta or haloumi cheese, 200g (7oz) (if using cheese, day 22)
- [ ] Hen's eggs, 4 (3 if making Egg noodles, day 21, 1 if making Vegetarian burgers, day 23)
- [ ] Live natural low-fat yoghurt, 1 large pot (if you have run out)
- [ ] Black olives, 8–10
- [ ] Smoked tofu, 100g (3½oz) if making Stir-fry tofu, day 19
- [ ] Tofu, 200g (7oz) (if making Vegetarian burgers, day 23)
- [ ] Rye bread, 1 loaf
- [ ] Chicken, 100g (3½oz) (if making Stir-fry chicken, day 19)
- [ ] Chicken or turkey, minced, 300g (10oz) (if making Chicken burgers, day 23)
- [ ] Salmon fillet, 150–200g (5–7oz) (if making Salmon cakes, day 21)

- [ ] White fish fillet, 250–300g (8–10oz) (if using fish, day 22)

DAY 20 DINNER OPTIONS
Salade niçoise
- [ ] Carrot, medium, 1
- [ ] Gem lettuce or similar, 1
- [ ] Green or runner beans, 100g (3½oz)
- [ ] Pepper, yellow, 1
- [ ] Spring onions, 1 bunch
- [ ] Tomatoes, medium, 2
- [ ] Fresh herbs of your choice, 1 bunch
- [ ] Hen's eggs 1 (2 if making vegetarian option)
- [ ] Black olives, 6–8
- [ ] Tuna steak, fresh, 1 or 1 large can of tuna in spring water (if making traditional Salad niçoise)
- [ ] *Chick-peas, 1x400g (13oz) can (if you have run out and are making Spicy chick-peas)

Leek & potato soup
- [ ] Leeks, large, 1
- [ ] Onions, medium, 1
- [ ] Sweet potato, medium, 1
- [ ] Dried sea vegetables, 1 small packet
- [ ] Quinoa, 100g (3½oz) (if you have run out)
- [ ] Light vegetable stock 250ml (8fl oz)

*All cans should be free from added salt and sugar

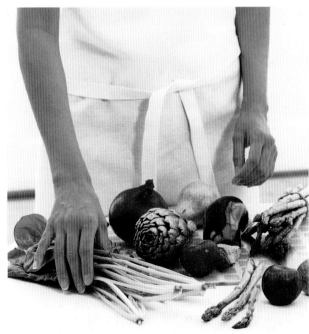

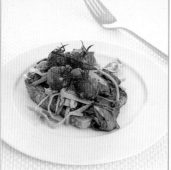

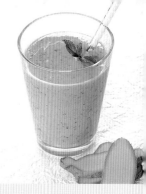

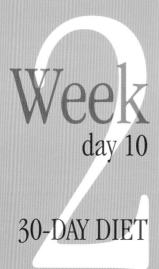

Week

day 10

30-DAY DIET

Breakfast

Hot lemon & ginger
drink *(p.84)*

Cereal or ham
breakfast *(below)*

Cereal recipes are listed on
pages 84, 86, 90, 92 and 94.

Sliced ham with tomatoes & spinach

4 cherry tomatoes

A drizzle of olive oil

45g (1½oz) baby spinach leaves

1 thin slice ham, cut into fine strips

1 slice rye or wholemeal toast

Preheat the oven to 180°C/350°F/
Gas mark 4. Put the tomatoes on a
baking tray, and drizzle over a little
olive oil. Roast for 10–15 minutes.
Meanwhile, steam the spinach.
Place the tomatoes, spinach and
ham on the toast and serve.

Morning snack

Choose either:

250ml (8fl oz) Vitamin juice
(if you have any portions left
over from week 1) and
1 oatcake with your choice
of spread *(below)*

OR

2 oatcakes or rye biscuits
with your choice of spread:

☐ Bean & mustard
   mash *(p.137)*

☐ Home-made houmous *(p.88)*

☐ Reduced-fat fromage frais
   & peppers *(below)*

☐ Spicy chick-pea
   spread *(p.137)*

Reduced-fat fromage frais & peppers

2 tablespoons low-fat fromage frais

2 peppers from a jar, chopped

A squeeze of lemon juice

Spread the fromage frais on two
oatcakes. Top with the peppers
and a little lemon juice. Store any
leftovers in the fridge for up to
two days.

The Food Doctor

Tip for the day ...

Look back to days 3, 4, 6, 7 and 9 for different cereal-based recipes if you don't want ham for breakfast this morning.

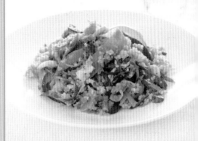

Lunch

Egg-fried quinoa

OR

Tuna or tofu salad with seeds

1 portion egg-fried rice reserved from dinner, day 9

OR

1 portion chopped raw vegetables reserved from dinner, day 9

1 tablespoon chick-peas, drained and rinsed

1 small can tuna, drained, or 150g (5oz) smoked tofu

A little dressing *(pp.173,175,177)*

If you are having egg-fried quinoa, serve it cold with a few mixed seeds scattered over the top if you wish. If you are having the tuna or tofu salad, mix all the ingredients together with the dressing and serve.

Afternoon snack

Choose either:

250ml (8fl oz) High-energy smoothie *(below)*

OR

2 oatcakes or rye biscuits with your choice of spread:

☐ Bean & mustard mash *(p.137)*
☐ Home-made houmous *(p.88)*
☐ Reduced-fat fromage frais & peppers *(see recipe, left)*
☐ Spicy chick-pea spread *(p.137)*

Afternoon snack recipe

All the smoothies listed in week 2 and beyond are complete foods and are good on their own for afternoon snacks. The quantities listed should make 500ml (17fl oz) – enough for two smoothies. If not, top up with a little apple juice. Always store the second portion in the fridge.

High-energy smoothie

½ avocado, stoned and peeled
A small handful fresh watercress
5cm (2in) fresh ginger, grated

Dinner

Baked trout or grilled haloumi *(p.130)*

Save a portion for lunch tomorrow

Serve your choice of baked trout or haloumi with stir-fried vegetables. If using haloumi, cook the stir fry first.

2 or 3 sprigs of mint
100ml (3½ oz) water
100ml (3½ oz) dry apple juice
Juice ½ lemon
150ml (¼ pint) live natural low-fat yoghurt

Blend all the vegetables, herbs, water and juices together. Stir in the yoghurt. Do not sieve the smoothie mix as this will remove valuable fibre. If you wish, serve the smoothie with an extra sprig of fresh mint as a garnish.

Week 2

day 11

30-DAY DIET

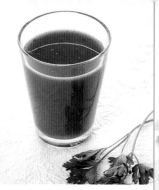

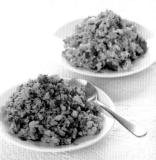

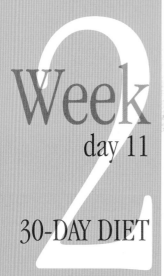

Breakfast

Hot lemon & ginger drink *(p.84)*

Scrambled eggs with toast or oatcakes & sesame seeds

1 teaspoon sesame seeds

2 medium hen's eggs

A dash semi-skimmed milk

A very small knob of butter

1 slice toasted rye or wholemeal bread, or 1 or 2 oatcakes, spread sparingly with butter

A sprig fresh parsley, chopped

Toast the sesame seeds in a small, dry pan over a medium-high heat. Toss the seeds frequently to develop an even colour. Whisk the eggs and milk. Melt the butter in a small pan over a medium heat and cook the eggs. Scatter the seeds and parsley on top of the eggs and serve with the toast or oatcakes.

Morning snack

Choose either:

250ml (8fl oz) Kick-start superjuice *(see recipe, right)*, and 1 oatcake spread with your choice of topping *(below)*

OR

2 oatcakes or rye biscuits spread with your choice of topping:

- ☐ Bean & mustard mash *(p.137)*
- ☐ Reduced-fat fromage frais & peppers *(p.114)*
- ☐ Red lentil & turmeric spread *(p.163)*
- ☐ Spicy chick-pea spread *(p.137)*
- ☐ Sweet potato & goat's cheese topping *(p.163)*

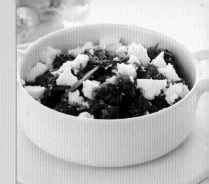

The Food Doctor

Tip for the day ...

If you are making Fruit compote (brunch) and Chicken brochettes (dinner) tomorrow, marinate the ingredients overnight tonight.

Lunch

Cold trout or haloumi & your choice of carbohydrate

1 portion cold trout or haloumi reserved from dinner, day 10

1 portion mixed salad or steamed vegetables

Your choice of carbs: 1 slice of rye or wholemeal bread or 2 oatcakes, rice cakes or rye biscuits, or 1 tablespoon rice or quinoa (leftover from a dinner)

A couple of tablespoons of reserved dill sauce or olive oil

A wedge of fresh lemon

Flake the cold trout or cube the haloumi and arrange on a plate with a salad or steamed vegetables and your choice of carbohydrate. Drizzle a little olive oil over the haloumi or the dill sauce over the trout, add a wedge of fresh lemon and serve.

Afternoon snack

Choose either:

250ml (8fl oz) High-energy smoothie (if you have portion 2 leftover from yesterday)

OR

2 oatcakes or rye biscuits spread with your choice of topping:

- [ ] Bean & mustard mash (p.137)
- [ ] Reduced-fat fromage frais & peppers (p.114)
- [ ] Red lentil & turmeric spread (p.163)
- [ ] Spicy chick-pea spread (p.137)
- [ ] Sweet potato & goat's cheese topping (p.163)

Dinner

Beetroot risotto with feta cheese & green salad (p.131)

Save a portion for lunch tomorrow

Cook the rice and the beetroot at the same time for speed – or alternatively you can use ready-cooked beetroot.

Morning snack recipe

With its mildly spicy undertones of cayenne and paprika, this energy drink is especially good if you are in need of a boost mid-way through the morning. The quantities listed here should make enough for two snacks; if not, top up with tomato juice.

Kick-start superjuice

150ml (¼ pint) carrot juice

100ml (3½fl oz) tomato juice (or ready-mixed vegetable juice)

1 tablespoon lemon juice

A small handful fresh parsley

½ teaspoon cayenne powder

½ teaspoon paprika powder

Put all the ingredients in a food processor and blitz for a few seconds until mixed.

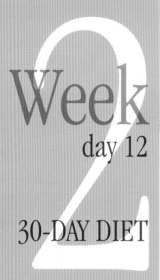

Week
day 12

30-DAY DIET

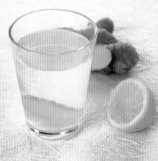

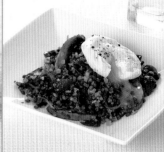

Breakfast

Hot lemon & ginger drink *(p.84)*

If you are having brunch today, eat a small snack at your usual breakfast time.

OR

Your choice of cereal or ham breakfast

Cereal recipes are listed on pages 84, 86, 90, 92 and 94; see page 114 for a ham breakfast recipe.

Morning snack

If you are not having brunch, have the second portion of Kick-start superjuice *(p.117)*, and 1 oatcake spread with a topping:

- [ ] Bean & mustard mash *(p.137)*
- [ ] Classic guacamole (below)
- [ ] Reduced-fat fromage frais & peppers *(p.114)*
- [ ] Red lentil & turmeric spread *(p.163)*
- [ ] Spicy chick-pea spread *(p.137)*
- [ ] Sweet potato & goat's cheese topping *(p.163)*

Classic guacamole

2 ripe avocados

2 tablespoons grated onion

1 tablespoon mixed pumpkin, sunflower and sesame seeds

1 small clove garlic, crushed

2 teaspoons lemon juice

2 teaspoons olive oil

A pinch cayenne pepper

A dash of Worcestershire sauce (to taste)

A dash of Tabasco (to taste)

Mash all the ingredients together in a small bowl and season with freshly ground black pepper. Cover tightly with cling film and store in the fridge for up to two days.

The Food Doctor
Tip for the day ...
You're now allowed a cup of decaffeinated coffee or tea each day if you wish. Ideally, just have one cup, or two cups maximum.

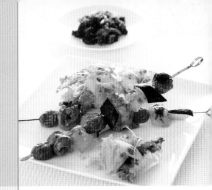

Brunch/Lunch

Brunch:
1 livening drink *(right)*,
either Fruit compote *(below)*
or 1 apple or pear and your
choice of brunch *(pp.138–139)*

Fruit compote

6 dried apricots and 5 dried
prunes, halved and soaked in 150ml
(¼ pint) peppermint tea

50ml (2fl oz) apple juice

½ crisp apple, cored and sliced

½ pear, cored and sliced

Soak the dried fruit overnight.
Strain the tea and mix with the
apple juice. Combine all the
fruits, pour the tea and juice mix
over and serve.

OR

Lunch:

Beetroot risotto

1 portion reserved Beetroot risotto from
dinner, day 11

Several sprigs watercress

1 hard-boiled egg, quartered

1 slice rye bread

Pile the risotto on top of the
watercress, top with the egg
and serve with the bread.

Afternoon snack

Choose either:

**250ml (8fl oz) High-energy
smoothie *(p.115)* or Fruit
smoothie *(p.107)* with 1
tablespoon of mixed seeds**

OR

**2 oatcakes or rye biscuits
sdwith your choice of spread:**

- [ ] Bean & mustard mash *(p.137)*
- [ ] Classic guacamole *(left)*
- [ ] Reduced-fat fromage frais & peppers *(p.114)*
- [ ] Red lentil & turmeric spread *(p.163)*
- [ ] Spicy chick-pea spread *(p.137)*
- [ ] Sweet potato & goat's cheese topping *(p.163)*

Dinner

Brochettes *(p.132)*

**Include the reserved portion
of Beetroot risotto if you
had brunch**

These brochettes are easy to make
and are perfect for cooking either
on a barbecue or under the grill.

Livening drinks

**These fresh tonics are a
great way to begin brunch.**

Orange tonic

**125ml (4fl oz) freshly
squeezed orange juice**

125ml (4fl oz) water

Mix the juice and water
together and serve chilled.

Fresh juice burst

125ml (4fl oz) chilled carrot juice

125ml (4fl oz) unsweetened or dry
apple juice

Juice ½ orange

Juice ½ lemon

A sprig of mint or lemon balm

Mix the ingredients together
and serve chilled with the sprig
of mint or lemon balm.

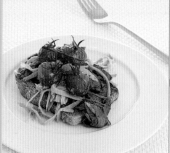
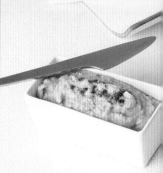

Week 2

day 13

30-DAY DIET

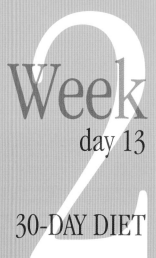

Breakfast

Hot lemon & ginger drink *(p.84)*

If you are having brunch today, eat a small snack at your usual breakfast time.

OR

Your choice of cereal or ham breakfast

Cereal recipes are listed on pages 84, 86, 90, 92 and 94; see page 114 for a ham breakfast recipe.

Morning snack

If you are not having brunch, have 2 oatcakes or rye biscuits with your choice of spread:

☐ Bean & mustard mash *(p.137)*

☐ Classic guacamole *(p.118)*

☐ Home-made houmous *(p.88)*

☐ Spicy chick-pea spread *(p.137)*

☐ Sweet potato & goat's cheese topping *(p.163)*

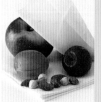

Fuel up frequently

If you have ever felt hungry soon after a meal, you may have found yourself eating more and more. Five small healthy meals, rather than the traditional "three square meals a day", will help you to control what you eat, keep any hunger pangs at bay

The Food Doctor
Tip for the day ...
For a spicy kick, try adding some lemon juice mixed with a teaspoon of olive oil and a few chilli flakes to any dish.

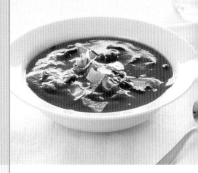

Brunch/Lunch

Brunch: 1 livening drink, either Fruit salad *(below)* or 2 apricots and your choice of brunch *(pp.138–139)*

Fruit salad
3 tablespoons fruit salad
2 tablespoons reduced-fat fromage frais
A sprinkling of mixed seeds

Put the fromage frais in a bowl, spoon over the fruit and seeds and serve.

OR

Lunch:
Salmon & steamed vegetables
1 salmon fillet, simply poached or grilled
Approx. 300g (10oz) steamed vegetables
Fresh dill sauce *(p.130)*
Your choice of carbohydrate

Mix up some more sauce if necessary. Serve the salmon with the vegetables, your choice of carbohydrate and the sauce on the side.

Afternoon snack

Choose either:

250ml (8fl oz) High-energy smoothie *(p.115)* or Fruit smoothie *(p.107)* with 1 tablespoon of mixed seeds

OR

2 oatcakes or rye biscuits with your choice of spread:
- Bean & mustard mash *(p.137)*
- Classic guacamole *(p.118)*
- Home-made houmous *(p.88)*
- Spicy chick-pea spread *(p.137)*
- Sweet potato & goat's cheese topping *(p.163)*

Dinner

Quick country soup or Four bean salad *(p.133)*

Save two portions of soup for lunch, days 14 and 17, or one portion of salad for lunch, day 14

Freeze the second reserved portion of soup until you need it on day 17.

and maintain your energy levels – hence the all-important fourth Food Doctor Principle, Fuel up frequently.

Ideally, you should eat a light meal every three hours or so. This is why it's important to eat morning and afternoon snacks every day in addition to breakfast, lunch and dinner. Even if you aren't hungry, you really should have something to eat, however small it might be, in order that your metabolic rate is maintained. All The Food Doctor Principles are listed on pages 14–41.

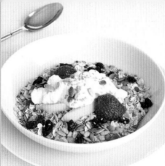

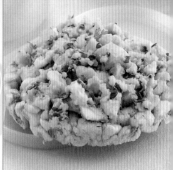

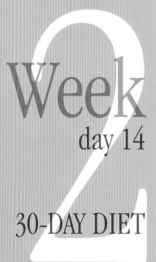

Week

day 14

30-DAY DIET

Breakfast

Hot lemon & ginger drink *(p.84)*

Ham or cereal breakfast *(below)*

Other cereal recipes are listed on pages 84, 86, 90, 92 and 94; see page 114 for a ham breakfast recipe.

Millet porridge

30g (1oz) millet flakes

150ml (¼ pint) water

2 tablespoons live natural low-fat yoghurt

1 pear, chopped, but not peeled

1 tablespoon pumpkin seeds

Gently simmer the flakes and water for 5 to 10 minutes until the water is absorbed. Stir in the yoghurt until creamy and serve with the chopped pear and pumpkin seeds on top.

Morning snack

Choose either:

250ml (8fl oz) Kick-start superjuice *(p.117)* and 1 oatcake spread with your choice of topping *(below)*

OR

2 oatcakes or rye biscuits spread with your choice of topping:

- [ ] Bean & mustard mash *(p.137)*
- [ ] Classic guacamole *(p.118)*
- [ ] Home-made houmous *(p.88)*
- [ ] Spicy chick-pea spread *(p.137)*
- [ ] The Food Doctor fresh pesto *(below)*

The Food Doctor fresh pesto

2 tablespoons toasted seeds *(p.93)* or 1 tablespoon each pumpkin and sunflower seeds

3 tablespoons olive oil

A small handful fresh watercress

2 teaspoons lemon juice

Combine the ingredients in a blender and blitz into a thick paste. Add more oil if the paste is too thick. Season with freshly ground black pepper.

The Food Doctor

Tip for the day ...

If you have any of The Food Doctor fresh pesto left over, it will keep well in the fridge for three or four days for snacks.

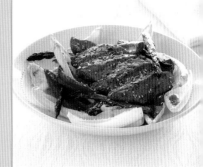

Lunch

Soup or salad & your choice of carbohydrate

1 portion Quick country soup or Four bean salad reserved from dinner, day 13

1 tablespoon mixed seeds

1 hard-boiled egg for the salad (optional)

Your choice of carbs: 1 slice of rye or wholemeal bread or 2 oatcakes, rice cakes or rye biscuits, or 1 tablespoon rice or quinoa (leftover from a dinner)

Heat the soup thoroughly and serve with the seeds scattered over the top, or have the remainder of the salad with the egg and mixed seeds. Add your choice of carbs and extra vegetables if you prefer.

Afternoon snack

Choose either:

250ml (8fl oz) Apple & mint smoothie *(below)* or High-energy smoothie *(p.115)*

OR

2 oatcakes or rye biscuits spread with your choice of topping:

- [ ] Bean & mustard mash *(p.137)*
- [ ] Classic guacamole *(p.118)*
- [ ] Home-made houmous *(p.88)*
- [ ] Spicy chick-pea spread *(p.137)*
- [ ] The Food Doctor fresh pesto *(see recipe, left)*

Dinner

Duck breast or smoked tofu salad *(p.134)*

Game such as duck is an excellent source of low-fat protein, and is high in iron. If you don't like duck, you can use chicken instead. Tofu is an excellent choice of vegetarian protein.

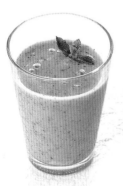

Afternoon snack recipe

This clean-tasting, deliciously refreshing recipe should make 500ml (17fl oz) – enough for two smoothies. If not, top up with apple juice. If you prefer the drink thick, increase the quantities slightly to ensure you have a second smoothie for tomorrow all prepared.

Apple & mint smoothie

1 crisp eating apple, cored and chopped

1 pear, cored and chopped
½ small cucumber
200g (7oz) live natural low-fat yoghurt
A small handful mint leaves
1 tablespoon pumpkin seeds
A squeeze lemon juice

Blend all the fruit, vegetables, herbs, seeds and juice together. Stir in the yoghurt. Do not sieve the smoothie as this will remove valuable fibre.

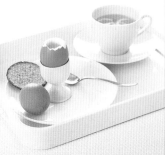

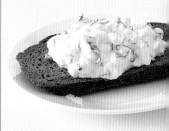

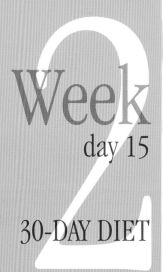

Week 2

day 15

30-DAY DIET

Breakfast

Hot lemon & ginger drink *(p.84)*

Egg or cereal breakfast

Egg recipes are listed on pages 88 and 116; cereal recipes are listed on pages 84, 86, 90, 92, 94 and 122.

Morning snack

Choose either:

250ml (8fl oz) Energizer juice *(see recipe, right)* and 1 oatcake spread with your choice of topping *(below)*

OR

2 oatcakes or rye biscuits spread with your choice of topping:

- [ ] Bean & mustard mash *(p.137)*
- [ ] Classic guacamole *(p.118)*
- [ ] Flavoured no-fat soft cheese spread *(p.84)*
- [ ] Home-made houmous *(p.88)*
- [ ] Spicy chick-pea spread *(p.137)*
- [ ] The Food Doctor fresh pesto *(p.122)*
- [ ] Sweet potato & goat's cheese topping *(p.163)*

The Food Doctor

Tip for the day ...

For an instant snack on the go, buy a pot of houmous and eat with raw vegetable crudités you've prepared at breakfast time.

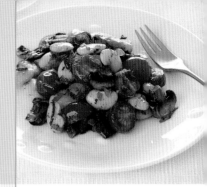

Lunch

Mixed sprouted seed salad with avocado & your choice of carbohydrate

3 tablespoons sprouted seeds *(p.181)*

½ avocado, peeled and cut into chunks

1 tablespoon each of at least two other raw vegetables (whatever you have in the fridge, e.g., peppers, celery, cucumber or cherry tomatoes)

Your choice of carbs: 1 slice of rye or wholemeal bread or 2 oatcakes, rice cakes or rye biscuits, or 1 tablespoon rice or quinoa (leftover from a dinner)

Mix all the ingredients together and serve with your choice of dressing and carbohydrate.

Afternoon snack

Choose either:

250ml (8oz) Apple & mint smoothie (if you have portion 2 leftover from yesterday, day 14) or High-energy smoothie *(p.115)*

OR

2 oatcakes or rye biscuits spread with your choice of topping:

☐ The Food Doctor pesto *(p.122)*
☐ Banana & fromage frais spread *(below)*

Banana & fromage frais spread

½ banana, mashed

1 tablespoon reduced-fat fromage frais

1 teaspoon sesame seeds

Mix the ingredients together and spread on 1 slice of wholemeal or rye bread or 2 oatcakes.

Dinner

Butter beans in tapenade with vegetables *(p.135)*

Save a portion of steamed vegetables for lunch tomorrow

Like other legumes, butter beans are high in fibre and an excellent source of vegetable protein.

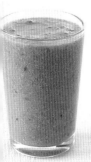

Morning snack recipe

The hint of fresh ginger in this refreshng juice is very beneficial for your digestion. The quantities listed here should make 500ml (17fl oz) – enough for two snacks; if not, top up with carrot or tomato juice. Store the second serving in the fridge until tomorrow afternoon.

Energizer juice

100ml (3½fl oz) carrot juice

100ml (3½fl oz) tomato juice

1 red pepper

Juice of 1 orange and lemon

2.5cm (1in) fresh ginger, grated

Put all the ingredients in a food processor and blitz for a few seconds until mixed.

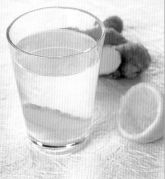
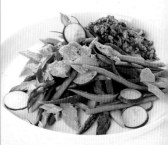

Week

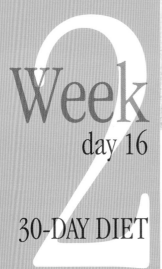

day 16

30-DAY DIET

Breakfast

Hot lemon & ginger drink *(p.84)*

Cereal or ham breakfast

Cereal recipes are listed on pages 84, 86, 90, 92, 94 and 122; see page 114 for the ham recipe.

Morning snack

Choose either:

250ml (8oz) Kick-start superjuice *(p.117)* or Energizer juice *(p.125)* and 1 oatcake spread with your choice of topping *(below)*

OR

2 oatcakes or rye biscuits spread with your choice of topping:

☐ Bean & mustard mash *(p.137)*

☐ Spicy chick-pea spread *(p.137)*

☐ Home-made houmous *(p.88)*

☐ Reduced-fat fromage frais & peppers *(p.114)*

☐ The Food Doctor fresh pesto *(p.122)*

☐ Flavoured no-fat soft cheese spread *(p.84)*

☐ Egg & crudités *(below)*

Egg & crudités

Approx 100g (3½oz) raw vegetables, such as carrots, peppers, cucumber, cherry tomatoes

1 hard-boiled egg, shelled

Rinse and cut the vegetables into bite-size pieces. Keep the egg and crudités in a sealed plastic container.

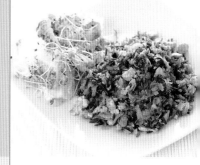

The Food Doctor
Tip for the day ...
The Egg & crudités snack listed here is another great snack if you are on the go: just keep it in your bag until needed.

Lunch

Tuna & vegetable salad & your choice of carbohydrate

½ large can tuna, drained

1 portion of steamed vegetables reserved from dinner, day 15

Your choice of dressing *(pp.173,175,177)*

Your choice of carbs: 1 slice of rye or wholemeal bread or 2 oatcakes, rice cakes or rye biscuits, or 1 tablespoon rice or quinoa (leftover from a dinner)

Mix the tuna with last night's steamed vegetables. Add some extra raw vegetables if you like and serve with your choice of dressing and carbohydrate.

Afternoon snack

Choose either:

250ml (8oz) Vegetable smoothie *(below)* or Apple & mint smoothie *(p.123)* OR

2 oatcakes or rye biscuits spread with your choice lof topping:

☐ Cottage cheese
☐ Chick-pea & banana spread *(see recipe, below)*

Chick-pea & banana spread

½ banana, mashed

3 tablespoons chick-peas, drained and rinsed

1 tablespoon reduced-fat fromage frais

A squeeze lemon juice

A pinch cinnamon (optional)

Put the ingredients in a blender and blitz until smooth. Enough for two snacks. Store in the fridge.

Dinner

Carrot & cardamom rice with a green leaf salad *(p.136)*

Save a portion of the rice for lunch tomorrow

Afternoon snack recipe

If you don't have all the right ingredients for this recipe, try adding whatever is to hand in the fridge such as cooked beetroot, watercress or celery (avoid raw root vegetables though). This recipe should make 500ml (17fl oz) – enough for two smoothies. If not, top up with carrot juice. If you prefer the drink thick, increase the quantities slightly to ensure you have a second smoothie all prepared for tomorrow's snack.

Vegetable smoothie

150g (5oz) cucumber

1 medium tomato

50g (2oz) red pepper

100ml (3½fl oz) carrot juice

Juice 1 lemon

3 tablespoons live natural low-fat yoghurt

Blend the vegetables and juice in a blender. Stir in the yoghurt. Do not sieve as this will remove valuable fibre.

Week 2 diary

If you found week 1 quite tough and restrictive in terms of what you could eat, you should find week 2 easier, as there are more snack options and foods to try. Write down which choices you've made, and any new symptoms or changes you've been noticing.

DAY 10
What I've enjoyed eating/How do I feel?

DAY 13
What I've enjoyed eating/How do I feel?

DAY 14
What I've enjoyed eating/How do I feel?

☐ **DAY 11**

What I've enjoyed eating/How do I feel?

☐ **DAY 12**

What I've enjoyed eating/How do I feel?

☐ **DAY 15**

What I've enjoyed eating/How do I feel?

☐ **DAY 16**

What I've enjoyed eating/How do I feel?

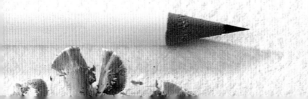

Baked trout or haloumi & stir-fried vegetables

Whether you choose the trout or haloumi
option, save a portion for lunch tomorrow.
Each recipe serves two.

ready in 30 minutes

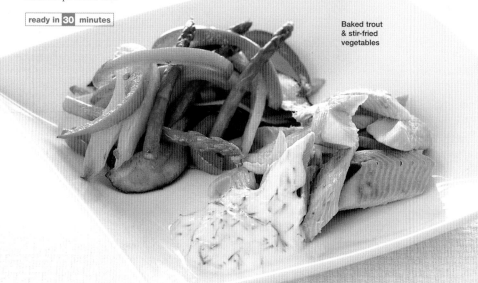

Baked trout
& stir-fried
vegetables

2 trout, gutted, about 200g (7oz) each with head and tail removed
(to allow for cold trout being left over for lunch tomorrow) or 200g
(7oz) haloumi, cut into thin slices

1 tablespoon each fresh parsley and coriander

Dill sauce for the trout:
2 tablespoons reduced-fat fromage frais
2 tablespoons horseradish sauce
1 tablespoon lemon juice
1 tablespoon fresh dill, chopped

Heat the oven to 150°C/300°F/Gas mark 2. Rinse the
fish and fill the cavity with herbs. Wrap each fish
loosely in foil and place on a baking tray. Cook for 15–
20 minutes until the flesh is opaque, but moist. Cook
the stir-fry and mix the sauce. Save a little sauce for
lunch tomorrow. Open the parcels, lift the skin from
the fish and ease the flesh from the bones. Turn the fish
over and repeat on the other side. Serve with the sauce
and stir-fry.

For the stir-fry:
300g (10oz) raw vegetables per person, cut into bite-
size pieces, or 1 packet ready-prepared vegetables

Optional sauce for the stir-fry:
2cm (¾in) ginger, grated
1 clove garlic, crushed
Grated zest 1 lime
4 tablespoons lime juice
2 tablespoons soy sauce
1 tablespoon balsamic vinegar
1 tablespoon olive oil

Cook the vegetables in a wok over a high heat with
a little water or lemon juice until al dente. Add the
sauce after cooking.

To make the haloumi:
Once the stir-fry is ready, grill the slices of haloumi
until golden. Serve while still hot.

Beetroot risotto with feta cheese & green salad

Supermarkets now sell fresh, ready-cooked beetroot if you want to save time making this dish. You can also cook the rice in advance. Save a portion for lunch tomorrow. Serves two.

500ml (17fl oz) light stock

150g (5oz) rice (red or brown)

1 clove garlic, peeled

1 stick cinnamon

150g (5oz) beetroot, rinsed, or use vinegar-free, ready-cooked beetroot

½ teaspoon caraway seeds, lightly toasted

1–2 tablespoons olive oil

100g (3½oz) spinach or kale, coarsely shredded with thick stems removed

1 medium onion, chopped

1 medium head of fennel, trimmed and cut into medium fine slices

2 teaspoons tamarind paste

150g (5oz) feta cheese, chopped or crumbled

Bring the stock to the boil and add the rice, garlic and cinnamon. Simmer gently, without a lid, for about 35 minutes or until the rice is tender. Drain, remove the cinnamon and mash in the garlic.

While the rice is cooking, cover the beetroot with very lightly salted boiling water and simmer until tender, about 30 minutes. Once cooked, it will be easy to slip off the skins under cold running water and then top and tail the beetroot.

As the rice and beetroot cook, heat a frying pan and lightly toast the caraway seeds. Remove the seeds and add a tablespoon of olive oil to the frying pan. Add the coarsely shredded spinach or kale and cook gently until the leaves have wilted. Remove from the pan and set aside. Add more oil and cook the onion and fennel until golden brown. Stir in the cooked shredded greens, the caraway seeds and tamarind paste. Combine with the rice and beetroot and season with freshly ground black pepper to taste.

Put aside one helping for tomorrow's lunch. Place the remaining risotto in a shallow baking dish and scatter over the feta cheese. Slip into a hot oven for 10 minutes. Serve with a green salad.

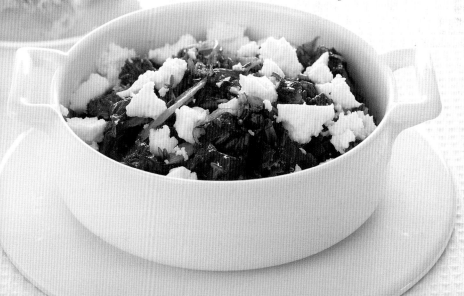

Chicken or mixed vegetable brochettes & salad

It's worth marinating the chicken overnight or preparing it in the morning to make the dish tastier. Include the Beetroot risotto if you didn't have it for lunch today. Serves two.

250–300g (8–11oz) chicken thigh fillets, cut into 2 or 3 chunks, or 8 button mushrooms (chestnut mushrooms have a good flavour)

12 baby tomatoes

1 medium courgette, cut into thick slices

1 yellow pepper, cut into chunks

For the marinade:

1 clove garlic, crushed

1 tablespoon dry apple juice

1 tablespoon soy sauce

1 tablespoon tamarind paste

1 tablespoon mustard

A squeeze of lime juice

Mix the marinade. If using chicken, put the chicken pieces and the marinade in a bowl, mix well and leave as long as you can.

Thread the vegetables – and chicken, if you are using it – alternately onto 4 metal or soaked wooden skewers. Brush with olive oil. If you are cooking just vegetables, brush some of the marinade over the prepared skewers. Either cook under a medium grill, or on a barbecue, until the vegetables are hot and turning golden or the meat is thoroughly cooked.

Serve with a green salad and any leftover Beetroot risotto. Heat the remaining marinade thoroughly and serve as a sauce on the side.

You can add different sources of protein to the Mixed vegetable brochettes: tofu or haloumi can be marinated in the sauce and grilled with the vegetables. Or serve the vegetables, and the sauce, with cooked quinoa (120g/4oz is enough for two servings), or Spicy chick-peas (p.187).

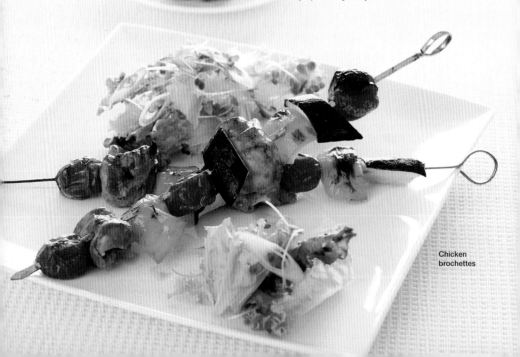

Chicken brochettes

Quick country soup or Four bean salad

Sea vegetables for the soup are available in good health food shops, or use shredded spinach or kale. Save a portion of salad for lunch tomorrow, and two portions of soup.

Quick country soup

Quick country soup

ready in **30** minutes

1 medium onion, finely chopped
2 tablespoons olive oil
400g (13oz) button mushrooms, sliced
500ml (17fl oz) passata or 1x400g (13oz) can tomatoes, zapped in a blender until smooth
500ml (17fl oz) vegetable stock
1 tablespoon tomato paste
Juice ½ lemon
½ teaspoon dried Herbes de Provence
2 tablespoons dried sea vegetables or 50g (2oz) washed shredded spinach

Soften the chopped onion in the olive oil in a saucepan. Add the mushrooms and more oil if necessary. Mix well and cook for about 5 minutes. Add the passata, stock, tomato paste, lemon juice, and dried herbs and simmer for 15 minutes or so. Stir in the sea vegetables or shredded spinach and cook for a further 5–10 minutes.

Serve with a scattering of grated parmesan or hard goat's cheese over the top if you wish.

Four bean salad

ready in **10** minutes

100g (3½oz) broad beans (frozen or fresh)
100g (3½oz) green beans, topped and tailed and cut in half
100g (3½oz) mangetout or fresh petis pois
100g (3½oz) red or orange pepper
1x400g (13oz) can beans, well rinsed and drained
2 spring onions, finely chopped
A handful of chopped herbs of your choice

For the dressing:
2 tablespoons lemon juice
2 tablespoons reduced-fat fromage frais
1 tablespoon dry apple juice
1 clove garlic, crushed
1 teaspoon Dijon mustard

Steam the beans and mangetout until *al dente* (about 3–4 minutes). Refresh under cold running water and drain. Mix the fresh beans, petit pois, pepper, canned beans, spring onions and herbs in a bowl. Mix the dressing, pour over the salad and stir well. Season with freshly ground black pepper. Top with some crumbled feta if you like, and serve.

Carrot & cardamom rice with a green leaf salad

You can cook the rice up to 24 hours in advance and keep it in the fridge if you think you will be pressed for time making dinner tonight. Serves two.

50g (2oz) red or brown rice
250ml (8fl oz) vegetable stock
2 tablespoons dried sea vegetables
2 hen's eggs
A little oil to cook the eggs
5 cardamom pods
1 tablespoon olive oil
1 small onion, chopped
100g (3½oz) carrot, coarsely grated
Grated rind 1 orange
Fresh parsley, chopped, to garnish

Simmer the rice in the vegetable stock for about 25 minutes, until just tender. Add the dried sea vegetables and stir for 2 minutes. If there is any liquid left, turn up the heat and boil hard until the liquid has evaporated. Set to one side.

In a non-stick pan, scramble the two eggs in a little oil. Then set the scrambled eggs to one side.

Slit each cardamom pod open, scrape the seeds into a pestle and crush with a mortar. Heat the oil in a frying pan and soften the onion for a few minutes. Add the crushed seeds and stir together, then add the grated carrot and orange rind. Cook for about five minutes until the carrot begins to soften. Stir in the cooked rice, fold in the scrambled egg, place the mix in a shallow baking dish, cover and cook for about 15 minutes in a hot oven. Serve with a garnish of parsley and a green leaf salad.

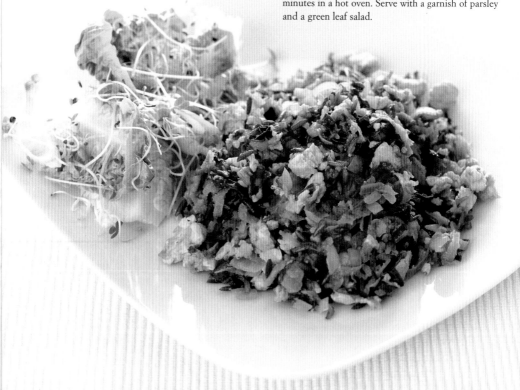

Snacks

Both these snacks will keep well in the fridge for up to five days, so if you make both recipes at the weekend you should have plenty of weekday snacks to hand.

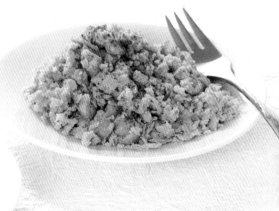

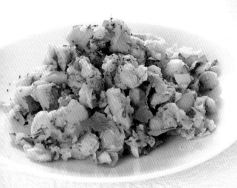

Bean & mustard mash

ready in **20** minutes

1x400g (13oz) can butter beans, drained and rinsed
Approx. 300ml (½ pint) vegetable stock
2 tablespoons olive oil
1 heaped teaspoon Dijon mustard or scant tablespoon tapenade
A small handful fresh parsley, chopped

Simmer the beans with enough vegetable stock to cover for about 15–20 minutes. Drain, reserving the stock. Put the beans in a bowl with the olive oil, mustard or tapenade and season with freshly ground black pepper. Mash the ingredients together until reasonably smooth. Stir in plenty of chopped parsley and more olive oil if necessary. Add a little of the reserved stock if the mash is too stiff. Store covered in the fridge.

Spicy chick-pea spread

ready in **10** minutes

2 tablespoons olive oil
1x400g (13oz) can chick-peas, drained and rinsed and patted dry on kitchen paper
1 teaspoon paprika

Heat the oil in a frying pan, add the chick-peas and cook, turning frequently over a medium heat until they begin to turn crispy. Tip onto a plate covered with absorbent kitchen paper to absorb any remaining oil. Put the chick-peas in a clean bowl and add the paprika. Mash the ingredients coarsely with a fork and keep in the fridge.

Brunch

Brunches are designed to be relaxed affairs, and these straightforward recipes will hopefully encourage you to sit down and enjoy your meal at leisure. All recipes serve two.

Eggs, spinach & smoked salmon

ready in **15** minutes

100g (3½oz) spinach, rinsed and cleaned well

1 generous tablespoon each reduced-fat fromage frais and live natural low-fat yoghurt

½ teaspoon grated ginger

2 hen's eggs

80g (2½oz) smoked salmon, cut into wide strips

A squeeze of lemon juice

A pinch of paprika

2 teaspoons toasted seeds *(p.93)*

If the spinach leaves are large, shred them coarsely. Steam for about 5 minutes until limp. Drain well and keep warm.

Combine the fromage frais, yoghurt and ginger. Poach the eggs as you like them.

Combine the smoked salmon and spinach with the lemon juice and season with freshly ground black pepper. Divide onto two plates. Top each with a poached egg and spoon over the yoghurt mixture. Sprinkle over the paprika and seeds.

Serve with pitta bread or a carbohydrate of your choice.

Smoked salmon pasta

ready in **20** minutes

100g (3½oz) corn pasta shells

A drizzle of olive oil

A drizzle of lemon juice

50ml (2fl oz) reduced-fat fromage frais

50ml (2fl oz) live natural low-fat yoghurt

1 tablespoon olive oil

100g (3½oz) smoked salmon

A small bunch fresh dill, chopped

Cook the pasta according to the instructions on the packet. Once cooked, strain and toss in a little olive oil and lemon juice.

Combine the fromage frais and yoghurt with the olive oil.

Cut the smoked salmon into strips. Combine the salmon with the pasta and yoghurt mix. Season with freshly ground black pepper and lemon juice to taste. Stir in the chopped dill, divide onto two plates and serve while warm.

Deluxe omelette

ready in **25** minutes

2 tablespoons white wine

2 tablespoons water

½ teaspoon Thai fish sauce

A small handful fresh tarragon sprigs, chopped

100g (3½oz) salmon fillet

3 tablespoons pinenuts

100g (3½oz) fresh asparagus (weight after snapping off the tough end of the stalk)

4 tablespoons reduced-fat fromage frais

Juice and rind ½ lime

4 hen's eggs

4 tablespoons live natural low-fat yoghurt

A little olive oil to cook the eggs

Pour the wine, water and fish sauce into a pan and add half the tarragon. Bring to the boil and put the salmon in, skin side down. Lower the heat to a gentle simmer and cook for 10 minutes or so until the salmon is just cooked through. Lift the fish from the pan, remove the skin and coarsely flake the fish.

Toast the pinenuts in a dry pan over a medium heat, tossing frequently, until they are brown on all sides.

Steam the asparagus until just cooked – about 5–6 minutes. Cut each asparagus stalk into 3 pieces.

Mix the fromage frais, lime juice and rind together in a bowl. Gently fold in the asparagus and fish.

To make the omelettes, beat the eggs, yoghurt and remaining tarragon in a bowl. Season with freshly ground black pepper and use half the mixture to make the first omelette.

Heat a little oil in a frying pan, pour in the egg mix and cook over a medium heat. When the omelette is set underneath, but still soft on top, spread half the filling on one half of the omelette, sprinkle half the nuts on top, and then carefully fold the plain half of the omelette over the filling. Leave to cook for a few more seconds, then lift it out and keep it warm in the oven while you cook the second omelette. Then serve.

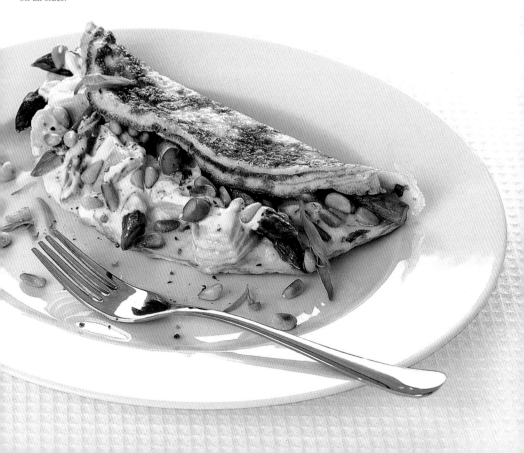

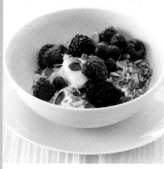

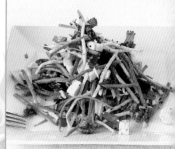

Week

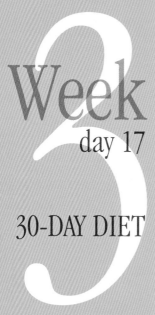

day 17

30-DAY DIET

Breakfast

Hot lemon & ginger drink *(p.84)*

Cereal or ham breakfast

Cereal recipes are listed on pages 84, 86, 90, 92, 94 and 122; see page 114 for a ham breakfast recipe.

Morning snack

Choose either:

250ml (8oz) Red energy juice *(right)* or Energizer juice *(p.125)*, and 1 oatcake spread with your choice of topping *(below)*

OR

2 oatcakes or rye biscuits with your choice of topping:

☐ Crab meat spread *(see recipe, below)*

☐ Red lentil & turmeric spread *(p.163)*

☐ Sweet potato & goat's cheese topping *(p.163)*

Crab meat spread

2 tablespoons crab meat (canned or fresh)

1 tablespoon low-fat fromage frais

A good squeeze of lemon juice

A little chopped parsley, coriander or rocket (if you have some to hand)

Mix all the ingredients together and spread on the oatcakes or rye biscuits.

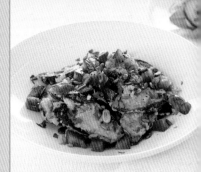

The Food Doctor

Tip for the day ...

Soak 8 dried apricots overnight in water if you want to make tomorrow afternoon's Digestive booster smoothie.

Lunch

Soup or tuna salad & your choice of carbohydrate

1 portion of Quick country soup reserved from day 13 or ½ remaining can of tuna (from lunch yesterday) with a mixed salad

Your choice of dressing *(pp.173,175,177)*

Your choice of carbs: 1 slice of rye or wholemeal bread or 2 oatcakes, rice cakes or rye biscuits

Heat the soup thoroughly and serve, or mix the remainder of the tuna with some salad vegetables and serve with your choice of dressing and carbohydrate.

Afternoon snack

Choose either:

250ml (8oz) Vegetable smoothie (if you have portion 2 leftover from yesterday) or Apple & mint smoothie *(p.123)*

OR

2 oatcakes or rye biscuits with your choice of topping:

☐ Banana & fromage frais spread *(below)*

☐ Sweet potato & goat's cheese topping *(p.163)*

Banana & fromage frais spread

½ banana, mashed

1 tablespoon reduced-fat fromage frais

1 teaspoon sesame seeds

Mix the ingredients together and spread on the biscuits.

Dinner

Courgettes in chick-pea sauce with quinoa & salad *(p.156)*

This dish, like all the dinners on the plan, includes low-saturated fat protein and encourages you to prepare vegetables in a new and fresh way.

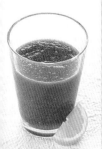

Morning snack recipe

Raw food always offers a greater level of nutrients, so this juice helps to provide you with a boost of nutritious energy. This recipe should make enough for two snacks.

Red energy juice

100ml (3½fl oz) carrot juice

75ml (3fl oz) dry apple juice

150g (5oz) cucumber

1 medium tomato

50g (2oz) red pepper

Juice 1 lemon

Put all the ingredients in a food processor and blitz for a few seconds until mixed.

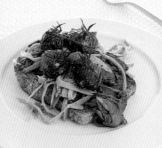

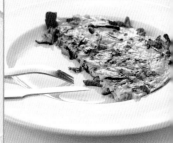

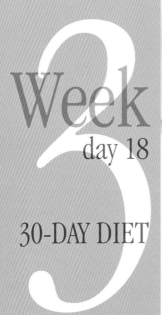

Week 3

day 18

30-DAY DIET

Breakfast

Hot lemon & ginger drink *(p.84)*

Cereal or ham breakfast

Cereal recipes are listed on pages 84, 86, 90, 92, 94 and 112; see page 114 for a ham breakfast recipe.

Morning snack

Choose either:

250ml (8oz) Red energy juice *(p.141)* and 1 oatcake generously spread with your choice of topping *(below)*

OR

2 oatcakes or rye biscuits spread with your choice of topping:

- [ ] Red lentil & turmeric spread *(p.163)*
- [ ] Sweet potato & goat's cheese topping *(p.163)*
- [ ] Crab meat spread *(p.140)*
- [ ] Tomato & bean mash *(below)*

Tomato & bean mash

12 cherry tomatoes
1 clove garlic, crushed
1 tablespoon olive oil
2 tablespoons barlotti beans
A little balsamic vinegar

Put the tomatoes and garlic in a roasting dish and drizzle the oil over the top. Roast in the oven at 200°C/400°F/Gas mark 6 for about 15 minutes. Mix in the beans and roughly break up. Add a dash of balsamic vinegar and pile onto the oatcakes, rye biscuits or a piece of wholemeal toast.

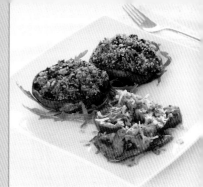

The Food Doctor
Tip for the day ...
If you want to make the Fruit compote for brunch tomorrow, soak the dried fruit in peppermint tea overnight tonight.

Lunch

Carrot & cardamom rice with salad & your choice of carbohydrate

1 portion carrot and cardamom rice reserved from dinner, day 16

1 mixed salad or sprouted seeds

A little olive oil

A squeeze of lemon juice

Your choice of carbs: 1 slice of rye or wholemeal bread or 2 oatcakes, rice cakes or rye biscuits

Put the reserved rice and salad on a plate. Drizzle with a little olive oil and the lemon juice. Serve with the carbohydrate of your choice.

Afternoon snack

Choose either:

250ml (8oz) Digestive booster smoothie *(below)*

OR

2 oatcakes or rye biscuits with Chick-pea & banana *(p.127)* or Banana & fromage frais *(p.141)*

OR

Dates & fromage frais

2 teaspoons reduced-fat fromage frais

A squeeze of lime juice

2 fresh organic dates, stoned and opened

6 pumpkin seeds

Mix the fromage frais with the lime juice, divide the mixture in half and spoon into each date with the pumpkin seeds.

Dinner

Baked mushrooms & salad *(p.157)*

Save a portion for lunch tomorrow if not eating brunch

Mushrooms – and especially exotic varieties – help to boost the immune system, and are packed with B vitamins, which help to lower cholesterol.

Afternoon snack recipe

The creamy, orange-tasting undertones of this luxurious smoothie give way to a lovely ginger aftertaste. The quantities listed should make 500ml (17fl oz) – enough for two smoothies. If not, top up with apple juice. Store the second portion in the fridge for tomorrow.

Digestive booster smoothie

8 dried apricots, soaked overnight in water

Juice 1 orange

Juice ½ lemon

2.5cm (1in) fresh ginger, grated

1 tablespoon sesame seeds

100ml (3½ fl oz) dry apple juice

150ml (¼ pint) live natural low-fat yoghurt

Blend all the fruits, ginger, seeds and juices together. Stir in the yoghurt. Do not sieve the smoothie as this will remove valuable fibre.

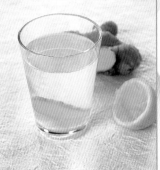
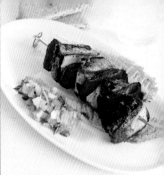

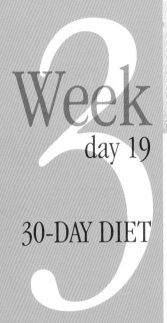

Week
day 19

30-DAY DIET

Breakfast

Hot lemon & ginger drink *(p.84)*

If you are having brunch today, eat a small snack at your usual breakfast time.

OR

Your choice of cereal or ham breakfast

Cereal recipes are listed on pages 84, 86, 90, 92, 94 and 122; see page 114 for a ham breakfast recipe.

Morning snack

If you are not having brunch, have 2 oatcakes or rye biscuits with your choice of spread:

- [ ] Crab meat spread *(p.140)*
- [ ] Egg & crudités *(p.126)*
- [ ] Red lentil & turmeric spread *(p.163)*
- [ ] Sweet potato & goat's cheese topping *(p.163)*
- [ ] The Food Doctor fresh pesto *(p.122)*
- [ ] Tomato & bean mash *(p.142)*

The Food Doctor

Tip for the day ...

Don't overlook the importance of a daily intake of fruits and vegetables. My plan supplies at least five portions a day.

Brunch/Lunch

Brunch:

1 tonic drink *(right)*, either Fruit compote *(p.118)*, Fruit salad *(p.120)*, 1 apple or pear or 2 apricots, and your choice of brunch *(pp.138–139, 164-165)*

OR

Lunch: Vegetable stir-fry with your choice of protein & carbohydrate

Your choice of protein, such as chicken, fish or tofu

Your choice of carbohydrate

Approx. 300g (4oz) raw vegetables per person, or 1 packet prepared vegetables

Stir-fry sauce *(p.171)*, optional

Cook the protein and prepare the carbohydrate first. Cook the vegetables in a wok over a high heat with a little water or lemon juice until *al dente*. If using the sauce, add it after cooking. Serve with the other prepared ingredients.

Afternoon snack

Choose either:

250ml (8oz) Digestive booster smoothie (if you have portion 2 leftover from yesterday, day 18) or Vegetable smoothie *(p.127)*

OR

Dates & fromage frais *(p.143)*

OR

2 oatcakes or rye biscuits spread with your choice of topping:

- [ ] Red lentil & turmeric spread *(p.163)*
- [ ] Sweet potato & goat's cheese topping *(p.163)*
- [ ] Banana & fromage frais *(p.141)*
- [ ] Chick-pea & banana spread *(p.127)*

Dinner

Stir-fry curry with smoked tofu or chicken *(p.158)*

Save a portion of lentils for lunch, day 22

Spices such as turmeric have a positive effect on your blood sugar levels, and therefore on your weight.

Tonics

Apple tonic
125ml (4fl oz) dry apple juice
125ml (4fl oz) water

Mix the juice and water together and serve chilled.

Cleansing tonic
125ml (4fl oz) tomato juice or passata (or 1x400g/13oz can tomatoes, blended)
125ml (4fl oz) dry apple juice
Juice ½ lemon
A dash of Tabasco sauce
2.5cm (1in) grated fresh ginger (optional)

Mix the ingredients together and serve chilled with a slice of lemon or lime.

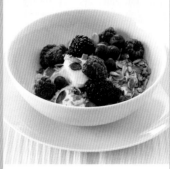
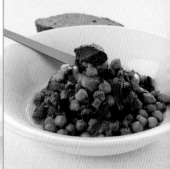

Week 3

day 20

30-DAY DIET

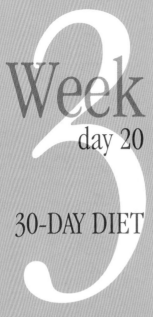

Breakfast

Hot lemon & ginger drink *(p.84)*

If you are having brunch today, eat a small snack at your usual breakfast time.

OR

Your choice of cereal or ham breakfast

Cereal recipes are listed on pages 84, 86, 88, 90, 92, 94 and 122; see page 114 for a ham breakfast recipe.

Morning snack

If you are not having brunch, have 2 oatcakes or rye biscuits with your choice of spread:

- [ ] Crab meat spread *(p.140)*
- [ ] Red lentil & turmeric spread *(p.163)*
- [ ] Sweet potato & goat's cheese topping *(p.163)*
- [ ] The Food Doctor fresh pesto *(p.122)*
- [ ] Tomato & bean mash *(p.142)*

The Food Doctor

Tip for the day ...

Aim to add one new food to your diet every week to benefit from a wide variety of flavours as well as nutrients.

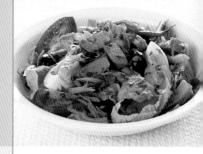

Brunch/Lunch

Brunch:

1 tonic drink *(p.145)*, either Fruit compote *(p.118)*, Fruit salad *(p.120)*, 1 apple or pear or 2 apricots, and your choice of brunch *(pp.138–139, 164–165)*

OR

Lunch:

Your choice of protein, vegetables and carbohydrate

Afternoon snack

Choose either:

250ml (8oz) Vegetable smoothie *(p.127)* or High-energy smoothie *(p.115)*

OR

Dates & fromage frais *(p.143)*

OR

2 oatcakes or rye biscuits spread with your choice of topping:

- ☐ Banana & fromage frais spread *(p.141)*
- ☐ Chick-pea & banana spread *(p.127)*
- ☐ Red lentil & turmeric spread *(p.163)*
- ☐ Sweet potato & goat's cheese topping *(p.163)*

Dinner

Leek & potato soup or Salade niçoise *(p.159)*

Save a portion of soup or salad for lunch tomorrow

Leeks and potatoes both have cleansing properties, while fresh tuna and eggs are ideal forms of lean protein.

Eat a wide variety of food

The foods we eat have the greatest impact on our outward appearance and our inner energy levels, so it's vital that we eat a wide variety of food to reap the nutritional benefits.

Most of us tend to limit the range of foods we buy to those we feel comfortable eating – which can then lead to boredom and a desire to reach for fast food, processed snacks and takeaways. One of the main aims of this plan is to encourage you to eat as many healthy foods as possible: all the recipes include nutrient-dense foods such as wholegrains, beans, pulses, nuts, seeds, oily fish and fresh seasonal vegetables. Some or most of the foods listed in this plan may be new to you, but keep trying them and you'll soon enjoy eating them. Eat a wide variety of food is Principle 3 of The Food Doctor principles *(pp.24–27)*.

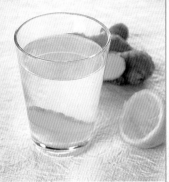

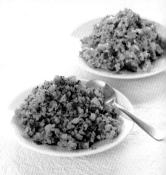

Week

day 21

30-DAY DIET

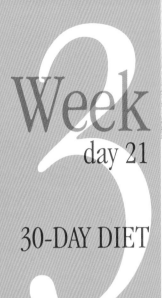

Breakfast

Hot lemon & ginger drink *(p.84)*

Cereal or ham breakfast

Cereal recipes are listed on pages 84, 86, 90, 92, 94 sand 122; see page 114 for a ham breakfast recipe.

Morning snack

Choose either:

250ml (8oz) Red energy juice *(p.141)*, Energizer juice *(p.125)*, and 1 oatcake spread with your choice of topping *(below)*

OR

2 oatcakes or rye biscuits spread with your choice of topping:

- [ ] Crab meat spread *(p.140)*
- [ ] Classic guacamole *(p.118)*
- [ ] Home-made houmous *(p.88)*
- [ ] Red lentil & turmeric spread *(p.163)*
- [ ] Sweet potato & goat's cheese topping *(p.163)*
- [ ] The Food Doctor fresh pesto *(p.122)*
- [ ] Tomato & bean mash *(p.142)*

The Food Doctor

Tip for the day ...

The most colourful fruits and vegetables supply an abundance of antioxidants, so try to buy this sort of fresh produce often.

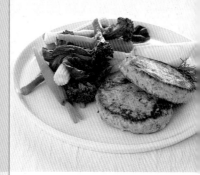

Lunch

Soup or salad & your choice of carbohydrate

1 portion Leek & potato soup or Salade niçoise reserved from dinner, day 20

2 tablespoons canned beans

Your choice of carbs: 1 slice of rye or wholemeal bread or 2 oatcakes, rice cakes or rye biscuits

Heat the soup thoroughly, or add some extra vegetables and tuna to the salad if needed, and serve with your choice of carbohydrate.

Afternoon snack

Choose either:

250ml (8oz) High-energy smoothie *(p.115)*, Vegetable smoothie *(p.127)* or Digestive booster smoothie *(p.143)*

OR

2 oatcakes or rye biscuits spread with your choice of topping:

- ☐ Banana & fromage frais spread *(p.141)*
- ☐ Chick-pea & banana spread *(p.127)*
- ☐ Classic guacamole *(p.118)*
- ☐ Red lentil & turmeric spread *(p.163)*
- ☐ Sweet potato & goat's cheese topping *(p.163)*

Dinner

Salmon cakes or Egg noodles with vegetables *(p.160)*

Eat protein with complex carbohydrates

Combining lean proteins such as chicken or fish with complex carbohydrates (that is, vegetables and wholegrains such as brown rice and rye bread) in the correct proportions at every meal ensures that your body receives a steady flow of energy, as the body converts these foods into glucose relatively slowly. Complex carbs also contain fibre, which promotes digestive health.

When we think of carbohydrates, we tend to think of starchy foods such as potatoes and white rice. These foods are broken down more quickly, so it's important to avoid them.

Eat protein with complex carbohydrates is the first of The Food Doctor principles *(pp.46–53)*.

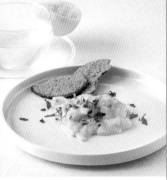
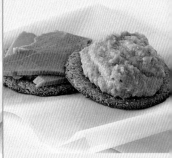

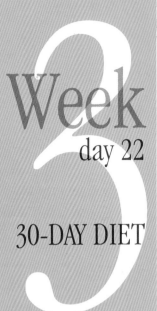

Week
day 22

30-DAY DIET

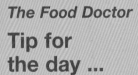

The Food Doctor
Tip for the day ...

If you are taking lunch to work tomorrow, cook a sweet potato tonight and cut it into bite-size chunks once it has cooled.

Breakfast

Hot lemon & ginger drink *(p.84)*

Cereal, egg or ham breakfast

Cereal recipes are listed on pages 84, 86, 90, 92, 94 and 122; egg recipes are on pages 88 and 116; see page 114 for a ham breakfast recipe.

Morning snack

Choose either:

250ml (8oz) Red energy juice *(p.141)* or Kick-start superjuice *(p.117)*, and 1 oatcake spread with your choice of topping *(below)*

OR

2 oatcakes or rye biscuits spread with your choice of topping:

- [ ] Crab meat spread *(p.140)*
- [ ] Feta cheese & roast pepper spread *(below)*
- [ ] Red lentil & turmeric spread *(p.163)*
- [ ] Sweet potato & goat's cheese topping *(p.163)*
- [ ] Tomato & bean mash *(p.142)*

Feta cheese & roast pepper spread

50g (2oz) roast pepper slices (from a jar)

50g (2oz) feta cheese

A few sprigs parsley

Chop the peppers finely. Combine all the ingredients in a bowl, season with freshly ground black pepper and mash roughly with a fork.

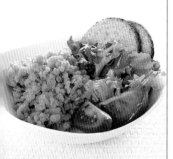
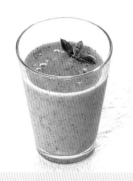
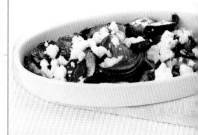

Lunch

Tomatoes with lentils

2 sliced tomatoes

1 portion reserved lentils
from dinner, day 19

1 handful green leaves

Your choice of dressing (pp.173,175,177)

Your choice of carbs: 1 slice of rye or
wholemeal bread or 2 oatcakes, rice
cakes or rye biscuits

Arrange the ingredients on a plate,
drizzle over a little of your chosen
dressing and serve with your
choice of carbohydrate.

Afternoon snack

Choose either:

250ml (8oz) Digestive booster
smoothie (if you have portion
2 leftover from yesterday) or
Apple & mint smoothie (p.123)

OR

Dates & fromage frais (p.143)

OR

2 oatcakes or rye biscuits with
your choice of topping:

- [ ] Banana & fromage frais
spread (p.141)
- [ ] Chick-pea & banana
spread (p.127)
- [ ] Classic guacamole (p.118)
- [ ] Feta cheese & roast pepper
spread (see recipe, left)
- [ ] Red lentil & turmeric (p.163)
- [ ] Sweet potato & goat's
cheese topping (p.163)

Dinner

Spicy roast ratatouille with fish or white cheese (p.161)

For extra flavour, add some
chopped fresh herbs – whatever
you have to hand or needs using
up from the fridge – just before
serving this dish.

Eat fat to lose fat

There's a clear distinction
between essential fats and
saturated fat. The body needs
essential fats in order to
function properly. Foods such
as avocados, nuts, oily fish,
and cold-pressed oils all
provide these necessary fats.

Saturated fat, on the other
hand, is a non-essential fat:
the body doesn't need it, even
though we often find ourselves
craving foods, such as crisps,
that contain saturated fat.

By cutting out saturated fats
and including more essential

fats in your diet, you can enjoy
the satisfaction that comes
with eating healthy foods
containing fat and minimize
any cravings for unhealthy
foods. Eat fat to lose fat is
principle 10 of the 10 Food
Doctor principles (pp.72–73).

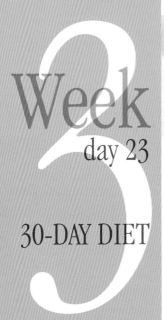

Week
3
day 23

30-DAY DIET

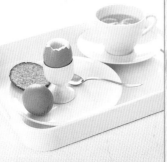

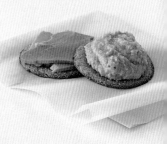

Breakfast

Hot lemon & ginger drink *(p.84)*

Cereal, egg or ham breakfast

Cereal recipes are listed on pages 84, 86, 90, 92, 94 and 122; egg recipes are on pages 88 and 116; see page 114 for a ham breakfast recipe.

Morning snack

Choose either:

250ml (8oz) Red energy juice *(p.141)*, or Energizer juice *(p.125)*, and 1 oatcake spread with your choice of topping *(below)*

OR

2 oatcakes or rye biscuits spread with your choice of topping:

- Bean & mustard mash *(p.137)*
- Classic guacamole *(p.118)*
- Crab meat spread *(p.140)*
- Feta cheese & roast pepper spread *(p.150)*
- Home-made houmous *(p.88)*
- Red lentil & turmeric spread *(p.163)*
- Reduced-fat fromage frais & peppers *(p.114)*
- Spicy chick-pea spread *(p.137)*
- Sweet potato & goat's cheese topping *(p.163)*
- The Food Doctor fresh pesto *(p.122)*
- Tomato & bean mash *(p.142)*

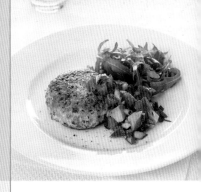

The Food Doctor
Tip for the day ...
Keep your choice of fruit and vegetables seasonal: feel free to substitute any vegetables with whatever is in season.

Lunch

Sweet potato with cottage cheese & spring onions

1 medium sweet potato
Your choice of dressing (pp.173,175,177)
2 tablespoons cottage cheese
2 spring onions, diced
1 handful green leaves
4 cherry tomatoes

Bake the sweet potato in the oven for 15–20 minutes at 180°C/350°F/ Gas mark 4. If you cooked the sweet potato last night, drizzle a little dressing over the dish before serving it.

Arrange the sweet potato on a plate, spoon over the cottage cheese, scatter the spring onions over the top and serve with the leaves and tomatoes on the side.

Afternoon snack

Choose either:

250ml (8oz) Apple & mint smoothie (if you have a portion leftover from yesterday)

OR

2 oatcakes or rye biscuits spread with your choice of topping:

- Sweet potato & goat's cheese topping (p.163)
- Banana & fromage frais (p.141)
- Chick-pea & banana spread (p.127)
- Feta cheese & roast pepper spread (p.150)

Dinner

Chicken or vegetarian burgers & salad (p.162)

To grind the seeds for the vegetarian burgers, use a blender or coffee grinder; the flat blades of a food processor may not grind the seeds finely enough.

Health check

Now that you've reached the end of week 3 you should be aware of some or all of the following improvements in your health and well-being:

- Increased energy
- Falling asleep more easily

- Restful, undisturbed sleep
- More alert on waking
- No more headaches
- Less irritable
- Thicker, healthier hair
- Stronger nails
- Clearer skin

- Sparkly eyes
- Improved digestion

Don't worry if you haven't experienced many of these effects yet: you may well find that it's in week 4 that you'll begin to feel your absolute best.

Week 3 diary

Now that you've moved on to week 3, you may find yourself wanting to return to some recipes that you've enjoyed. Note down any adaptations you make to these recipes and on which days you've eaten them. Record any improvements in your health too.

☐ **DAY 17**
What I've enjoyed eating/How do I feel?

- -
- -
- -
- -
- -
- -
- -
- -

☐ **DAY 20**
What I've enjoyed eating/How do I feel?

- -
- -
- -
- -
- -
- -
- -

☐ **DAY 21**
What I've enjoyed eating/How do I feel?

- -
- -
- -
- -
- -
- -
- -

DAY 18

What I've enjoyed eating/How do I feel?

DAY 19

What I've enjoyed eating/How do I feel?

DAY 22

What I've enjoyed eating/How do I feel?

DAY 23

What I've enjoyed eating/How do I feel?

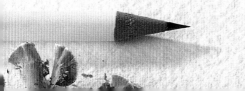

Courgettes in chick-pea sauce, quinoa & salad

DINNER DAY 17

If you have time and want to substitute the quinoa for another protein, serve this dish with a small turkey escalope. Serves two.

ready in 20 minutes

120g (4oz) quinoa (or 175g/6oz if you are cooking enough for dinner tomorrow)

250ml (8fl oz) light vegetable stock (or 300ml/12fl oz if you are cooking enough quinoa for dinner tomorrow)

2 tablespoons olive oil

400g (13oz) courgettes, sliced diagonally

1 good-sized tomato, chopped

1 handful fresh coriander or parsley, chopped

2 tablespoons toasted seeds *(p.93)*

For the sauce:
1x400g (13oz) can chick-peas, drained and rinsed (use half the can and store the rest in the fridge for snacks)

1 clove garlic, crushed

1 tablespoon lemon juice

¼ teaspoon Tabasco

½ teaspoon cumin powder

2 tablespoons live natural low-fat yoghurt

Cook the quinoa in the stock for 15 minutes or until the quinoa is soft and the liquid is absorbed. If you made extra quantities, put aside one third of the cooked quinoa for tomorrow night's supper.

Meanwhile, put all the sauce ingredients into a blender and blitz until smooth.

Heat the olive oil in a large frying pan or wok, add the courgette slices and cook until browned on both sides. Add the sauce and sizzle for a couple of minutes, until the sauce is piping hot.

Divide the courgettes between two plates, top each serving with the chopped tomatoes and herbs, and add the quinoa. Sprinkle the toasted seeds over the top of the dish and serve.

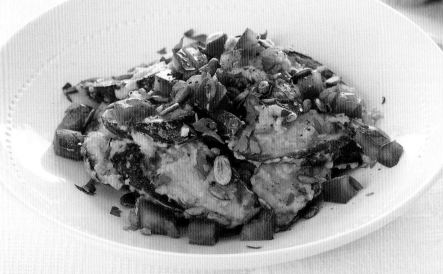

Baked mushrooms & salad

If you didn't reserve a cooked portion of quinoa from last night, tonight's supper will only take 15 minutes longer than suggested to prepare. Serves two.

ready in 25 minutes

1 portion of cooked quinoa reserved from last night
(or cook 50g/2oz quinoa in 100ml/3½fl oz light stock)

4 large mushrooms (approx. 100g/3½oz per person)

1 tablespoon olive oil, plus extra to drizzle

100g (3½oz) onion, finely chopped

2 cloves garlic, crushed

8–10 black olives, stoned and finely chopped

Grated zest 1 lemon

3 good sprigs of parsley, finely chopped

A drizzle of olive oil

For the salad:
2 large slicing tomatoes

A dressing of your choice
(pp.173,175,177)

1 spring onion, finely chopped, or sprouted seeds

If you need to cook some quinoa, gently simmer it in the stock for about 15 minutes or until it is soft and the stock is absorbed.

Cut the thick stems out of the mushrooms with a sharp knife, leaving an indentation. Chop the stems up finely.

Heat the oil in a frying pan, add the onion and soften it gently. Add the mushroom stems, garlic and olives, and cook together for a few minutes. Stir in the cooked quinoa, lemon and the parsley.

Preheat the oven to 180°C/350°F/Gas mark 4. Lay the mushroom caps in a shallow baking dish, skin side down. Pile the stuffing evenly over each mushroom, patting it down firmly. Drizzle with a little olive oil, cover with foil and bake for 15–20 minutes, until the mushrooms are soft and the flavours have combined.

Serve with a salad of sliced tomatoes drizzled with a dressing of your choice, and topped with the spring onion or sprouted seeds.

Stir-fry curry with smoked tofu or chicken

If you want to save time tonight, substitute a can of lentils for the dried red lentils and buy a pack of ready-prepared raw vegetables. Serves two.

Stir-fry curry with
smoked tofu

ready in **30** minutes

1 small onion, finely chopped

3 tablespoons olive oil

½ teaspoon curry powder

½ teaspoon turmeric powder

100g (3½oz) red lentils (or
1x400g/13oz can lentils)

200ml (l7fl oz) vegetable stock
(or 50ml/2fl oz for canned lentils)

250g (8oz) mixed vegetables,
chopped into bite-size pieces

1 tablespoon curry paste or
powder (quantities to taste)

100g (3½oz) chicken
or smoked tofu

Juice 1 lime

50ml (2fl oz) water

A small bunch fresh
coriander, chopped

2 lime wedges

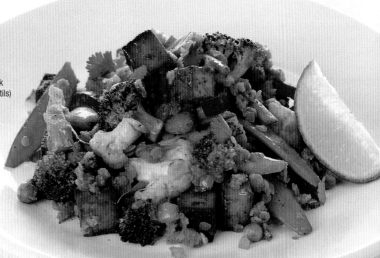

Soften the chopped onion in a tablespoon of olive oil, stir in the spices and cook for a couple of minutes. Add the lentils and stock. If you are using dried lentils, simmer them very gently in the stock for about 15 minutes until the lentils are soft but still keep their shape. The stock should all be absorbed. Put aside.

If you are using vegetables such as green beans, the stir-frying can be more even if the beans are blanched for a couple of minutes to start the cooking process: put in a small pan, cover with cold water, bring to the boil, simmer for 2 minutes and then drain.

Heat a tablespoon of olive oil in a wok, add the curry paste and stir. Add the chicken or tofu and stir until the chicken is cooked or the tofu is browned and has absorbed the curry flavours. Lift from the wok and put to one side. Add a further tablespoon of olive oil and a little more curry paste or powder (to taste), toss in the vegetables and stir to absorb the flavours. Add the lime juice and water and cook for a further 5–10 minutes until the vegetables are hot and *al dente*. Add the chicken or tofu and half the cooked lentils. Serve topped with chopped coriander and lime wedges.

Refrigerate the leftover lentils to make snacks *(p.163)*.

Leek & sweet potato soup or Salade niçoise

DINNER DAY 20

If you want to make a vegetarian Salade niçoise, omit the tuna, use two eggs and add Spicy chick-peas *(p.187)*. Both recipes serve two.

Leek & sweet potato soup

ready in **30** minutes

1 medium onion, finely chopped

2 tablespoons olive oil

1 good-sized leek (about 200g/7oz cleaned weight), finely sliced

1 medium sweet potato (200g/7oz), peeled and coarsely grated

1 teaspoon ground cumin

1.5 litres (2 pints) well-flavoured stock

1 tablespoon dried sea vegetables (optional)

100g (3½oz) quinoa

250ml (8fl oz) light stock

1 clove garlic, peeled and left whole

Soften the onion in a tablespoon of olive oil in a large saucepan. Add the leek and potato and cook for 2 minutes. Add the cumin and pour in the stock. Simmer for 10–15 minutes. Stir in the dried sea vegetables, if using. Simmer the quinoa in the stock with the garlic. When soft (after about 15 minutes), lift out the garlic, pour the quinoa and any remaining stock into the soup and serve. You can mash the garlic into the soup if you like.

Salade niçoise

ready in **15** minutes

100g (3½oz) green or runner beans, trimmed and halved

1 fresh tuna steak (approx. 200g/7oz) or 1 can of tuna, preferably in spring water, drained

1 little gem lettuce or similar green-leaved lettuce (or use 50–100g/2–3½oz mixed green leaves)

2 medium tomatoes, cut into quarters

½ yellow pepper

1 medium carrot, coarsely grated

2 spring onions, finely sliced

6–8 black olives, pitted

Your choice of dressing *(pp.173, 175, 177)*

1 hard-boiled egg, shelled and quartered, or 2 eggs and Spicy chick-peas for a vegetarian option

A handful chopped fresh seasonal herbs

Steam the beans until *al dente* (about 3–5 minutes). If using fresh tuna, cook the fish as for day 4 *(p.101)*.

Tear the lettuce leaves coarsely into a salad bowl. Toss in the beans, tomatoes, pepper, carrot, spring onions and olives. Add the dressing and mix. Top with the egg, tuna and herbs, or two eggs, Spicy chick-peas and herbs for a vegetarian dish.

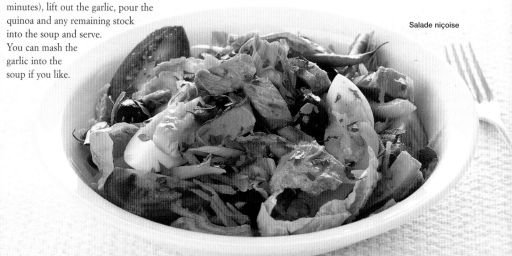

Salade niçoise

Salmon cakes or Egg noodles with vegetables

Choose from either the Salmon cakes or the Egg noodles for a satisfying, high-protein evening meal. Both recipes serve two.

Salmon cakes

ready in **15** minutes

150–200g (5–7oz) salmon fillet, skin removed *(p.75)*
1 medium shallot or 6 small spring onions, chopped
1 slice rye bread – about 25g (1oz)
1 egg white (reserve the yolk and add it to your scrambled egg if you are having it for breakfast tomorrow)
A squeeze of lemon juice
Zest ½ lemon
1 teaspoon tomato purée
A pinch of dried dill or ½ teaspoon chopped fresh dill
1 teaspoon olive oil
Approx. 300g (11oz) mixed vegetables per person, chopped, or 1 packet ready-prepared vegetables

Put the salmon, shallot or onions and bread into a food processor and zap to a paste. Tip into a bowl and combine with the egg white, lemon juice and zest, the purée, herbs and black pepper. Wet your hands and form two burger shapes from the mix. The thinner the cakes, the quicker they cook.

As you steam the vegetables, heat a teaspoon of olive oil in a non-stick frying pan and press the fishcakes into the oil. Cook gently for 3–4 minutes on each side – they should be golden on the outside and just cooked through the middle. Serve with wedges of lemon and the steamed vegetables.

Egg noodles

ready in **10** minutes

3 medium eggs
3 small spring onions, trimmed and finely sliced
1 tablespoon live natural low-fat yoghurt
½ teaspoon cumin
1 teaspoon olive oil

Put all the ingredients together in a bowl, season with freshly ground black pepper, and whisk well.

As you steam the vegetables, make three flat omelettes from the egg mix. Heat a little oil in a non-stick omelette pan. Pour in one third of the mix and spread it evenly around the pan. Allow to set and lightly brown on one side, flip over and brown the other side (or slip under a hot grill for a couple of minutes). Turn the omelette out onto a plate and keep it warm while you make the others. When they are all cooked, roll up each omelette and slice across to make ribbons.

Serve the egg ribbons on the steamed vegetables. Sprinkle a tablespoon of toasted mixed seeds *(p.93)* over the top if you prefer.

Salmon cakes with vegetables

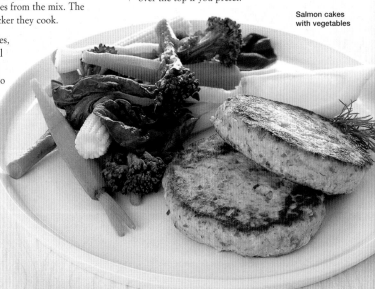

Spicy roast ratatouille with fish or white cheese

If you use feta cheese, you can add extra protein by stirring in some chick-peas or beans before you grill the dish. Serves two.

3 cloves garlic, skin left on

1 aubergine, sliced

1 medium courgette, sliced

1 medium red onion, cut into wedges

2 beefsteak tomatoes, cut into wedges

1 teaspoon dried Herbes de Provence

½ teaspoon chilli powder, or a chopped green chilli (or in quantities to your own taste)

100ml (3½fl oz) olive oil

A squeeze of lemon juice

250–300g (8–10oz) white fish fillet (such as cod, orange roughy, halibut, haddock) or 200g (7oz) haloumi cheese or feta cheese, cubed or crumbled

2 tablespoons canned chick-peas or canned beans (optional)

Preheat the oven to 200°C/400°F/Gas mark 6.

Leaving the skin on the garlic, cut off the tips. Put all the vegetables in a roasting pan together with the herbs, chilli and oil. Add a good grinding of black pepper. Cook in the hot oven for about 30 minutes, turning once or twice and adding a squeeze of lemon juice.

Squeeze a little lemon juice over the fish and cook it under a medium grill, or add the chick-peas (if using), sprinkle feta cheese over the roast vegetables, slip under a medium-hot grill for a few minutes and serve.

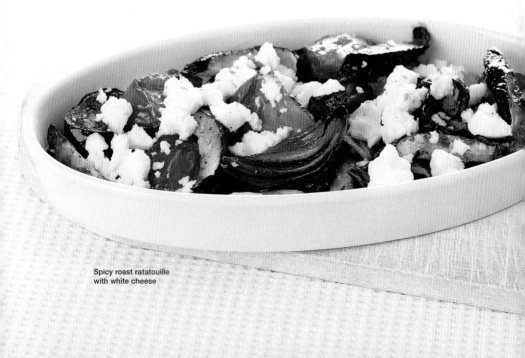

Spicy roast ratatouille
with white cheese

Chicken or Vegetarian burgers & salad

If you're making Vegetarian burgers, the raw mix may appear too wet to use. However, the egg binds the ingredients together as they cook, and after the burgers are turned over.

ready in **20** minutes

Chicken burgers

300g (10oz) minced chicken or turkey (or use chicken thigh fillets and process the meat in a food processor)
2 teaspoons tamarind paste
Rind ½ lemon
½ teaspoon soy sauce
1 spring onion, chopped very finely
1 tablespoon fresh parsley or coriander, finely chopped
A large pinch chilli powder or 1 fresh chilli, chopped (optional)
1 tablespoon olive oil

Combine the minced meat with all the other ingredients except the oil in a bowl. Add a little chilli powder or fresh chopped chilli if you like it hot. Divide the mixture into 2 burgers.

Heat a tablespoon of olive oil in a frying pan, preferably non stick, over a medium-high heat. Drop in the burgers and brown one side for a couple of minutes, then turn and brown on the other side. Turn down the heat a little to prevent any burning, and cook each side for a further 4–5 minutes so that the meat is thoroughly cooked.

Serve with a green salad and a dressing of your choice *(pp.173,175,177)*.

Vegetarian burgers

200g (7oz) firm tofu
2 spring onions, shredded lengthways and finely sliced
4 shiitake mushrooms, stalks removed and finely diced (or use small brown or button mushrooms)
25g (¾oz) carrots, finely grated
2.5cm (1in) fresh ginger root, finely grated
2 teaspoons tamarind paste
1 teaspoon soy sauce
5 tablespoons mixed or toasted seeds *(p.93)*
1 tablespoon fresh parsley or coriander, finely chopped
1 hen's egg, lightly beaten
1 tablespoon olive oil

Drain the tofu and firmly pat dry using absorbent kitchen paper. Combine all the ingredients except the oil in a bowl and mix. Divide into 4 burgers.

Heat a frying pan, preferably non stick, with a little olive oil over a medium-high heat. Brown each side for about 4 minutes, turning only once. Use a spatula to pat the mixture together after you turn each burger over.

Serve with a green salad and a dressing of your choice *(pp.173,175,177)*.

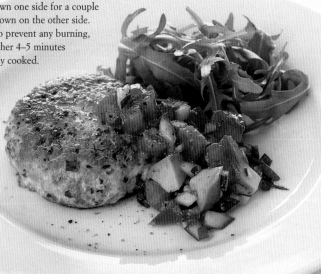

Chicken burgers
with green salad

Snacks

These snacks are tasty, filling and high in protein. They're also versatile enough to be used as a side dish with a meal if you wish. Keep in the fridge for up to five days.

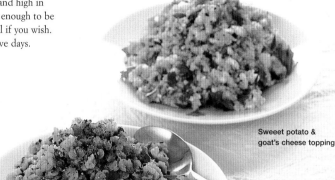

Red lentil &
turmeric spread

Sweeet potato &
goat's cheese topping

Red lentil & turmeric spread

1 tablespoon olive oil

1 medium onion, finely chopped

1 clove garlic, chopped

1 bay leaf

2 teaspoons ground turmeric

2 teaspoons curry powder

½ teaspoon chilli paste, or 1 small fresh chilli, chopped

2 teaspoons black mustard seeds

½ teaspoon cumin seeds

150g (5oz) red lentils

300ml (½ pint) vegetable stock

1–2 tablespoons fresh coriander, finely chopped

Heat the oil in a small saucepan and gently cook the onion, garlic and bay leaf until the onion is soft, but not coloured. Stir in the turmeric, curry powder, chilli paste or fresh chilli, and mustard and cumin seeds and cook gently for 3–4 minutes to allow the onion to absorb the flavours.

Add the lentils and stock. Stir and simmer gently for about 15 minutes until the lentils are very tender and the stock is absorbed. Mash the ingredients coarsely, stir in the fresh coriander and season with some freshly ground black pepper. Keep covered in the fridge.

Sweet potato & goat's cheese topping

200g (7oz) sweet potato, peeled and coarsely chopped

2 garlic cloves in their skins, tips chopped off

1 tablespoon olive oil

75g (2½oz) soft goat's cheese, roughly cubed

Lemon juice, to taste

1–2 tablespoons fresh coriander, chopped

Preheat the oven to 350C/180F/Gas mark 4.

Put the chopped sweet potato and garlic cloves in a baking dish. Toss the pieces in the oil, cover the dish and put it in the preheated oven. Bake for about 25 minutes, or until the sweet potato pieces are soft. Allow to cool, then squeeze the soft garlic cloves out of their skins and tip into a bowl with the sweet potato. Add the goat's cheese and mash together until well blended, but not reduced to a smooth purée. Add the lemon juice, season with freshly ground black pepper to taste and add the fresh coriander. Store, covered, in the fridge.

Brunch

These brunch recipes are all quick and easy to make. Buckwheat wraps, a great form of carbohydrate, are a tasty alternative to toast, and versatile enough to be used for other meals too. All recipes serve two.

Poached egg country style

ready in **10** minutes

2 hen's eggs
1 tablespoon olive oil
120g (4oz) mushrooms, sliced (brown mushrooms give a better flavour)
2 medium tomatoes, sliced
100g spinach, washed and shredded
2 slices of wholemeal or rye toast

Heat a large frying pan of water and cook the poached eggs as you like them. Heat the olive oil in a frying pan, add the mushrooms and cook over a gentle heat until they are soft and just turning brown. Add the tomatoes and spinach. Heat until the spinach has wilted and the tomatoes are hot.

Heap the mushroom mix onto lightly buttered toast and top with the poached eggs. Season with a good grinding of black pepper and serve.

Mixed grill wrap

ready in **20** minutes

2 medium tomatoes, quartered
2 medium mushrooms, quartered
1 medium pepper (yellow makes a nice contrast in colour), cut into thin slices
2 tablespoons olive oil
100g (3½oz) liver (chicken, calf, lamb or venison)

For the buckwheat wraps:
100g (3½oz) buckwheat flour
1 large hen's egg
300ml (½ pint) milk and water mixed (or all water)
½ teaspoon dried Herbes de Provence
1 teaspoon olive oil

For the sauce:
3 teaspoons soy sauce
3 teaspoons Dijon mustard
1 tablespoon lemon juice

To make the wraps, put the flour into a large bowl. Make a well in the middle and break the egg into the well. Using a whisk, gradually add the fluid, whisking until the mix is like thin cream. Add the herbs and season with black pepper.

Heat the oil in an omelette or pancake pan. Add about 75ml (3fl oz) of the mixture and cook for a few minutes. Flip over and brown the other side. When cooked, turn onto an upturned plate, cover with another plate and make the other wraps. The mix should make 4 wraps; freeze the excess wraps for up to one month, or store in the fridge for up to two days.

Put the tomatoes, mushrooms and pepper into a grill pan and toss them in a tablespoon of olive oil. Season with freshly ground black pepper. Grill under a medium grill for about 10 minutes, turning frequently, until the vegetables are soft.

Heat another tablespoon of oil in a frying pan and gently cook the liver for 4–6 minutes, depending on the thickness of the meat. It should be nicely brown on the outside, but still slightly pink in the middle. Once cooked, cut the liver into several small slices. Mix the sauce ingredients together and pour into a jug.

Put a wrap back in the pan, heat one side gently, turn over and fill half the wrap with half of the grilled vegetables. Top with half of the liver and pour over a little of the sauce. Fold the wrap in half and leave in the pan for a couple of minutes to heat through. Make another mixed-grill wrap and serve.

Warm lentil & poached egg salad

ready in **15** minutes

1 tablespoon olive oil
1 small onion, finely chopped
1 small carrot, finely chopped
1 small celery stick, finely chopped
1 red pepper, deseeded and roughly chopped
100g (3½oz) flat mushrooms, sliced
150g (5oz) canned puy or brown lentils, drained and rinsed
2 hen's eggs
50g (2oz) fresh spinach
1 tablespoon balsamic vinegar

Heat the oil in a saucepan and soften the onion, carrot, and celery over a low heat. Cook for 5 minutes. Add the pepper and mushrooms and cook for a further 5 minutes.

Add the lentils to the pan. Stir all the ingredients together and allow the lentils to heat through thoroughly.

Heat a large frying pan of water and poach the eggs. While the eggs cook, add the spinach to the lentil mix and cook until the spinach has wilted.

Stir in the vinegar, spoon into two bowls and season with freshly ground black pepper. Top each bowl with a poached egg and serve.

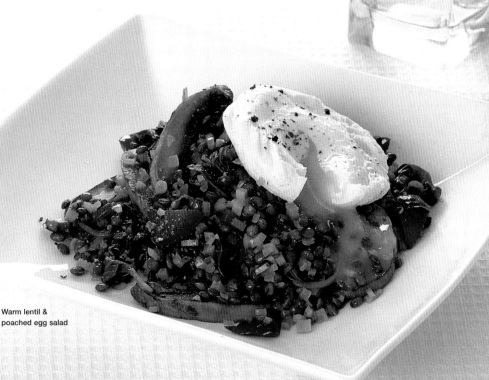

Warm lentil &
poached egg salad

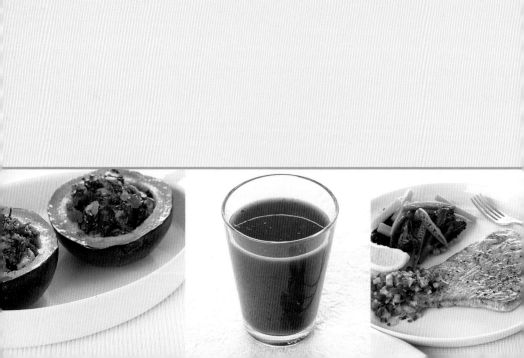

Week 4 & beyond:eat better forever

Welcome to the final week of The Food Doctor Diet plan. You may well find that this week is easier than the previous weeks because it provides you with ample choice while still providing simple yet delicious meals and snacks.

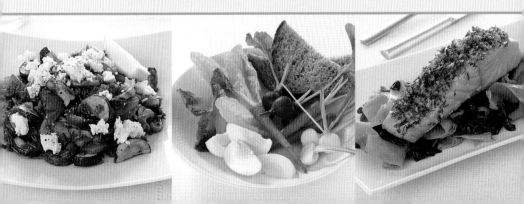

Eat better forever: Ian's advice

When you started this plan, you may have thought that the end was a long way off, but now that you are entering the final week you should be finding that my eating plan is second nature. This week is the blueprint for how you will eat in the future.

My aim has been to lead you through a month-long programme that will set you up and leave you feeling your best so you can carry on eating healthily from now on. This last week really underlines how you will be eating after this month has passed.

Week 4 differs from the previous weeks in that you have far more freedom to decide what you want to eat. It's up to you to choose which Food Doctor breakfasts, snacks and lunches you'd like each day. Despite the choices, supper recipes are still provided and this week's shopping list will help you organize yourself for these meals. Feel free to swap things around to suit yourself within the rules of combining food groups.

Boosting your exercise routine

Now that you have more energy, you may want to exercise more, so eat a Food Doctor snack just before and after a work-out. Remember that you're not trying to burn off calories by eating too little, so if you increase your energy output, eat a little more food. This avoids creating a gap between energy intake and expenditure, which could alert the metabolic rate to a potential famine. If you don't have time to exercise, keep moving. Have a good week and enjoy this last stage of the plan.

Feel free to **swap** things around to **suit yourself** within the **rules** of the plan

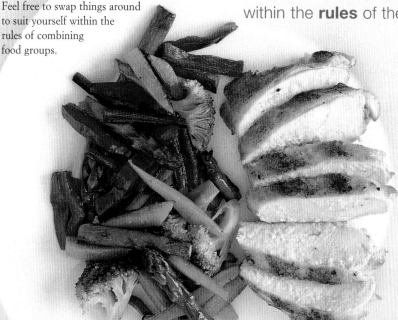

Shopping list for week 4, days 24–30

This shopping list includes approximate quantities for seven dinner recipes only. It does not include ingredients for your choice of Food Doctor breakfasts, snacks, brunches or lunches.

- [ ] Lemons, 3
- [ ] Limes, 1
- [ ] Oranges, 1
- [ ] Broad beans, 100g (3½oz)
- [ ] Broccoli, 250g (8oz)
- [ ] Carrots, approx. 300g (10oz)
- [ ] Courgettes, medium, 2
- [ ] Fennel, 1
- [ ] Mixed raw vegetables, approx. 600g (1lb 3½oz) or equivalent weight of ready-prepared vegetables in packets
- [ ] Mixed salad ingredients: enough for 4 portions
- [ ] Mushrooms (brown), 60g (2½oz)
- [ ] Onions, medium, 1
- [ ] Peppers, red (bell, jalapeno or romano), large, 1, OR 1 jar red peppers
- [ ] Red onions, medium, 1
- [ ] Spinach fresh, 450g (15oz)
- [ ] Spring onions, 1 bunch
- [ ] Sweet potatoes, medium, 1
- [ ] Tomatoes, medium, 1
- [ ] Coriander, fresh, 1 packet
- [ ] Dill, fresh, 1 bunch
- [ ] Ginger, fresh, 1 large piece (if you have run out)
- [ ] Parsley, fresh, 1 bunch
- [ ] Rosemary, fresh, 2 sprigs
- [ ] Feta cheese, 1 packet
- [ ] Haloumi, 1 packet (if making Haloumi & mushrooms, day 25)
- [ ] Hen's eggs, 4 (plus 2 if making Ginger eggs, day 28)

- [ ] Live natural low-fat yoghurt, 1 large pot (if you have run out)
- [ ] Tofu, 1 packet (if making Tofu stir-fry, day 29)
- [ ] Chicken breasts, 2, approx. 300g (10oz) (if making Chicken stir-fry, day 29)
- [ ] Salmon fillets, 2, 200–300g (7–10oz) (if making Ginger salmon, day 28)
- [ ] White fish fillets (sole, orange roughy, cod, haddock), 200–300g (7–10oz) (if making Fish & mushrooms, day 25)
- [ ] Mixed roast peppers in oil, 250g (8oz) jar, 1
- [ ] Dry apple juice, 1 carton
- [ ] Sundried tomatoes, 60g (2½oz)
- [ ] Camargue (red) or brown risotto rice, 1 packet (if you have run out)
- [ ] Red kidney beans, 1x400g (13oz) can (if you have run out)
- [ ] Vegetable stock, 550ml (19fl oz)

DAY 27 DINNER OPTIONS
Tuscan bean soup
- [ ] Carrots, medium, 1
- [ ] Celery, 2 sticks
- [ ] Leeks, large, 1
- [ ] Onions, small, 1
- [ ] Mixed beans, 1x400g (13oz) can
- [ ] Dried sea vegetables, 1 small packet (optional)

- [ ] Raw cashews, 1 small packet (if you have run out)
- [ ] Vegetable stock, 1 litre (1¾ pints)

Mixed bean salad
- [ ] Carrot, medium, 1
- [ ] Celery, 1 stick
- [ ] Cucumber, ½
- [ ] Pepper (red/yellow/orange), 1
- [ ] Tomatoes, medium, 3
- [ ] Mixed beans, 1x400g (13oz) can
- [ ] Dried sea vegetables or seaweed, 1 small packet

Week

days 24–25

30-DAY DIET

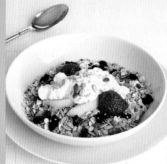

Breakfast

Your choice of Food Doctor cereal or ham breakfast

Cereal recipes are listed on pp.84, 86, 90, 92, 94 and 122; a ham recipe is listed on p.114

Morning snack

Your choice of juice and 1 oatcake, or 2 oatcakes or rye biscuits, spread with a protein topping such as:

☐ Bean & mustard mash (p.137)

☐ Home-made houmous (p.88)

☐ Reduced-fat fromage frais & peppers (p.114)

☐ Spicy chick-pea (p.137)

☐ The Food Doctor fresh pesto (p.122)

RECIPES

Breakfast

Your choice of Food Doctor cereal or ham breakfast

Morning snack

Your choice of juice and 1 oatcake, or 2 oatcakes or rye biscuits, spread with a protein topping such as:

☐ Egg & crudités (p.126)

☐ Flavoured no-fat soft cheese (p.84)

☐ Red lentil & turmeric spread (p.163)

☐ Sweet potato & goat's cheese topping (p.163)

The Food Doctor
Tip for the day ...

Carry some unsalted nuts or seeds and a piece of fruit in your bag or briefcase so you always have an accessible snack.

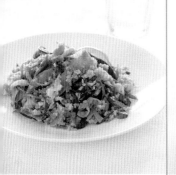
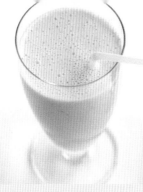

Lunch

Your choice of protein, vegetables and carbohydrates *(see p.180)*

Afternoon snack

Your choice of smoothie and 1 tablespoon of mixed seeds, or Dates & fromage frais *(p.143)* or 2 oatcakes or rye biscuits, spread with a protein topping such as:

☐ Banana & fromage frais spread *(p.141)*
☐ Chick-pea & banana spread *(p.127)*
☐ Classic guacamole *(p.118)*
☐ Cottage cheese

Dinner

Mexican bean omelette or frittata & salad *(p.188)*

Lunch

Your choice of protein, vegetables and carbohydrates *(see Lunch ideas, p.180)*

Afternoon snack

Your choice of smoothie and 1 tablespoon of mixed seeds, or Dates & fromage frais *(p.143)* or 2 oatcakes or rye biscuits, with:

☐ Feta cheese & roast pepper *(p.150)*
☐ Tomato & bean mash *(p.142)*

Dinner

Fish or haloumi, mushrooms & stir-fry *(p.189)*

Stir-fry sauces

Making your own stir-fry sauces is quick and easy (bought sauces are usually high in salt and sugar).

Fresh lime sauce
2.5cm (1in) fresh ginger, grated
1 clove garlic, crushed
Rind 1 lime, grated

4 tablespoons lime juice
2 tablespoons soy sauce
1 tablespoon balsamic vinegar
1 tablespoon olive oil

Spicy sauce
2 tablespoons five-spice paste

2 tablespoons soy sauce
1 tablespoon apple juice
1 clove garlic, crushed
1 tablespoon balsamic vinegar
1 tablespoon lemon juice

For both recipes, mix ingredients and add to the stir-fry after cooking.

Week 4

days 26–27

30-DAY DIET

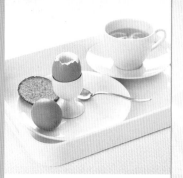

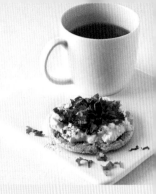

Breakfast

If you're not having brunch, make eggs for breakfast

Morning snack

Your choice of juice and 1 oatcake, or 2 oatcakes or rye biscuits, spread with a protein topping such as:

- [ ] Bean & mustard mash *(p.137)*
- [ ] Cottage cheese
- [ ] Crab meat spread *(p.140)*
- [ ] Home-made houmous *(p.88)*
- [ ] Reduced-fat fromage frais & peppers *(p.114)*
- [ ] Spicy chick-pea *(p.137)*

RECIPES

Breakfast

If you're not having brunch, choose a ham or cereal recipe for breakfast

Morning snack

Your choice of juice and 1 oatcake, or 2 oatcakes or rye biscuits, spread with a protein topping such as:

- [ ] Egg & crudités *(p.126)*
- [ ] No-fat soft cheese *(p.84)*
- [ ] Red lentil & turmeric *(p.163)*
- [ ] Sweet potato & goat's cheese topping *(p.163)*

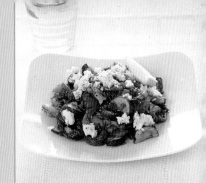

The Food Doctor

Tip for the day ...

If you're having brunch this weekend, remember to have a small snack first thing in the morning instead of breakfast.

Brunch/Lunch

See pages 138–139 and 164–165 for ideas on what to make for brunch, and pages 118–119 and 144–45 for suggestions on what to eat and drink with your main brunch dish

OR

Look at pages 180–181 for ideas of what to have for lunch

Afternoon snack

Your choice of smoothie and 1 tablespoon of mixed seeds, or Dates & fromage frais *(p.143)* or 2 oatcakes or rye biscuits, spread with a protein topping such as:

- [ ] Banana & fromage frais spread *(p.141)*
- [ ] Chick-pea & banana spread *(p.127)*
- [ ] Cottage cheese
- [ ] Classic guacamole *(p.118)*

Dinner

Mediterranean risotto *(p.190)*

Brunch/Lunch

Your choice of brunch or lunch (above)

Afternoon snack

Your choice of smoothie and 1 tablespoon of mixed seeds, or Dates & fromage frais *(p.143)* or 2 oatcakes or rye biscuits, with a protein topping such as:

- [ ] Feta cheese & roast pepper spread *(p.150)*
- [ ] Tomato & bean mash *(p.142)*

Dinner

Tuscan bean soup or Mixed bean salad *(p.191)*

Salad dressing

Like stir-fry sauces, bought salad dressings are usually high in salt and sugar, and even saturated fat. Try this salad dressing, and also those listed on pages 175 and 177, as alternatives. This recipe makes 100ml (3½fl oz).

Store any extra dressing in a screw-top container in the fridge. It should keep for up to five days.

Lemon & carrot juice dressing
50ml (2fl oz) carrot juice
3 tablespoons olive oil

1 tablespoon live natural low-fat yoghurt
1 tablespoon lemon juice
½ teaspoon red chilli paste

Mix all the ingredients well, season with ground black pepper and drizzle over a salad before serving.

Week 4
days 28–29

30-DAY DIET

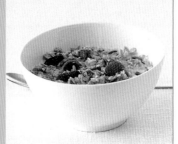

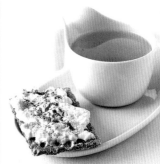

Breakfast

Your choice of Food Doctor
Diet plan breakfast

Morning snack

Your choice of juice and
1 oatcake, or 2 oatcakes or
rye biscuits, spread with a
protein topping such as:

- [ ] Bean & mustard *(p.137)*
- [ ] Cottage cheese
- [ ] Home-made houmous *(p.88)*
- [ ] Reduced-fat fromage
      frais & peppers *(p.114)*
- [ ] Spicy chick-pea *(p.137)*
- [ ] The Food Doctor
      fresh pesto *(p.122)*

Breakfast

Your choice of Food Doctor
Diet plan breakfast

Cereal recipes are listed on
pages 84, 86, 90, 92, 94 and
122; egg recipes are on pages
88 and 116; see page 114
for a ham breakfast recipe.

Morning snack

Your choice of Food Doctor
Diet plan snack

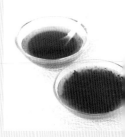

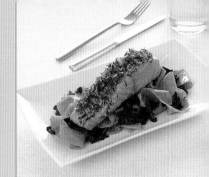

The Food Doctor
Tip for the day ...
Prepare the ingredients and marinate your choice of chicken or tofu in the evening on day 28, or in the morning on day 29.

Lunch

Tuscan bean soup or Mixed bean salad reserved from day 27

Afternoon snack

Your choice of smoothie and 1 tablespoon of mixed seeds, or Dates & fromage frais *(p.143)* or 2 oatcakes or rye biscuits, with a protein topping such as:

☐ Banana & fromage frais spread *(p.141)*
☐ Chick-pea & banana spread *(p.127)*
☐ Classic guacamole *(p.118)*

Dinner

Salmon or eggs with spinach & sweet potato *(p.192)*

Lunch

Your choice of Food Doctor Diet plan lunch, or:

Baked sweet potato & steamed spinach with spicy chick-peas *(p.187)*. Add extra steamed vegetables if necessary

Afternoon snack

Your choice of smoothie and 1 tablespoon of mixed seeds, or Dates & fromage frais *(p.143)* or 2 oatcakes or rye biscuits with:

☐ Feta cheese & roast pepper spread *(p.150)*
☐ Tomato & bean mash *(p.142)*

Dinner

Chicken or tofu & broccoli stir-fry *(p.193)*

Salad dressing recipes

Store any extra salad dressing in separate screw-top containers in the fridge for up to five days.

Olive dressing
1 heaped teaspoon tapenade
4 tablespoons olive oil

2 tablespoons lemon juice
1 tablespoon orange juice

Oriental dressing
3 tablespoons olive oil
1 tablespoon soy sauce

1 tablespoon lime juice
½ teaspoon five-spice paste

For both the salad dressing recipes, mix all the ingredients together well. Drizzle some dressing over a salad just before serving.

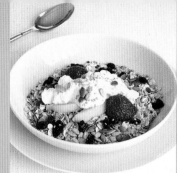
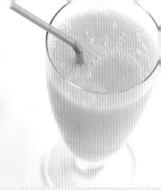

Week 4

day 30

30-DAY DIET

Breakfast

Your choice of Food Doctor
Diet plan breakfast

Morning snack

Your choice of juice and
1 oatcake, or 2 oatcakes
or rye biscuits, spread with
a protein topping such as:

- [ ] Egg & crudités *(p.126)*
- [ ] Flavoured no-fat
  soft cheese *(p.84)*
- [ ] Red lentil & turmeric
  spread *(p.163)*
- [ ] Sweet potato & goat's
  cheese topping *(p.163)*

The Food Doctor

Tip for the day ...

Now that you are
at the end of the
30-day Food Doctor
Diet plan, read up
about Principle 8,
Follow the 80:20
rule *(pp.36–37)*.

Salad dressing recipe

**Store any extra dressing in
a screw-top container in the
fridge for up to five days.**

Classic French dressing
2 tablespoons olive oil
1 teaspoon cider vinegar

1 flat teaspoon Dijon mustard
½ teaspoon red chilli paste

Mix all the ingredients
together well and drizzle
some dressing over a salad
just before serving.

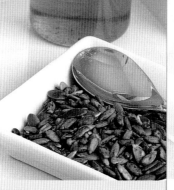

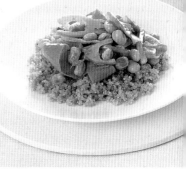

Lunch

Chicken or tofu reserved
from day 29 with mixed leaf
salad & tomatoes

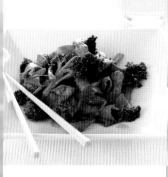

Afternoon snack

Your choice of smoothie and
1 tablespoon of mixed seeds,
or Dates & fromage frais *(p.143)*
or 2 oatcakes or rye biscuits,
spread with a protein topping
such as:

- [ ] Banana & fromage frais
  spread *(p.141)*
- [ ] Chick-pea & banana spread
  (p.127)
- [ ] Cottage cheese
- [ ] Classic guacamole *(p.118)*

Dinner

Fennel, carrot, broad bean
& quinoa risotto with green
salad *(p.194)*

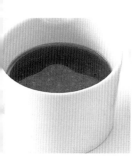

Congratulations!

You've reached the end of
The Food Doctor 30-day
Diet plan, which is great
news. I hope that you have
not only lost weight and feel
healthier, but that you are
confident about eating
healthily on the Plan for Life.

Lunch ideas

Week 4 is all about starting to make your own meal choices. It's up to you which protein, vegetables and starchy carbohydrates you choose at lunchtime, so here are some suggestions.

Lunches to go

Easy proteins are a hard-boiled egg, canned tuna, smoked fish, cold chicken, seeds and chick-peas. Include a slice of rye or wholemeal bread with these lunch choices:

● 50g (2oz) sprouted seeds, ½ avocado, sliced, 1 chopped tomato, 1 tablespoon mixed seeds, 30g (1oz) feta and a dressing (*pp.173,175,177*).

● 50g (2oz) raw grated carrot or sweet potato, 50g (2oz) sprouted seeds tossed in a dressing of 1 tablespoon yoghurt, 1 tablespoon fromage frais, 1 tablespoon horseradish. For protein add 1 hard-boiled egg or tuna, smoked mackerel or other smoked fish.

● 4 tablespoons mixed beans or chick-peas, green leaves, raw vegetables (chopped tomatoes, cucumber, peppers, celery) and a dressing (*pp.173,175,177*).

● ½ can tuna with canned artichoke hearts, some mixed peppers from a jar, and a dressing (*pp.173,175,177*).

● If there's nothing in the house, buy your lunch from a supermarket: ready-prepared raw vegetables with some smoked fish and a dressing.

● If your supermarket has a salad bar, choose a mix of two or three salads (only one should contain pasta, couscous or rice).

● Buy some baby tomatoes and a filled wholemeal sandwich, and throw away half the bread.

Lunches at home

● Bake a small sweet potato or ordinary potato, add some mixed green leaves and 2 tablespoons of cottage cheese topped with spring onions.

● Grill sliced mushrooms and tomatoes and heat 2 tablespoons of sweet corn from a can. Mix together and pile on a slice of wholemeal toast, topped with a poached egg.

● Soften a small chopped onion in a frying pan, add a small can of chopped tomatoes, crushed garlic and chopped fresh herbs and add a can of drained and rinsed chick-peas. Simmer for 5 minutes. Add lemon juice, black pepper and ground cumin to taste.

● 75g (2½oz) prawns, 75g (2½oz) peas, ½ chopped red pepper (or use some from a jar) mixed with the juice of ½ lemon and 2 tablespoons olive oil and chopped fresh herbs. For extra flavour add a little horseradish sauce. Toast a slice of wholemeal or rye bread, drizzle with a little olive oil, pile on the prawn mix and top with some sliced spring onion.

● Make a quick stir-fry using any vegetables you have in the fridge, topped with seeds and your chosen protein (feta, tofu, cold chicken, tuna, egg, etc.). Serve with wholemeal noodles.

● Make a frittata using 2 eggs, 1 tablespoon live natural low-fat yoghurt, a small chopped onion and any fresh vegetables or peppers from a jar.

Salads

To make a healthy salad, follow these simple rules:

● 300g (10oz) vegetables per person (choose at least 5 different vegetables in a wide variety of colours)

● Mix cooked vegetables with raw (steam beans, mangetout and asparagus; red or white cabbage, broccoli, cauliflower, courgettes, grated carrot, grated sweet potato, grated celeriac, mushrooms, baby sweet corn, sprouted seeds and shelled peas are all good raw).

● Try different kinds of leaves; the paler the lettuce, the less nutrients there are.

● Sprout your own seeds for a constant supply of ultra-fresh vegetables. Put a shallow layer of seeds (alfalfa, aduki beans, etc.) in a glass jar, cover with water and cover the lid with a piece of muslin. Stand for 1 hour, then drain the water through the muslin. Rinse and drain quickly daily until the seeds have sprouted.

Stir-fries

● Use 300g (10oz) mixed vegetables per person, cut into bite-size pieces or ribbons so they cook at the same rate. If you buy a pack of ready-prepared vegetables, add some fresh vegetables too.

● Lightly blanch vegetables such as green beans and asparagus first to allow them all to cook at the same time.

● Sprouted seeds (bought or your own) add good flavour and are super-nutritious.

● Avoid olive oil; cook the vegetables in a little water or lemon juice.

● If you use seed oils, add after cooking, as the cooking process will damage them.

● Add a sauce of your choice after cooking *(p.171)*.

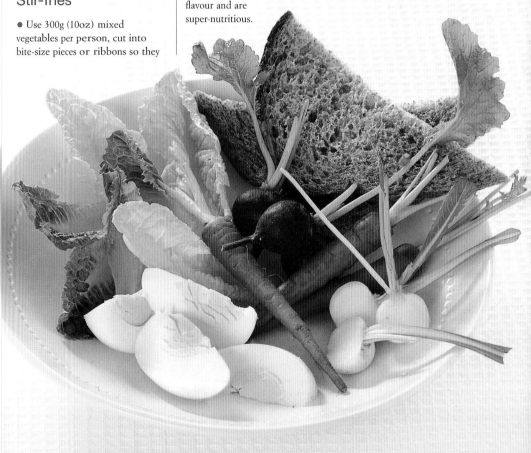

Salmon or eggs with spinach & sweet potato

DINNER DAY 28

If you wish, save a portion of the spinach and sweet potato stir-fry, store it in the fridge and have it with your choice of protein and carbohydrate for lunch tomorrow. Serves two.

ready in 30 minutes

For the ginger topping:
2cm (¾in) cube ginger, peeled

2 small spring onions, chopped

2 sprigs dill (or 1 teaspoon dried)

Zest and juice 1 lime

2 salmon fillets (approx. 100–150g/3½–5oz each) or 2 hen's eggs

150g (5oz) sweet potato

250g (8oz) spinach leaves, washed

1 tablespoon olive oil

1 clove garlic, crushed or chopped

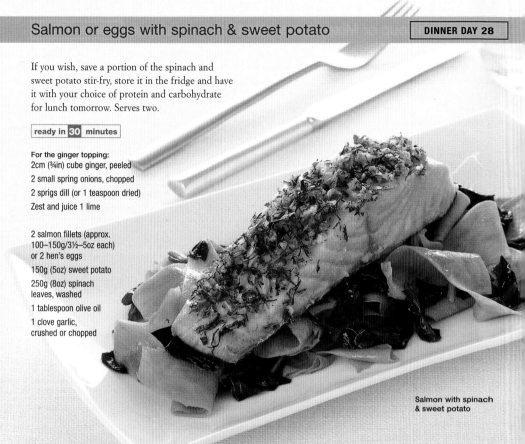

Salmon with spinach & sweet potato

Either prepare the ginger topping by blitzing the ingredients in a food processor, or by hand: grate the ginger, very finely chop the onions and dill, grate the lime zest, and mix together.

Preheat the oven to 160°C/320°F/Gas mark 3. If using salmon, lightly oil an ovenproof dish and put in the salmon fillet skin side down. Top with the ginger mix. Cover with foil and cook for about 15 minutes, until just opaque.

If using eggs, break the eggs into 2 lightly oiled ramekin dishes. Top with the ginger mix. Bake

for about 10 minutes, or until the eggs are cooked as you like them.

Meanwhile, peel the sweet potato and cut into long ribbons using a potato peeler. Coarsely shred the spinach. Heat the oil in a frying pan or wok, add the garlic and sweet potato and gently stir-fry for about 5 minutes, until the sweet potato is hot but still crunchy. Add the spinach and cook for a further 2–3 minutes until the spinach is wilted.

Serve the vegetables topped with the salmon or eggs.

Chicken or tofu stir-fry

Reserve a portion of tonight's meal for lunch tomorrow if you wish. If you're short of time, use a packet of ready-prepared vegetables instead of the carrot and broccoli. Serves two.

1 tablespoon olive oil

2 chicken breasts (approx. 150g/5oz each), cut into strips, or 200g (7oz) firm tofu, cut into cubes

250g (8oz) broccoli, broken into bite-sized florets

150g (5oz) carrot, cut into matchsticks or sliced into ribbons

A drizzle of sesame oil

For the marinade:
2 tablespoons soy sauce

1 teaspoon tamarind paste

1 teaspoon five-spice paste

1 clove garlic, crushed

1 tablespoon dry apple juice

1 teaspoon cider vinegar

Mix together the marinade ingredients and leave the chicken or tofu in the marinade for a minimum of 15 minutes, and preferably as long as possible, while you prepare the vegetables.

Heat the olive oil in a wok, add the chicken or tofu pieces and brown lightly. Remove with a slotted spoon. Add the vegetables and a tablespoon of the marinade, and cook until the broccoli is just soft – the carrot will probably still be al dente. Add the chicken or tofu pieces and the rest of the marinade, bring to the boil and serve drizzled with a little sesame oil.

Chicken stir-fry

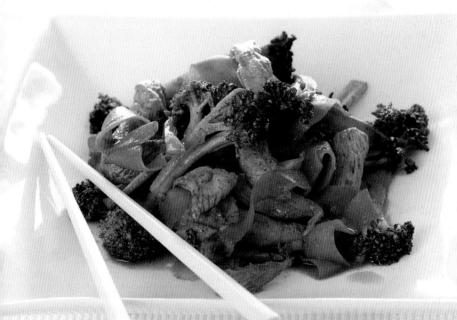

Roast vegetable quinoa & salad

DINNER DAY 30

If you can't get hold of broad beans or fennel, this recipe works well with whatever vegetables are in season. Serves two.

ready in 30 minutes

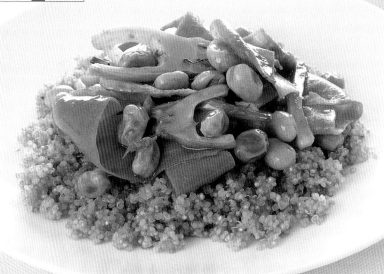

1 head fennel (150g/5oz), finely sliced lengthways

1 tablespoon olive oil

120g (4oz) quinoa

250ml (8fl oz) light vegetable stock

1 clove garlic, peeled

150g (5oz) carrot, cleaned and sliced into ribbons using a potato peeler

100g (3½oz) broad beans (weight after shelling, or use frozen)

Zest 1 orange

For the dressing:

2 tablespoons sesame oil

2 tablespoons orange juice

1 heaped teaspoon mango powder (or juice ½ lemon)

Preheat the oven to 180°C/350°F/Gas mark 4. Put the fennel in a roasting pan, drizzle over the olive oil and toss well. Cook in the oven for 15 minutes or so. Meanwhile, simmer the quinoa in the stock with the garlic for about 15 minutes, or until the quinoa is just tender and the stock is absorbed. If the garlic is tender, mash it into the quinoa.

Add the carrots and broad beans to the fennel, toss well with the orange zest and season with a good grinding of black pepper. Cook for a further 10 minutes until the vegetables are cooked, but still retain some bite.

Mix the sesame oil, orange juice and mango powder or lemon juice together. Pile the quinoa onto two plates, top with the vegetables and pour over the dressing. Serve with a small mixed leaf salad.

Salsas

These salsas are a deliciously tasty addition to any meal; serve them with lunch or dinner dishes. Any leftovers can be kept in the fridge for up to three days. Each salsa serves two.

Green salsa

`ready in` **5** `minutes`

½ green pepper, very finely diced
½ small cucumber, finely diced
1 small spring onion, trimmed and finely chopped
A small handful fresh parsley, very finely chopped
1 tablespoon lemon juice
1 tablespoon olive oil
½ teaspoon soy sauce

Combine all the ingredients in a bowl. Season with some freshly ground black pepper and serve in a small side dish or bowl.

Red salsa

`ready in` **30** `minutes`

½ small red onion, finely chopped
1 medium-sized ripe tomato, skinned and chopped
½ red pepper, chopped
½ small cucumber, chopped
A couple of good sprigs of fresh basil, finely chopped (for preference, use red basil)
1 spring onion, finely chopped
1 tablespoon lime juice
1 tablespoon olive oil
1 teaspoon soy sauce

Combine all the ingredients in a bowl. Season with some freshly ground black pepper and serve in a small side dish or bowl.

If you wish, you could also zap all the ingredients together in a food processor, but take care not to process them to a purée.

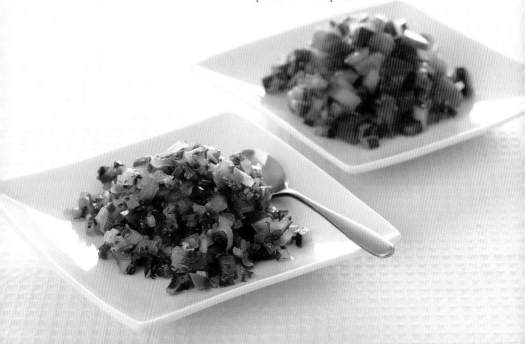

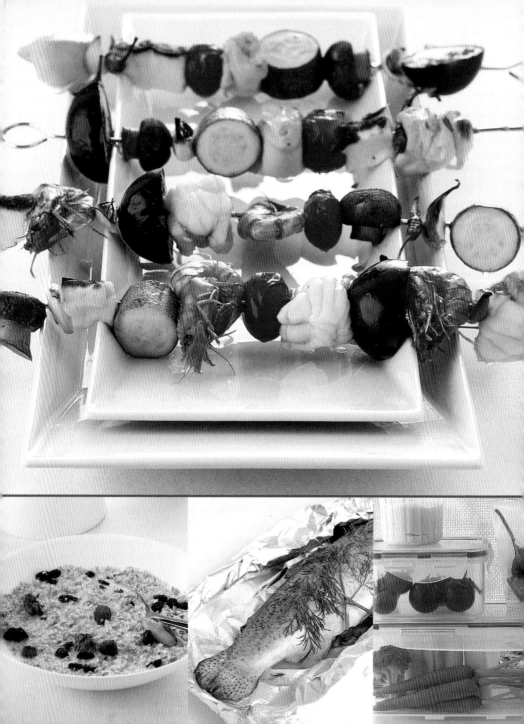

Plan for life

The Plan for Life is a simple, sustainable eating programme that is designed to be adapted to your individual lifestyle. Once you begin to incorporate the ten basic Food Doctor principles *(see pp.14–41)* into your own routines you may want to plan ahead a little to ensure you have the appropriate foods for the right meals, but hopefully this plan will soon become second nature to you.

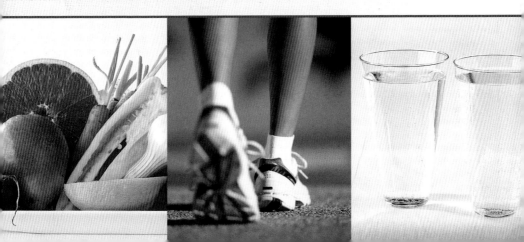

Planning meals

Any diet plan should be a sensible one that incorporates all the best that food can offer, from nutrients and fibre to flavour and taste. I believe that the process of safe, sustainable weight loss and healthy eating advocated by the Plan for Life will help you to look and feel your best.

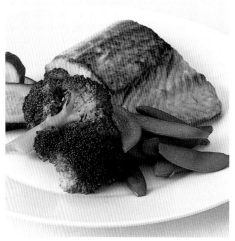

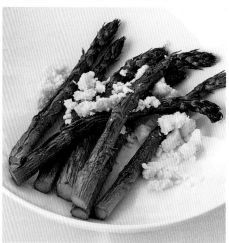

This part of the book explains the practice behind the theory of the Plan for Life. The information in this section reminds you of the main aims for each mealtime – what you should be eating, and when – in order to sustain your energy levels and maintain a healthy digestive system.

To help you remember the food groups in The Food Doctor plan, which consist of complete proteins, starchy complex carbohydrates and complex carbohydrates in the form of vegetables, look at my food equations. These equations will help you to think carefully about which categories your food choices fall into, and whether they are really healthy enough to be part of this eating plan.

The selections of suggested meal and snack options will provide a springboard to encourage you to think for yourself when deciding what you should eat at mealtimes. These suggestions combine the food groups in the ratios that I feel are ideal for maximizing energy, reducing hunger and promoting weight loss. Feel free to substitute any protein for another according to your preference, and always include vegetables at lunch and dinner and with snacks to ensure that you don't end up on a very high-protein diet.

The Plan for Life should suit almost every lifestyle. It has been designed to reduce your levels of hunger, it's easy to follow and you don't have to buy obscure foods. By sticking to it 100 per cent of the time and exercising regularly, you'll achieve maximum weight loss. However, if this proves hard to sustain, why not think of this plan as a life-changing experience that will improve your health and self-image while still giving you a chance to eat what you like once in a while?

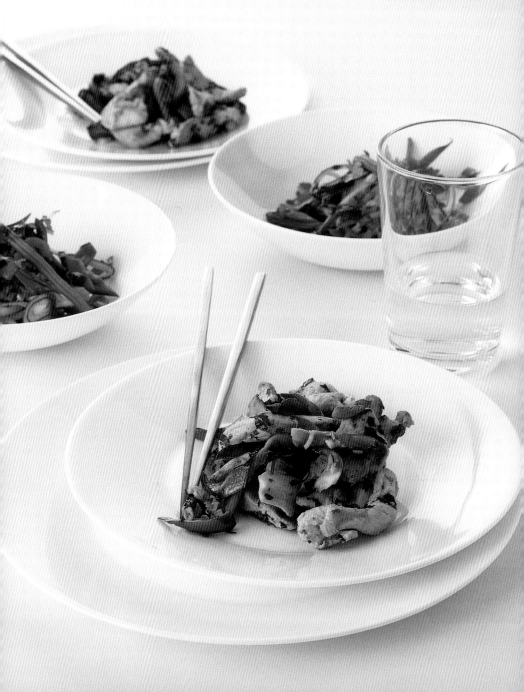

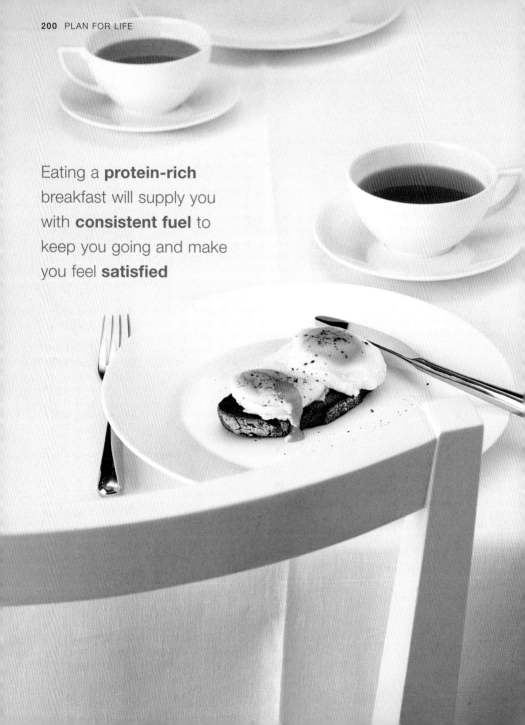

Eating a **protein-rich** breakfast will supply you with **consistent fuel** to keep you going and make you feel **satisfied**

Breakfast

We have already examined the principle of eating breakfast and how it sets the scene for rest of the day *(see pp.30–31)*, but let's look more closely at how this theory works and why it is such a fundamental and important principle to establish.

The food you eat is broken down by your digestive system into its component parts – glucose, vitamins, minerals, and so on. It is glucose that creates energy and acts as the fuel for every cell, so the breakfast you eat is responsible for providing you with energy for a significant part of the morning. In order to lose weight you must eat the right ratio of food groups *(see p.16)* to ensure that glucose is released gradually into the bloodstream. This steady release limits the production of insulin, which must be minimized if body fat is to be reduced accordingly.

What is a healthy breakfast?

Having established that breakfast must include some foods that are broken down slowly by the body, the reality is that conventional breakfast foods usually comprise caffeine and simple carbohydrates, which supply a quick energy surge and little more. The image of a "healthy" breakfast of cereal, toast, orange juice and black coffee is, in fact, based on the theory of calorie counting, and does not include any protein. I can almost guarantee that this type of breakfast will not meet your energy requirements for the morning: as the glucose created from this food runs out, your body interprets this signal as hunger and you begin an eating cycle of desire and denial.

Eating a protein-rich breakfast will supply you with consistent fuel to keep you feeling satisfied so that you don't become overly hungry. Remember that this is a protein-rich breakfast, not a pure protein one, so include some complex carbohydrates too. This sort of meal isn't always as instant as a packet of cereal, so turn to pages 204–205 for some ideas and then put aside a few extra minutes each day to make a proper breakfast.

THE FOOD DOCTOR BREAKFAST EQUATION

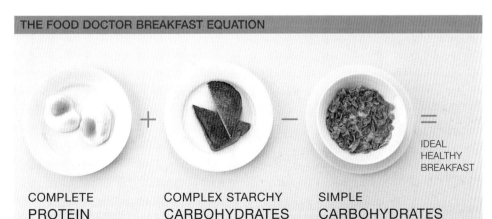

IDEAL
HEALTHY
BREAKFAST

COMPLETE PROTEIN
such as poached eggs or nuts and seeds

COMPLEX STARCHY CARBOHYDRATES
whole grains such as wholemeal bread or oats

SIMPLE CARBOHYDRATES
such as highly sugared, processed cereal

A good breakfast ...

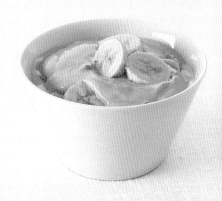

Those rumours you heard about how essential this meal is were true: it really is important to start the day well with a healthy breakfast.

The usual choice

Peach and papaya smoothie How can a drink made almost entirely from fruit be improved upon? It depends on your choice of fruit. This smoothie also lacks protein, so it's important to make some additions.

Strawberry yoghurt with banana Surely a yoghurt and some fresh fruit is a healthy option? Well, yes, but only if you choose the right yoghurt and fruit and improve the ratio of protein to complex carbohydrate. Yoghurt alone won't provide enough protein, and you should check the label for sugars or other additives alongside the flavouring. Don't forget too, that some fruits are better than others at providing steady glucose conversion throughout the morning.

Cereal and milk A processed breakfast cereal with milk, even if you've chosen a high-fibre cereal such as bran flakes, is not a good choice, as your protein quota is unfulfilled and the processed cereal will convert into glucose rapidly to give only short-term energy. Many commercial cereals are laden with sugars, fats and salt, too.

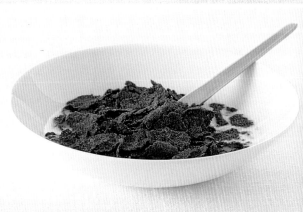

can be even better

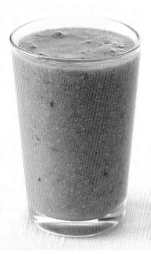

The Food Doctor choice

Cut out added extras such as honey and fruit juice, which can send the GI score soaring.

- Choose fruits with a low GI score, such as plums, strawberries, blackberries and pears.

- In place of the fruit juice, use full-fat milk to create the right consistency.

- Add some seeds and soft tofu to the blender to increase the protein content.

- See my smoothie recipes on pp.240–241.

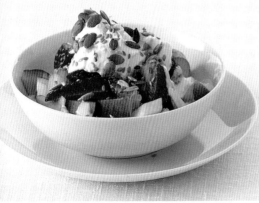

Bananas are a poor-choice carbohydrate as they have high GI scores and provide only short-term energy. Plain yoghurt is less likely than flavoured versions to contain any hidden "extras".

- Choose fruit with a low GI score, such as apples, apricots, strawberries and pears.

- Sprinkle some seeds and/or nuts on your yoghurt to ensure that it meets the protein requirements and keeps you feeling full.

- Add your own flavourings, such as a pinch of cinnamon with a mixture of fresh apple and hazelnuts, to ring the changes.

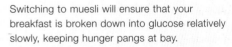

Switching to muesli will ensure that your breakfast is broken down into glucose relatively slowly, keeping hunger pangs at bay.

- Ensure your muesli is rich in nuts and seeds to bump up the protein quotient.

- Check that you don't have too much dried fruit and hidden sugars in any commercial muesli you buy.

- Make your own muesli. It can easily be stored for up to four weeks in an airtight container.

Breakfast suggestions

Many of us tend to view breakfast as a time-consuming event that keeps us from starting the day, but it is important to remember that this meal is vital if you want to maintain high energy levels through the morning. These suggestions are easy to prepare, yet are satisfying and taste good.

By now you should be familiar with the principle that protein combined with complex carbohydrates will provide a healthy, energy-giving meal *(see pp.14–17)*. This is a crucial requirement for the first meal of the day. For example, if you have a piece of fish left over from your supper the night before and you want to eat it for your breakfast, there is nothing to say that you shouldn't have it. It's not a typical choice, perhaps, but it fits in with The Food Doctor plan. You must eat some complex carbohydrates with the fish, so you could either have a mouthful or two of vegetables, a couple of rice crackers or a piece of rye toast. Here are some simple suggestions which may inspire you.

Hot breakfasts

Two eggs scrambled, poached or soft-boiled with a slice of rye toast or rice crackers
Eggs supply the protein in this meal, while the toast or crackers provide the complex carbohydrates. If you would like to try poached eggs with asparagus and mushrooms, turn to the recipe section *(see p.237)*. If you don't have time to cook in the morning, hard-boil some eggs the night before and leave them to cool. At breakfast time chop up the eggs, add chopped fresh herbs such as dill or tarragon and eat them with a piece of toast or two oatcakes.

Porridge A sustaining meal of porridge will provide you with some of the necessary fibre required for a healthy digestive system. Add protein in the form of a tablespoon of live natural yoghurt and mix in some chopped pear to provide more complex carbohydrates (this also gives it added taste) – or try a recipe for apple porridge *(see p.86)*.

Fish with grilled or steamed vegetables or a piece of rye or wholemeal toast
Fish is delicious as well as quick and simple to cook, and provides your body with valuable nutrients at the start of the day.

Uncooked breakfasts

Sugar-free cereal, such as flaked corn, with sunflower seeds
When you shop for a packaged cereal, check the ingredients label first to ensure that it does not contain any sugar. If you combine a serving of the cereal with some hazelnuts and sunflower seeds, topped with a tablespoon of live natural yoghurt and a teaspoon of sultanas, the cereal and sultanas will provide your complex carbohydrates and the nuts, seeds and yoghurt will supply your protein.

BENEFICIAL NUTRIENTS

The best way to maximize your nutritional benefits is to eat as many unprocessed foods as possible. This is because the nutrient levels of, for example, whole grains remain intact as long as they have not been refined in any way. In contrast, the grains contained in processed cereals have been refined to such a degree that it's very possible the nutrient levels in these products are depleted. So, when deciding what to eat for breakfast, remember that the fibre content and level of B vitamins in whole grains such as oats are potentially higher than those of processed cereals. In fact, oats contain most of the B vitamins, which have numerous functions in the body. These include being involved in the production of energy and in helping to maintain stable moods, which can, in turn, help to reduce your cravings for sugar and caffeine.

Nut and seed muesli

A simple recipe to mix up your own muesli should be one that includes whole grains, nuts and seeds to provide an ideal combination of the food groups. It may be worth making up a quantity of muesli in advance and storing it in a sealed plastic container ready for those mornings when you don't feel like doing anything more than pouring your breakfast into a bowl, adding some milk and eating it straight away.

Natural yoghurt with apple

For a tasty, quick breakfast, try mixing one chopped apple with two tablespoons of live natural yoghurt and sprinkling over a tablespoon each of flaked almonds and pumpkin or sesame seeds. The yoghurt, nuts and seeds provide the protein while the apple provides the complex carbohydrates and fibre.

Tofu smoothie

Try a smoothie for a change. Use a food processor to blend 50g (2oz) of soft tofu, one chopped apple and a tablespoon of either sunflower, pumpkin or sesame seeds with your preferred choice of full-fat milk – cows', goats', sheep's, rice or soya milk. Add a couple of drops of vanilla essence or a teaspoon of unsweetened cocoa powder if you like the taste, blend for a few seconds more and then drink the smoothie.

Try a **refreshing smoothie** made with **tofu, fruit and seeds** for a perfectly balanced breakfast

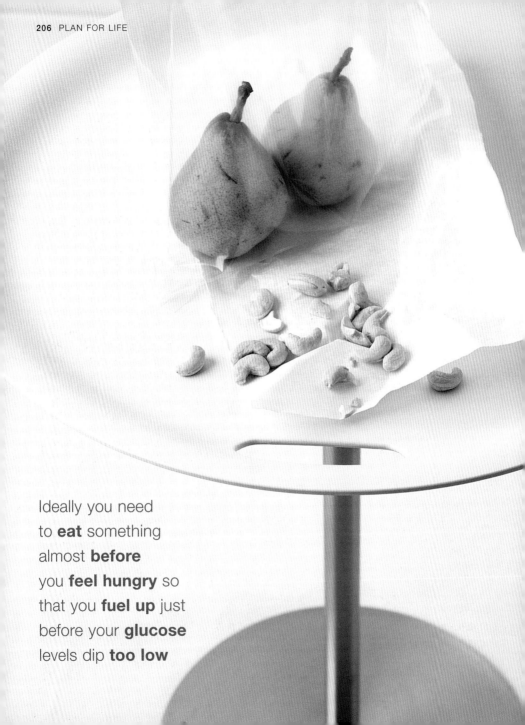

Ideally you need to **eat** something almost **before** you **feel hungry** so that you **fuel up** just before your **glucose** levels dip **too low**

Snacks

By the middle of the morning or afternoon, the energy created from your last protein-rich meal will have been used up by your body for various functions – anything from breathing and thinking to walking and exercising. At this point it's time to refuel again.

Assuming that you ate your breakfast at about 8am, you should eat a mid-morning snack between 10.30am and 11am. Likewise, if you ate lunch at 1pm, have a mid-afternoon snack at about 4pm. Ideally, you should eat something almost before you feel hungry so that you fuel up just before your glucose levels dip too low; don't wait until you feel ravenous.

Which snacks are best?

The snacks you choose needn't be a time-consuming culinary feast. For example, when I suggest eating some crudités and a dip, don't assume that you must cut the vegetables perfectly and arrange them on a plate with the dip in the centre. You can just as easily stand in the kitchen, dip a carrot into an opened tub of dip and munch it. After all, it's the combination of the complex carbohydrate and protein that is important, not how it is

presented. However you decide to eat your snack, do remember not to rush it and to chew each mouthful well.

If you go out to work, try to plan ahead by taking something simple with you in your bag, such as a tupperware box of chopped raw vegetables and a few cubes of hard cheese. You only need eat a few mouthfuls to make a satisfying snack.

Energy bars and drinks

Energy bars are not an ideal option. Many are sold as "healthy" but they are not as wholesome as they seem. Look at the labels of energy bars or drinks and you will see that they all contain sugar in varying amounts. Also check whether the protein content of an energy bar is anywhere near the correct Food Doctor ratio of around 40 per cent. Ideally, opt for the suggested snacks on pp. 210–211 instead.

THE FOOD DOCTOR SNACK EQUATION

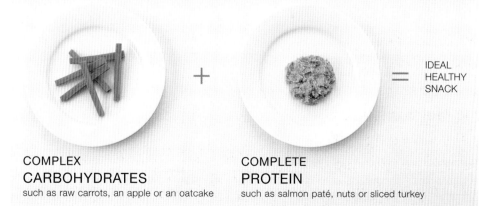

IDEAL
HEALTHY
SNACK

**COMPLEX
CARBOHYDRATES**
such as raw carrots, an apple or an oatcake

**COMPLETE
PROTEIN**
such as salmon paté, nuts or sliced turkey

Quick and easy snacks ...

Snacks keep the body supplied with a steady energy supply. If you snack regularly, you'll be less likely to over-eat at meal-times or make poor food choices due to hunger.

The usual choice

Dried fruits and an "energy bar" I can almost sense your disappointment at being told this isn't a perfect choice though it might seem very healthy. There are still a few substitutions you could make, however, to turn this into a truly healthy snack.

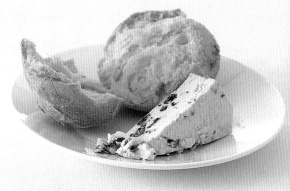

Bread and cheese Many of us find it hard to resist a chunk of fresh bread and cheese: with a few careful substitutions The Food Doctor Diet allows you to continue enjoying such pleasures, while still controlling your weight.

Low-fat biscuits Surely dieters can eat biscuits if they are labelled low in fat? Unfortunately not. To create flavour, low-fat options are often packed full of sugar and sweeteners, guaranteed to trigger insulin production. However convenient this option seems, there is always a price to pay.

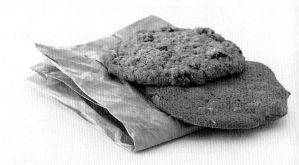

and how to improve them

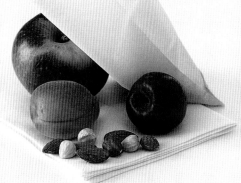

The Food Doctor choice

Many energy bars are packed with sugars and cheap ingredients instead of the nuts and seeds required to supply protein. Dried fruits are a poor-choice carbohydrate as they have a high GI rating.

- Choose fresh fruits that have low GI scores, such as apples, plums, pears or apricots.

- Instead of an energy bar, eat five or six hazelnuts or other nuts with your piece of fruit.

- As a tasty alternative protein source to nuts, try some mixed sunflower and pumpkin seeds.

White bread is a poor choice as it is low in fibre and has a high GI value. Instead, try rye bread or oatcakes as this allows you to vary your grain intake, or sourdough if you want to avoid yeast.

- Cottage cheese, possibly flavoured with some fresh herbs or spring onions, makes a tangy alternative topping.

- Goat's cheese is relatively low in fat and makes a good substitute for cow's-milk cheeses.

- Avoid blue and aged cheeses because they contain mould that can lead to excess yeast formation in the intestines.

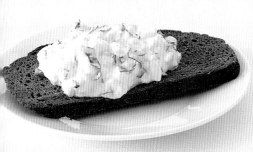

If convenience is the key, try to avoid the sweet biscuit section of a shop and buy some oatcakes instead. They are just as easy to eat on the go. Team them with some protein for the ideal snack.

- The quickest accompaniment to your crackers is to layer some lean ham on top.

- Houmous is a great protein option. If you have time, make it yourself so it's additive-free.

- Chopped cucumber mixed with linseeds, mint and natural yoghurt makes a healthy topping.

Snack suggestions

Snacking is an important element of the Plan for Life, and every mid-morning and mid-afternoon snack must include a combination of the right food groups (as the equation on page 207 shows). The timing of each snack is also significant, as are the amounts you eat.

If you take care not to leave too long a gap between your previous meal and your next snack, the chances are that you won't be tempted to overeat or make poor choices about what your snack should consist of.

Snacks should be easy and quick to prepare, although you may sometimes have to be a little creative with your ingredients. If you are out and about during the day, take a piece of fruit and a packet of mixed seeds or nuts in your bag – an apple and five nuts should make an ample snack. Even if you don't feel very adventurous about what to eat, make sure that your snack is healthy and simple to make, that it consists of the correct proportion of protein and complex carbohydrates and it is something that you enjoy eating.

Easy options

A piece of fruit with raw nuts

Choose an apple or a pear to eat with five or six Brazil nuts or almonds. Nuts make an excellent standby as you can buy them in small packets to keep at home or in your bag, briefcase or rucksack. It is important that you don't eat too many nuts – limit yourself to an average of five or six a day – and that you eat complex carbohydrates, such as a piece of fruit, at the same time. You may prefer to substitute nuts with a handful of mixed sesame, pumpkin and sunflower seeds.

Soya nuts are now becoming widely available in shops and health-food stores, and, as they contain far less fat than other nuts, they make an excellent high-protein alternative. They may also be a good choice if you enjoy a little more variety.

Nut butter on two rice cakes, oatcakes, or a small piece of rye bread

Nut butters, such as peanut, cashew or almond butter, are another good standby, but ensure that the products you buy are free of sugar and that you don't eat too much at once. A thin scraping of your choice of nut butter on a rice cake, oatcake or piece of rye bread should suffice.

A tablespoon of dip with a few raw vegetables

Choose a dip such as guacamole, tzatziki, houmous or fish paste. If you would like to make your own houmous, see page 88 for a recipe. Chop up a couple of raw vegetables, such as a carrot, a stick of celery, some chicory, cucumber, a few broccoli florets or green beans, and use the pieces to scoop up the dip and eat it. If you go out to work, make things even easier for yourself by chopping up the vegetables at home first and storing the pieces in a sealed plastic bag. Keep the bag in a fridge at work if you can.

Guacamole on two oatcakes or rye crispbread

See page 118 for an easy recipe for homemade guacamole. If you add lemon juice to the ingredients when you make the dip, it will keep in the fridge for up to 24 hours.

TAKING SUPPLEMENTS

Although supplements can play a significant role in maintaining our health, I feel that many of us take too many of these products without knowing exactly what they do or how they interact. Since the Plan for Life is designed to enhance your digestion and improve the absorption of nutrients, I would prefer that your vitamins and minerals come directly from your food intake. There are one or two supplements that might make a small difference to your well-being, but most of your success will come from your dietary and lifestyle changes, not from a bottle of capsules. Rather than waste money on supplements that may not be necessary, make a one-off appointment with a nutritionist who will be able to tell you which supplements, if any, may suit your requirements.

Assemblies

Choose any **one** of the following complex carbohydrate bases:

1 piece of rye toast or bread
2 oatcakes
2 rice cakes
2 corn cakes

Top it with your choice of any **one** of the following protein sources:

Cheese – any type, although cottage cheese is the best choice. Avoid blue and aged cheeses.

Fish – a paté or spread made with any oily fish, such as mackerel, salmon, tuna or sardine.

Eggs – a chopped hard-boiled egg combined with finely chopped herbs such as parsley, dill or tarragon.

Chicken or turkey slices – use skinless poultry. If you buy pre-sliced products from the shops, ensure that they are sugar-free.

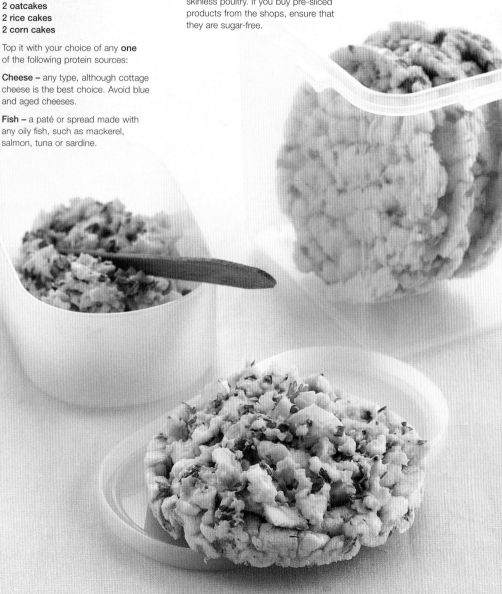

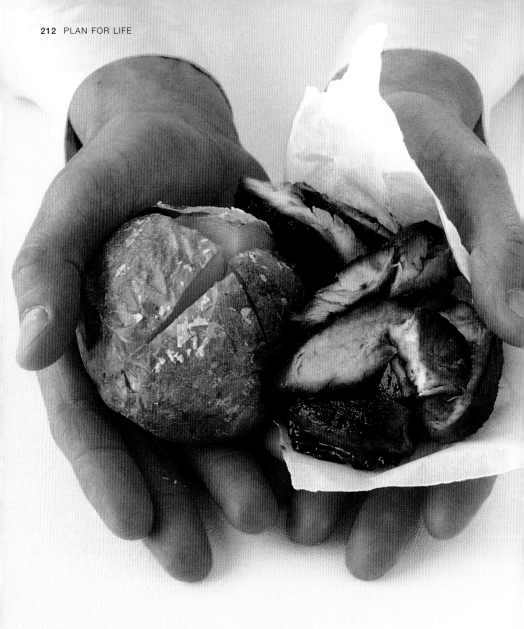

If you open your **hands** and **hold your palms** together, the **surface area** you see is the sort of **plate size** I have in mind

Lunch

When it comes to lunch, the most important thing to remember is that you should eat the right combination of complete protein, complex carbohydrates and fibre. The other rule to bear in mind is that you need to eat slightly larger quantities of food than you would at breakfast or dinner.

Your mid-morning snack should have kept your glucose levels even until lunchtime, so at about 1pm it will be time to fuel up again. For this meal the quantities are slightly larger than those of breakfast or dinner, although it is important that you do not overeat.

How much do I eat?

If you hold out one hand and open it, the portion of protein you should eat is a little smaller than the size of your palm. Complex carbohydrates make up the remaining 60 per cent of the food on your plate. To gauge

how much food that should be, open out both hands and hold your palms together side by side – the surface area you see is the sort of plate size that I have in mind. As long as your food isn't piled too high, you should be eating more or less the right amount of food.

If you have the time and you enjoy cooking, then by all means make the effort to prepare your food; given that digestive enzymes respond to visual stimuli, this process can aid digestion. However, lunch doesn't have to be a beautifully prepared meal: you can

easily cook a chicken breast, or bring a cold, cooked piece of chicken in to work from home, and add a small jacket potato and vegetables or some brown rice salad. Not quite the visual feast you might hope for, but it can taste just as good and supply all the energy and nutrients you need through much of the afternoon.

If you usually buy sandwiches for your lunch, I suggest that you buy sandwiches for only two days of the week and prepare homemade lunches for the remaining days. On pp.216–217 are some ideas for lunches to eat at home, at work and on the move.

THE FOOD DOCTOR LUNCH EQUATION

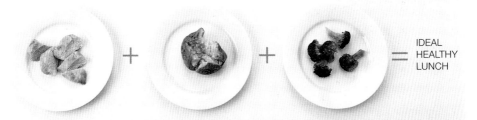

IDEAL
HEALTHY
LUNCH

COMPLETE PROTEIN
such as chicken, tofu or eggs

COMPLEX STARCHY CARBOHYDRATES
such as a jacket potato, brown rice, or wholewheat pasta or bread

COMPLEX VEGETABLE CARBOHYDRATES
such as broccoli, asparagus or cabbage

Lunch on the run ...

Good intentions are all very well, but what happens when you're buying lunch to go? Remember the ratios and you can easily create a healthy option.

The usual choice

Salad How can you go wrong with a salad? Well, if you just eat a plain lettuce salad, you're missing out on essential food groups and not fuelling your body properly. Add some protein to complete the ratio of foods.

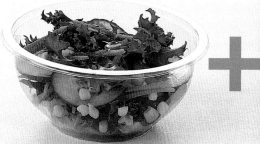

Sandwich Surely a sandwich packed with salad leaves is a healthy option? No, since it lacks a good balance of protein and complex carbohydrate. By asking for extra filling or removing one layer of bread from your sandwich, you can redress the ratio of food groups and turn your sandwich into a healthy choice.

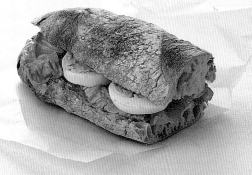

Vegetable soup and a roll This is an excellent choice for a perfect lunch on the run – if you choose the right foods in the right proportions. This choice needs additional protein and fibre to turn it into the perfect meal.

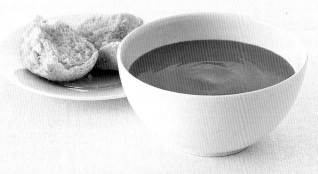

making it healthier

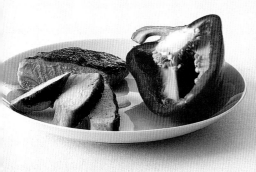

The Food Doctor choice

A salad can become a smarter choice if you know your vegetables. Eat those that are rich in vitamin C and other antioxidants, such as red peppers, raw carrots, watercress and tomatoes.

- Add a brown rice salad: it is high in B vitamins, so makes a good choice of lunch-time starchy complex carbohydrate.

- Protein such as chicken or tuna boosts the mineral content of your meal and makes it convert more slowly into glucose.

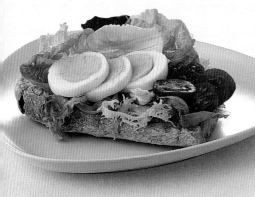

White bread is a poor choice as it is low in fibre and thus has a high GI value. Instead, try rye bread as it is dense and allows you to vary your grain intake, or sourdough if you want to avoid yeast (I believe we eat more yeast products than we should).

- Add tomato for extra fibre and antioxidants.

- Chicken, tuna, egg or smoked salmon are all good sources of protein for sandwich fillings.

- Remember to minimise mayonnaise and butter. Use seasoning instead: a layer of mustard on the bread adds flavour and a moist texture.

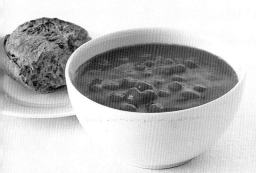

Favour vegetable-based soups over those based on cream or potatoes, and just add fibre and protein to make soup a smart option.

- Add some chick-peas or other pulses to boost the protein ratio of your soup, or add some tofu, shredded ham or sliced chicken breast.

- Stir in a small can of sweetcorn or some baby spinach leaves to give your soup extra fibre.

- Swap the white roll for a wholemeal or rye option to avoid high-GI refined flour products.

Lunch suggestions

Lunch is often a potentially rushed and perhaps functional meal, especially if you are working or busy with your day. Yet however little time you have, it is vital that you put aside ten minutes or so to relax and eat your lunch calmly and slowly.

Taking just a short amount of time to eat your lunch properly and chew your food well will help to improve the process of digestion, thus allowing you to derive the maximum benefit from the good food you are eating. This process also helps you to reduce your stress levels in the middle of a busy day.

Away from home

For many people, lunch is the one meal of the day that is eaten away from home and if this is the case for you, it may help to organize in advance what you will eat so that your meals fit in with the Plan for Life programme. You might prefer to plan for the whole week, writing down a rough idea of what you intend to eat each lunchtime. Tie your lunch plan in with dishes that you will make for your evening meals so that you can cook extra quantities to take into work the following day. Here are some ideas to inspire you.

Meal options

Roast cod with pesto, steamed cauliflower and French beans
Lay the fish on a lightly oiled baking tray, spread a tablespoon of fresh pesto over the fish, season with freshly ground black pepper and roast in a medium-hot oven for ten minutes or so. See page 122 if you would like a recipe to make your own pesto.

Fresh soup with rye or soda bread
Make your own soup using lentils or beans and vegetables, or refer to the recipes on pages 76–77 and 246–247. Pea and ham or chicken and vegetable soup make a well-balanced protein and carbohydrate meal in a bowl.

One grilled turkey breast, tuna fillet or a hard-boiled egg
Serve with a salad that contains five different vegetables and salad leaves.

Chick-peas and sliced red pepper
Add pine nuts, a green salad and a salad dressing.

Salade niçoise
Include your choice of tuna, black olives and green beans.

Chicken Caesar salad
Mix pieces of cold, grilled chicken breast with a large green salad and a dressing.

Goats' cheese salad
Add the cheese to a large mixed salad with a dressing.

Smoked mackerel fillet
Serve cold with a large green salad and half a sliced avocado.

Mixed lettuce salad
Add sliced turkey, fresh asparagus and feta cheese.

Poached or hard-boiled egg
Serve with a mixed bean and rice salad and sliced tomatoes.

Sardines, either fresh or tinned
Serve on rye toast with chopped dill.

One poached chicken breast
Serve with a mixed salad, roast vegetables or tabouleh.

One small baked potato
Add a portion of tinned or fresh tuna fish, salmon, sardines, chicken or baked beans to provide the protein, and serve with a large mixed salad.

Sandwich selections

Choose **one** of the following breads:

Gluten-free
Wholemeal
Granary
Rye

Fill the sandwich with your choice of these proteins and some salad. Use minimal quantities of butter, mayonnaise and cream cheese:

Cheese – any type, although cottage cheese is the best choice. Avoid blue and aged cheeses.

Egg – use chopped fresh herbs as a flavouring instead of salt.

Chicken or turkey slices – use skinless poultry. If you buy pre-sliced products from the shops, ensure that they are sugar-free.

Smoked salmon – add a squeeze of fresh lemon juice for added taste.

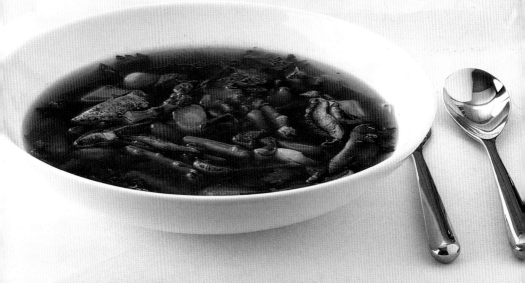

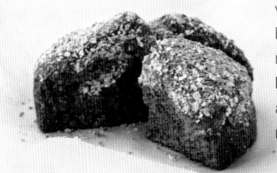

Soups made from vegetables, lentils or beans and chicken make a **well-balanced** protein and carbohydrate **meal in a bowl**

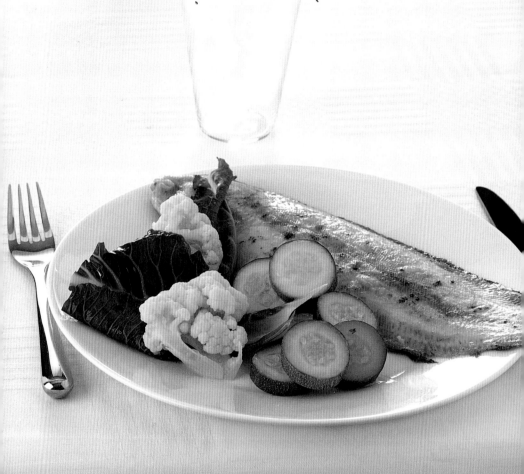

Choosing to **eat later** on in the evening, perhaps just a couple of hours before you go to bed, means that you should **omit starchy carbohydrates** and **increase** the complex carbohydrates from **vegetables** instead

Dinner

In the modern world, dinner has become the main meal of the day. It's the one meal we don't have to rush and is usually eaten in the company of family or friends. This all means we have come to expect more from our evening meal than just eating to keep our energy levels even.

Breakfast and lunch are usually functional meals, but dinner is almost an event by comparison, especially if you eat together as a family or with friends. It is at this time that your good intentions to eat sensibly may falter or be forgotten entirely.

If your last snack was at 4pm, you should aim to eat dinner at 7–7.30pm. Try not to eat any later, but if you do then still eat a snack at this time – a few nuts and an apple or a raw carrot and houmous should be enough.

Many dieters will be familiar with the theory that carbohydrates, especially those containing grains, should be limited in the evenings.

It isn't necessary to avoid carbohydrates on The Food Doctor plan as long as you eat relatively early. However, if you choose to eat later on in the evening – perhaps just a couple of hours before you go to bed – omit the starchy complex carbohydrates and increase the amount of complex vegetable carbohydrates instead. This means that you include just protein and vegetables at dinner.

If you have an evening meal with family or friends and you can't adhere closely to The Food Doctor plan, go ahead and eat, but avoid starchy carbohydrates containing saturated fats. For example, if your meal consists of steak, fries and salad, omit the fries and eat a large portion of salad and raw vegetables with your steak instead. This will make the meal healthier than it was, even though the steak contains saturated fat.

Plan ahead
Whatever you prepare, consider making a little extra for the next day. Cooking an extra chicken breast or another portion of fish at the same time will make your next meal or snack that much easier to prepare.

THE FOOD DOCTOR DINNER EQUATION

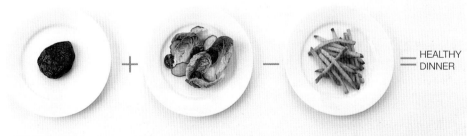

COMPLETE PROTEIN
such as steak, chicken or fish

COMPLEX VEGETABLE CARBOHYDRATES
such as salad and raw vegetables

COMPLEX STARCHY CARBOHYDRATES
such as French fries containing saturated fat

HEALTHY DINNER

Delicious dinners ...

Applying The Food Doctor principles to a main meal is simple: just remember the ratios *(see pp. 14–21)* and you can't go wrong.

The usual choice

Grilled lamb chop with roasted vegetables This is a delicious way to eat vegetables, especially with some herbs, such as rosemary. The ratio of protein to carbohydrate is also fine, but the choice of meat could be better.

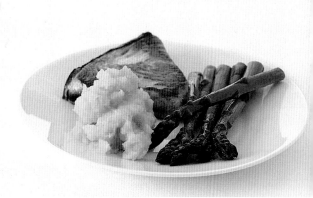

Seared tuna with mashed potato and steamed asparagus These foods are all healthy, nutritious and good Food Doctor choices. Mashed potato is a traditional comforting favourite and, if this meal were to be eaten at lunch-time, it would be fine. However there is a rule regarding eating starchy carbohydrates; don't do it after 7pm.

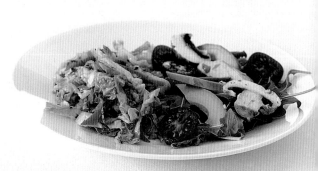

Vegetable stir-fry with avocado and watercress salad Stir-fries and salads are great ways of eating different varieties of vegetables with all their nutrients still intact. They are also quick options. However, there is something missing that stops this from being a healthy and complete meal.

can be diet-friendly too

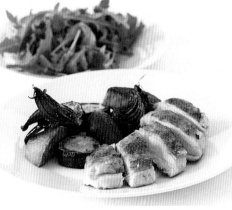

The Food Doctor choice

Although grilling is a healthy option, a lamb chop is a relatively fatty meat cut. Red meat contains a higher amount of saturated fats than white meat.

- A grilled chicken breast has a much lower saturated fat content than lamb. Chicken is versatile and can easily be spiced up too.

- There is a great range of fish available and many have the added bonus of being rich in essential fats. Try red or grey mullet, sardines or swordfish, either grilled or baked.

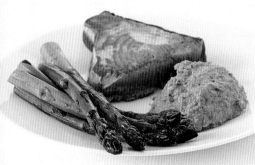

To make this the perfect evening meal, substitute pea and ginger mash *(see p.243)* for the starchy mashed potato.

- Try some of the other delicious mashes *(see pp.242–243)*. They all contain some protein too, so remember that when gauging portion sizes and ensure you have enough complex carbohydrate.

- Instead of the pea mash you could try some steamed green vegetables or a vegetable side-dish. As long as the protein: complex carbohydrate ratio is right, feel free to experiment.

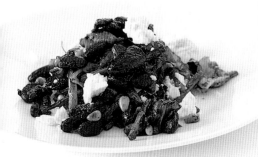

The missing element from the dinner on the left was protein. Without it you won't be receiving the slow-release glucose it contains and you may find yourself hungry again before bed-time.

- This feta, tomato and bean stir-fry is a delicious alternative. The feta, pine-nuts, and kidney beans together provide the requisite protein.

- Try a salad with a protein element, such as avocado and quinoa or root vegetable and goat's cheese.

Dinner suggestions

If you have time in the evenings and you enjoy preparing and cooking food, be as creative as you can with the meals that you eat. If time is short, however, or if your energy levels are low, then reach for store-cupboard ingredients or heat up some homemade soup from the freezer.

There are no prizes for guessing that, just like breakfast and lunch, dinner should combine protein and complex carbohydrates. If you eat your dinner later in the evening, remember to omit the starchy complex carbohydrates as you won't use the energy they provide.

First, select your protein. Choose from any one of the proteins listed on pages 18–19. These include cod, halibut, chicken, turkey or eggs.

Then choose your vegetables. It's all too easy to keep eating the same vegetables, so try to vary your selections (see pages 20–21).

Rather than flavour your food with salt, I suggest that you use herbs and spices to enhance the taste of your meal and make it more interesting (see below).

Meal suggestions

Gingery roast vegetables
Select vegetables such as squash or pumpkin, Florence fennel, onions, tomatoes and courgettes, cut into chunky cubes and put in a shallow dish. Drizzle with olive oil and add a teaspoon of grated ginger. Roast in a medium-hot oven for 45 minutes and then serve with crumbled feta cheese, goats' cheese or slices of mozzarella scattered over the top.

Mixed vegetable soup
Using the tomato and rosemary soup recipe on page 51 as a base, add pieces of raw chicken, fish, or a can of kidney beans or black-eyed beans when you pour in the stock. If you make fish or bean soup, prepare a larger batch and freeze extra portions.

Grilled Dover sole
Serve with green beans, steamed cauliflower and hollandaise sauce.

Whole roast trout
Place the cleaned fish in a shallow baking tray, season with freshly ground black pepper, add a knob of butter and scatter over flaked almonds. Cook in a medium-hot oven for 15 minutes or until the flesh is flaky. Serve with sautéed mushrooms and Florence fennel.

Spicy chicken
Mix a teaspoon each of ground coriander, cumin seeds, crushed garlic and water into a paste. Stuff the inside of a whole chicken with the spicy mixture. Drizzle over a little olive oil, season with freshly ground black pepper and roast the chicken in a medium-hot oven for one hour. Keep a portion of chicken aside for a cold meal the next day and serve the rest with grilled vegetables.

Mixed fish stew
See page 323 for a recipe. Serve with lightly steamed vegetables.

Baked mustard mackerel
Mix a tablespoon of sugar-free grain mustard with fresh lemon juice and spread it over the fish. Bake in a medium-hot oven for ten minutes or so. Serve with a green salad and fresh tomato relish.

Quick options
Stir-fried tofu
Add freshly grated ginger, chillies and red and yellow peppers.

HERBS & SPICES
Food can taste very different depending on which flavourings you use. Try every herb you can, either fresh or dried, and select those you like best. Spices can also make a meal more interesting. Try not to overdo fermented sauces such as vinegar and soy sauce (which is also highly salted), and instead try a little teriyaki sauce.

General – mint, marjoram, anise, cinnamon, caraway, rosemary, thyme, basil, sage, bay, nutmeg, sorrel, parsley.

Asian – lemon grass, chillies, coriander (seeds or leaves), garlic, lemon, pepper, ginger, sweet basil.

Indian – curry powder or paste, five-spice paste, garam masala, cumin seeds, cardamom pods, ginger, garlic.

Stir-fried mixed vegetables with chicken or prawns

Stir-fry the prawns or pieces of raw chicken first, then add chopped carrots, courgettes, asparagus, baby corn and herbs of your choice.

Roast asparagus

Place the asparagus in a baking dish, drizzle with olive oil and season with freshly ground black pepper. Cook for 10–15 minutes, then crumble feta cheese over the top and serve.

Chick-pea and tomato stew

Use ingredients from your store cupboard for this recipe. Warm a can each of chick-peas and tomatoes in a medium-sized saucepan over a low heat and add chopped fresh or dried basil and parsley. Scatter pumpkin seeds over the top and serve with a selection of grilled vegetables.

Egg salad

Cut two hard-boiled eggs into quarters and serve with cherry tomatoes and a large green salad.

Greek salad

Combine fresh tomatoes, feta cheese and black olives and serve with a large green salad.

Stir-fried squid

Stir-fry the chopped squid quickly in sunflower oil. Add chopped spring onions and pak choi and squeeze over fresh lemon juice just before serving.

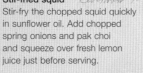

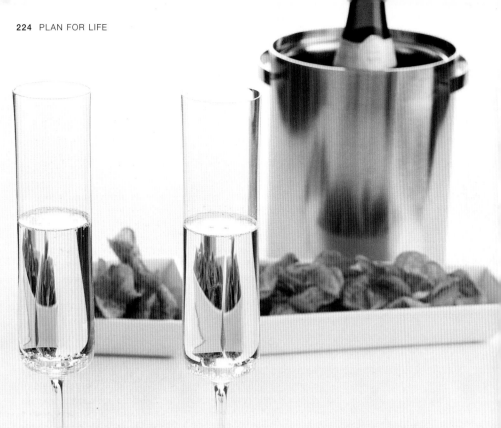

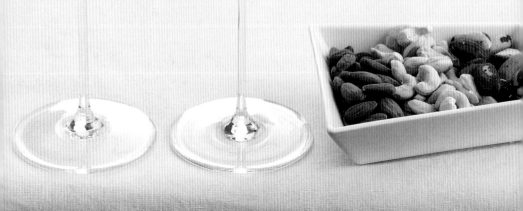

Don't worry too much about the occasional feast on **party food**, but try to eat something before you go so that you aren't overly **hungry** when you arrive

Special situations

Life isn't always predictable and, even when you know what your day is likely to hold, there will always be occasions when you will have to adapt The Food Doctor plan to work for you. Here are a few tips on how to cope with special situations and unexpected food choices.

Eating out

As long as you fully understand the principle of combining proteins with carbohydrates (*see pp. 14–21*), then eating out will be a lot easier than you may think.

The foods to avoid are those that are almost all pure carbohydrates, such as pizza, pasta, risotto, rice or noodles. For example, in a Chinese restaurant you could choose to order vegetables, fish and a little steamed rice rather than noodles and fried rice. This selection will help you to maintain a beneficial ratio of protein and complex carbohydrates.

Before you go out, it's a good idea to eat a small snack, even if it's just half a hard-boiled egg, to keep your glucose levels up so that when you come to order you aren't hungry enough to make poor food choices.

Finally, do be aware that restaurants use significantly more fat in dishes than you would use at home when making a similar dish.

Evening drinks

Going out for a drink straight after work can easily result in excessive alcohol intake, followed by a fatty, carbohydrate-loaded takeaway meal later in the evening. There is no reason why you shouldn't do this from time to time, but if it's become

a regular occurrence then evenings such as these could be responsible for some of the increased weight that you want to lose.

The best way to minimize the damage is, as always, to eat a snack before you go out. Look at the suggested snacks on pages 210–211 for some ideas, but if you don't have time for a small snack then eat a few raw, unsalted nuts or olives with your drink and avoid all other bar snacks.

Parties

Party foods like savoury crackers and crisps are mostly simple carbohydrates, so they will soon leave you feeling hungry for more. But parties are to be enjoyed, so don't worry too much about the occasional party feast. Have a snack, such as a piece of rye bread with cheese, beforehand so that you aren't too hungry when you arrive. Eating this sort of snack also helps to reduce the rate at which your body absorbs alcohol – because once you have had too much to drink, who cares about losing weight?

On the move

If you are away from home all day and on the move, I suggest that you eat a substantial breakfast and have

a packet of raw, unsalted nuts or seeds in your bag or briefcase to eat as your mid-morning snack. When it comes to lunch, have a sandwich by all means but buy one with added filling or discard half the bread to make one generously filled sandwich, so that the ratio of carbohydrates (in this case, bread) to protein (a filling such as meat or fish) is favourable.

Obviously it isn't always going to be easy, so the success of The Food Doctor plan depends on your ability to plan ahead a little. Make provisions for yourself so that you don't get caught in a situation where you have no choice but to eat the wrong foods. If this does happen – and of course it will sometimes – then just get back into line with the plan when you have your next meal.

Travelling

Whether you travel on a long aeroplane flight or take a short train ride, you may find it harder to eat food that fits easily into The Food Doctor plan. So, once again, try to plan ahead a little if you can.

If you are travelling by train, eat something before you leave the house. If the journey is a long one, you will probably need to take some food with you. A pot of houmous and some crudités in a sealed plastic container will make a convenient snack, while a wholemeal or rye bread sandwich generously filled with protein (such as tuna or egg) makes an easy meal.

A plane journey can prove more problematic. This may be one of those situations when you will have to accept that you just can't stick to your chosen food plan. If you are on a short flight, then you should be able to find something healthy to eat at the airport before you fly. If you are on a long flight, you may find that you are in luck and the main meal includes a lean protein. If not, don't worry about it, go ahead and eat what you are given and revert to the Plan for Life principles after you land. You can always take along a few apples and a packet of raw nuts such as cashews or almonds so that you can at least have a protein and carbohydrate snack as usual.

Holidays

Many people try to lose weight before they go on a beach holiday, only to put it all back on again while they are away. I am sure that most of us have heard people say to each other, "Go on, you're on holiday", and indulge in foods that won't do anyone any favours. Since The Food Doctor plan is a way of life, you shouldn't find yourself in this predicament. Many of my clients choose to follow the Seven-day Diet (see pp.42–65) before their holiday to ensure that they feel their best, and then eat sensibly while they are away.

If you are staying in a hotel that includes a continental breakfast as part of the room rate, you may have to invest in an extra breakfast dish

to make sure you eat enough protein. Continental breakfasts consist purely of refined carbohydrates, and if you are intending to spend a lazy day on the beach you won't utilize the extra glucose generated by eating this kind of food. Instead, order eggs or cheese and a piece of bread or toast. This choice is far more likely to help you maintain your preferred weight during the holiday.

When it comes to lunchtime, limit your alcohol intake and ensure that you include some fish, meat or poultry in your meal. The same is true for dinner.

As it's likely that you will be eating your evening meals later than you would at home, it's a good idea to have some fruit – preferably hard fruits such as apples – available to keep you going. Keep a supply of raw, unsalted nuts too, but don't eat a whole packet at once.

You might also want to take some healthy snacks on long car journeys for yourself and any children travelling with you. A couple of plastic containers filled with a few slices of raw vegetables, grapes, cherry tomatoes and pieces of hard cheese should help them – and you – avoid the last-minute lure of fast food and all the unnecessary fats and sugars that these meals contain.

Eating with kids

Many clients tell me that they gain weight because they either pick at their children's food or eat with them at their favourite fast-food restaurants. It's all too easy to forget about fuelling up yourself while you worry about the kids

and then suddenly feel hungry as they start to eat. As with all situations, it's best to plan ahead a little. If you pick the children up from school, eat a snack at home first, even if it's just a couple of mouthfuls or leftovers from your lunch. This will help you to resist the fatty, sugary foods that children seem to love. Alternatively, if you want to eat with the children, find something healthy that you can all eat: instead of burgers and fries, choose lean proteins, such as tuna or chicken, and some vegetables.

How do I cope with eating family meals?

If you have a family, think through your collective favourite foods, the sorts of dishes you make or buy that always go down well. Bearing in mind the principles of the Plan for Life, do such meals still fit in? Your family can continue to eat what they want, but you shouldn't forgo all of the foods that you have previously prepared to family acclaim.

Eating different meals to those of your family can sometimes create real problems, so the answer lies in which foods you leave out rather than what you replace them with. For example, if the family meal is pasta with a tomato sauce and vegetables, make sure that you have just a small spoonful of pasta and a much larger portion of vegetables. If you cook a roast chicken with all the trimmings, avoid the bread sauce and roast potatoes and enjoy the chicken and vegetables instead. You may have to make certain sacrifices, but your meals needn't be dull or unsatisfying.

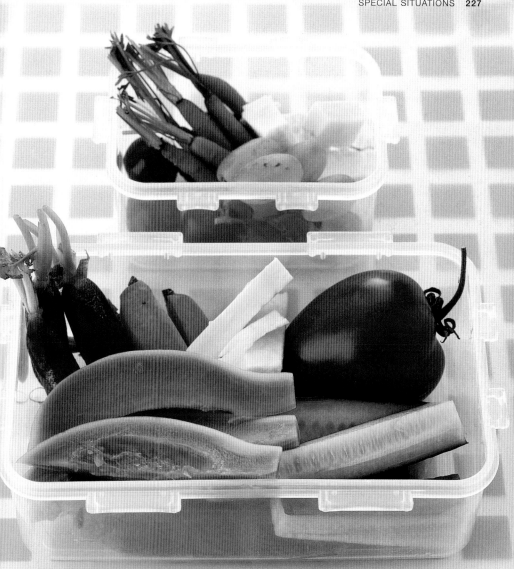

Take some **healthy snacks** in the **car** for yourself and
your children when you **travel** to avoid the lure of fast food

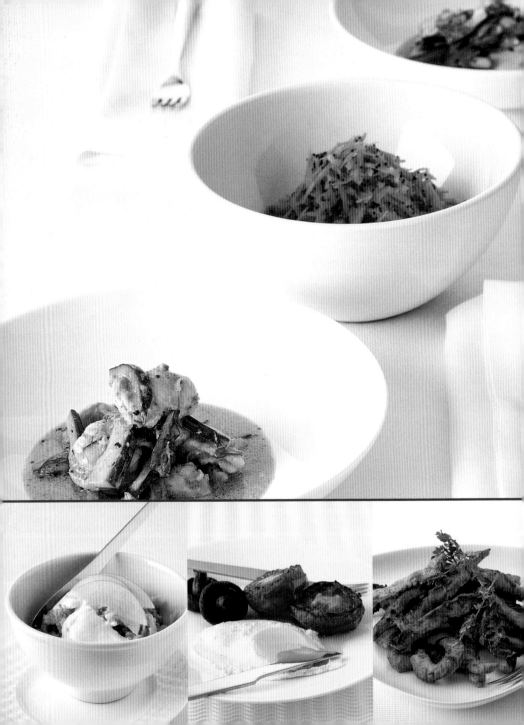

Recipes

Some of the recipes in this section are very basic and can be made in just a few minutes, while others need a little more preparation and cooking time. This will hopefully give you enough choice to suit your cooking skills and level of interest, and inspire you to try some new and original ideas. Remember that shopping for and cooking with the freshest, healthiest ingredients you can find are crucial to the success of The Food Doctor principles. For those of you who are still reluctant to cook for yourself, try the simplest of recipes to begin with.

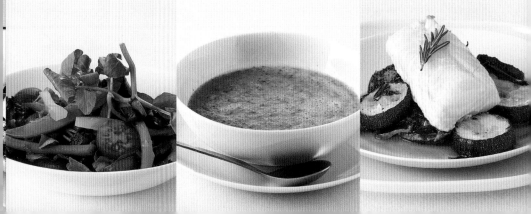

Blueberry cheese ⓥ

Fromage frais is a good choice for breakfast because it has a higher proportion of protein to carbohydrate than yoghurt. Mix with blueberries and seeds for an instant, delicious meal. Serves two.

ready in **1** minute

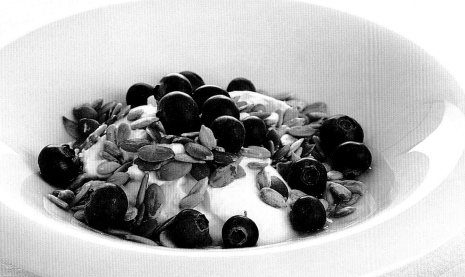

6 tablespoons reduced fat fromage frais

6 tablespoons mixed seeds (pumpkin, sesame, sunflower, hemp, ground linseeds – choose at least two)

4 tablespoons blueberries

Divide the fromage frais between two bowls. Top each serving with 3 tablespoons of seeds and 2 tablespoons of blueberries and serve.

Note: there are various mixes of seeds available, including The Food Doctor range.

Ham and cheese corn fritters

When you need something substantial on a cold morning, this tasty, protein-rich dish is excellent. You can experiment with other toppings, such as scrambled egg, or smoked salmon. Serves two.

ready in **10** minutes

2 corn fritters *(see p.237)*
2 tablespoons reduced-fat fromage frais
2 extra thin slices good-quality smoked ham, cut in strips
2 medium tomatoes, chopped
A few toasted sesame seeds

Spread the warm fritter with the fromage frais. Top with the ham, tomato and the toasted seeds and serve.

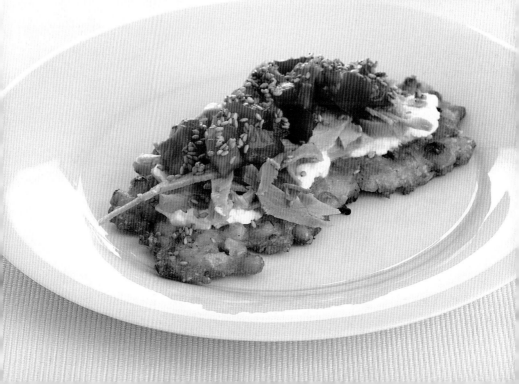

Easy egg breakfasts

Eggs are packed with vitamins, folate and calcium, are high in protein and have minimal saturated fat, so they are an ideal start to your day. In fact, these recipes are so versatile and tasty that you can have them as a light lunch or for supper as well. All recipes serve two.

Keep some **fresh eggs** in the **fridge**, as they are an **excellent** source of **protein**

Poached egg on asparagus and mushrooms

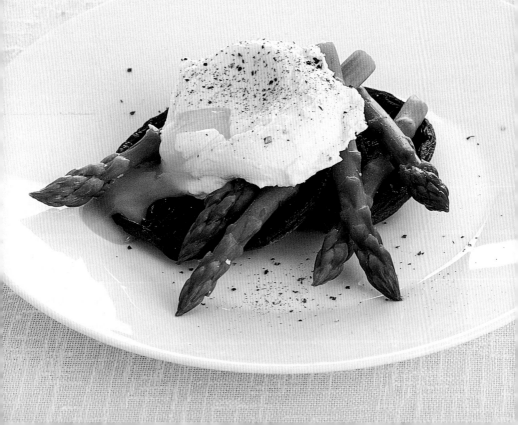

Poached egg on asparagus & mushrooms ⓥ

ready in **15** minutes

50g (2oz) medium-sized brown mushrooms
100g (3½oz) asparagus tips
A drizzle of olive oil
1 tablespoon cider vinegar
2 eggs
Freshly ground black pepper

Preheat the oven to 180°C/350°F/ Gas mark 4.

Slice the mushrooms diagonally to make large flat slices. Place them on a baking tray and drizzle a tiny amount of olive oil over each slice so that they are lightly coated. Bake in the oven for 10 minutes.

Put the asparagus into a small saucepan, pour boiling water on top and simmer for about a minute or so until the tips are *al dente*. Drain.

Heat a large pan of water and add the vinegar. Once the water is simmering, crack the eggs into the water or into poaching rings and cook until the egg whites are set. Remove with a slotted spoon.

Arrange the mushrooms on a plate, layer the asparagus over them and top with the poached egg. Season with black pepper and serve with wholemeal toast or corn fritters *(see right)* if needed.

Eggy bread with seeds ⓥ

ready in **10** minutes

2 eggs
2 tablespoons The Food Doctor Original Seed Mix, coarsely ground, or grind 2 tablespoons mixed pumpkin, sunflower, linseeds and sesame seeds
Freshly ground black pepper
A drizzle of olive oil
2 thick slices of wholemeal, rye or gluten-free bread
2 medium tomatoes

Lightly beat the eggs, seeds and black pepper together and pour the mixture onto a deep dinner plate. Soak the bread well in the egg mix.

Lightly oil a non-stick frying pan and, once the pan is hot, lift the egg-soaked bread and place in the pan to gently brown on both sides. If there is any egg mix left on the plate, pour it on top of the bread while the first side is browning.

If you have time, roast the tomatoes otherwise chop them coarsely, pile them on top of the eggy bread and serve.

Poached egg on a corn fritter ⓥ

ready in **15** minutes

2 eggs
1 tablespoon cider vinegar

For the corn fritters (makes 4):
100g (3½oz) maize flour
1 fresh egg
1 tablespoon olive oil
75ml (3fl oz) milk or water
70g (2½oz) canned sweetcorn (without added sugar), drained and rinsed
½ teaspoon ground caraway seeds or ground fennel seeds
Freshly ground black pepper

To prepare the corn fritters, put the flour in a bowl and make a well in the middle. Break the egg into the well and pour in the olive oil. Beating continually, add the milk gradually to give a smooth, thick batter. Stir in the sweetcorn and spices and season with black pepper.

Brush a non-stick frying pan with a little olive oil and pour in a quarter of the mixture. The batter should be thick enough not to run when poured. Brown one side over a medium heat, flip over and brown the other. Once cooked, keep warm.

Poach the eggs *(see left)* and serve on the fritters.

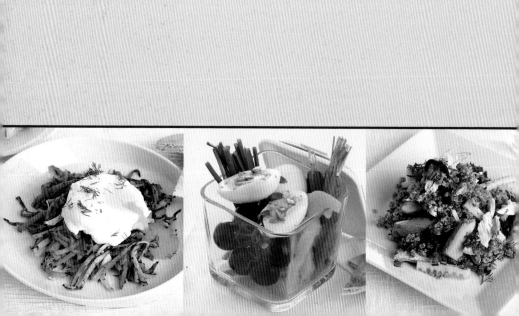

Food fast

When time is short, these recipes demonstrate just how simple
it is to apply my principles and cook delicious, healthy meals quickly.

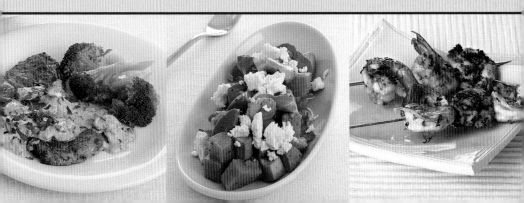

Simple smoothies

For breakfasts and snacks on the go, nothing beats an energy-boosting smoothie. This eclectic range of smoothie recipes caters to all tastes. From the sweet Tropical carrot smoothie to the tangy High-energy smoothie, all these drinks are vitamin-packed and filling. Serves two.

Carrot & caraway smoothie ⓥ

`ready in 3 minutes`

2 tablespoons The Food Doctor Fennel and Caraway Seed mix, or use ½ teaspoon each fennel and caraway seeds and 2 tablespoons mixed pumpkin and sunflower seeds

150ml (¼ pint) natural low-fat yoghurt

150ml (¼ pint) carrot juice

½ avocado

Juice 1 lemon

Juice 1 orange

Grind the seed mix in a seed or coffee grinder.

Put all the ingredients into a blender and whizz together for a few seconds before serving.

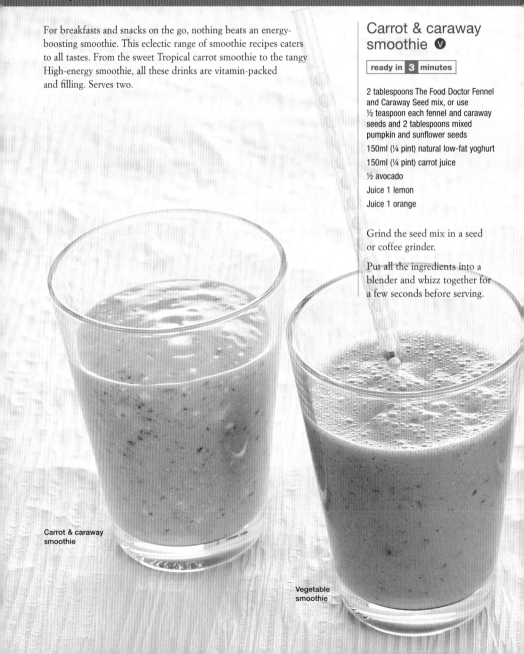

Carrot & caraway
smoothie

Vegetable
smoothie

Vegetable smoothie Ⓥ

ready in **2** minutes

150g (5oz) cucumber
1 medium tomato
50g (2oz) red pepper
100ml (3½fl oz) carrot juice
75ml (3fl oz) apple juice
Juice 1 lemon
3 tablespoons live natural
low-fat yoghurt

Whizz the vegetables with the carrot and fruit juices in a blender for a few seconds. Do not sieve as this will remove valuable fibre. Stir in the yoghurt and serve.

Tropical carrot smoothie Ⓥ

ready in **3** minutes

150ml (¼ pint) live natural
low-fat yoghurt
150ml (¼ pint) carrot juice
1 good, peeled chunk each mango
and papaya
Seeds and flesh 1 passion fruit, scooped
out of the skin (avoid the pith)
1 small cube fresh ginger, grated
25g (¾oz) raw unsalted cashew nuts

Combine all the ingredients in a blender and whizz together until smooth. Add more carrot juice if the mixture is too thick, and serve.

High-energy smoothie Ⓥ

ready in **10** minutes

½ avocado, stoned and peeled
150ml (¼ pint) live natural
low-fat yoghurt
100ml (3½fl oz) good-quality apple juice
100ml (3½fl oz) water
A small handful watercress leaves
2–3 springs fresh mint
Juice ½ lemon
A few drops Tabasco

Put all the ingredients, except the Tabasco, in a blender and whizz together until smooth. Add a dash of Tabasco to taste and serve.

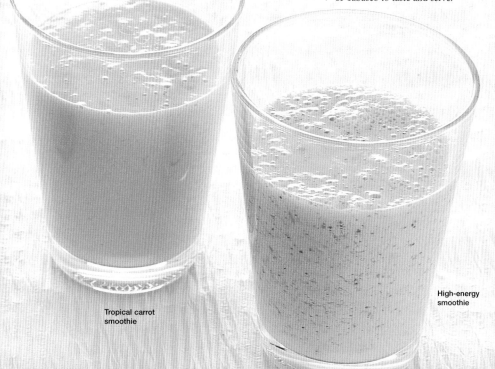

High-energy
smoothie

Tropical carrot
smoothie

The Food Doctor bagel toppings

These savoury toppings taste delicious on The Food Doctor High Bran and Seed Bagels, or on oatcakes or rye bread. Keep them in plastic containers in the fridge. You can also use these toppings as a side dish with grilled meat or fish. Each recipe makes enough for two bagels.

Feta cheese & roast pepper mash ⓥ

ready in **5** minutes

50g (2oz) roast pepper slices (from a jar)
50g (2oz) feta cheese
Freshly ground black pepper
A few sprigs fresh parsley, chopped

Chop the peppers finely. Combine all the ingredients in a bowl and mash them roughly with a fork. Keeps in the fridge for two days.

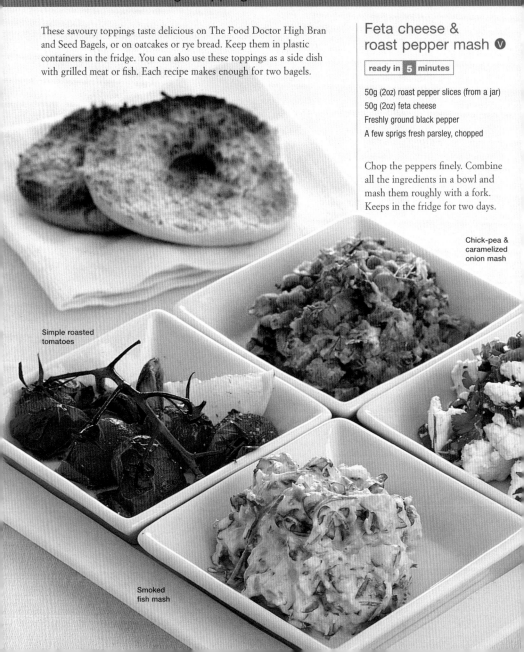

Chick-pea & caramelized onion mash

Simple roasted tomatoes

Smoked fish mash

Smoked fish mash

ready in **5** minutes

50g (2oz) hot smoked fish
(supermarkets often sell cheap off-cuts
of mackerel, trout and salmon, etc.)
2 tablespoons reduced-fat fromage frais
A good handful watercress, chopped
1 tablespoon fresh dill, chopped
Juice ½ lemon
Freshly ground black pepper

Mash all the ingredients together
using a fork and season with a
generous grinding of black pepper.
You can also use this mash like a
dip and scoop it out of a bowl with
oatcakes or rye crackers. Will keep
fresh for 24 hours in the fridge.

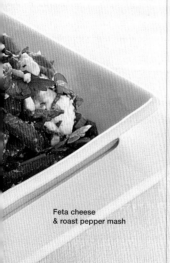

Feta cheese
& roast pepper mash

Chick-pea & caramelized onion mash ⓥ

ready in **20** minutes

1x400g (13oz) can organic chick-peas
1 garlic clove
2 sprigs fresh sage
A pinch bouillon powder
(or ¼ stock cube)
1 medium onion, finely sliced
3 tablespoons olive oil
1 teaspoon ground caraway seeds
1 tablespoon live natural low-fat yoghurt
2 tablespoons lemon juice
2 tablespoons fresh dill, chopped
Crumbled feta cheese as a garnish

Drain and rinse the chick-peas. Put
them in a saucepan with the garlic,
sage and bouillon powder, pour in
just enough water to cover the
chick-peas and bring to the boil.
Simmer gently for 15 minutes.

Meanwhile, heat a tablespoon of
olive oil in a saucepan, add the
onion and cook gently until soft.
Raise the heat to brown the onions
a little. Stir in the ground caraway
over a low heat, adding a little
more oil if it all binds too thickly.

Drain the chick-peas and remove
the herbs and garlic. Mash the
chick-peas with a fork or potato
masher, adding the olive oil and
yoghurt to soften the consistency.
Stir in the onions, lemon juice and
fresh dill. Pile onto two bagels with
a little feta cheese crumbled on top.

Pea, ginger and tapenade mash

ready in **15** minutes

5 teaspoons green tapenade
150g (5oz) frozen peas, thawed
1cm (½in) piece fresh root ginger,
peeled and finely grated
2 tablespoons olive oil
Juice of ½ orange
Grated zest of ½ orange and ½ lemon
2 spring onions, finely chopped
1 garlic clove, finely chopped
60g (2oz) tofu (silken, preferably)
Juice of ½ lemon
Freshly ground black pepper
Live natural yoghurt (optional)
1 tablespoon chopped fresh mint

Make the tapenade by combining
150g (5oz) chopped green olives,
6–7 anchovy fillets and a scant
tablespoon of capers. Add olive
oil and lemon juice to taste.

Put the peas, ginger, olive oil,
orange juice, zests, spring onions
and garlic in a heavy-based pan.
Bring to the boil, reduce the heat
and simmer gently for 10 minutes,
until the peas are well cooked.

Pour the mixture into a blender,
add the tofu and blend to make
a slightly rough mash. Alternatively,
mash together in the pan. Turn the
mash into a bowl and stir in the
tapenade, lemon juice and pepper
to taste. If it seems too thick, stir
in a little more oil and/or some
yoghurt. Finally, stir in the mint.

Lunch boxes

These salads are designed to be made the previous night or the morning before you go to work so that you can just reach for a nutritious meal at lunchtime. All recipes serve two, so you should be able to save yourself time by making enough lunch for two consecutive days.

Lentil & sprouted seed salad ⓥ

ready in **15** minutes

100g (3½oz) dried red lentils, or 4 tablespoons canned lentils, rinsed and drained

200ml (7fl oz) vegetable stock *(see p.296)*

1 avocado, peeled and sliced

Fresh lemon juice to taste

100g (3½oz) sprouted seeds, rinsed and drained

100g (3½oz) cucumber, cut into thick matchstick pieces

½ red pepper, sliced

French dressing to taste

2–3 tablespoons fresh herbs, chopped

If you have time, put the dried lentils in a saucepan, add the stock and simmer for 5–10 minutes until soft but not collapsed. Rinse and drain. Otherwise, spoon the canned lentils into a bowl.

If you make this salad the night before, leave slicing the avocado and sprinkling it with lemon juice until the morning.

Add the sprouts, cucumber and red pepper to the lentils. Add French dressing to taste and toss well. Fold in the avocado and fresh herbs of your choice and pack the contents into a lunch box. For a change, add some hot smoked fish too.

Tomato, bulgar wheat & spinach salad ⓥ

ready in **15** minutes

100g (3½oz) bulgar wheat, plus boiling vegetable stock to cover

2 tablespoons olive oil

1 garlic clove, finely chopped

100g (3½oz) baby spinach leaves, washed

Grated fresh nutmeg to taste

Juice 1 lemon

Freshly ground black pepper

12 baby tomatoes, halved

12 pitted black olives

100g (3½oz) feta cheese, cubed

Pour boiling stock over the bulgar wheat until it is just covered. Leave to stand for 10 minutes, then strain and squeeze it through a fine sieve.

Heat the oil in a frying pan and add the garlic. Soften over a low heat for 2 minutes. Add the spinach and stir over a medium heat until the spinach is wilted. Grate a little nutmeg over the spinach.

Combine the bulgar wheat and spinach with its oil in a bowl. Toss well, add the lemon juice and season with black pepper. Gently fold in the tomatoes, olives and feta cheese.

Put into a lunch box and go. The flavours improve if left for a couple of hours or more before eating.

Bean & feta salad ⓥ

ready in **5** minutes

1x400g (13oz) can mixed beans, rinsed and drained

½ cucumber, coarsely chopped with the skin left on

2 medium tomatoes, each cut into six pieces

French dressing to taste

Freshly ground black pepper

100g (3½oz) feta cheese, cubed

2–3 tablespoons fresh mixed herbs of your choice, chopped (parsley, mint, chives, coriander or basil, depending on what is available)

1 flat bread *(see p.298)*, 2 oatcakes or 1 piece rye bread per person

Mix the beans, raw vegetables, French dressing and black pepper together in a bowl. Fold in the feta cheese and chopped herbs.

Put the contents into a lunch box and eat with the rye bread, oatcakes or flat bread if you have some stored in the fridge or freezer.

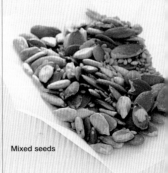

Mixed seeds

High-energy salad Ⓥ

`ready in 10 minutes`

4 eggs

2 medium tomatoes, quartered

4 closed white mushrooms, sliced

1 yellow pepper, cut into strips

2 raw baby carrots, washed

75g (2½oz) raw, bite-sized broccoli florets

75g (2½oz) raw, bite-sized cauliflower florets

4 tablespoons The Food Doctor Rosemary & Garlic Seed Mix, or use 4 tablespoons mixed pumpkin, sesame, sunflower and linseeds with ½ teaspoon garlic, chopped

1 flat bread *(see p.298)* or 1 corn fritter *(see p.233)* per person

Boil the eggs for 10 minutes until they are hard-boiled. cool them in cold water, then shell them and cut them in half.

Mix the other ingredients together, pack into a lunch box and place the eggs on top. Eat with the flat bread or corn fritter. Using the spiced Food Doctor seeds means that there is no need for dressing.

You can add any raw vegetables of your choice to change the mix, but keep the quantities high to give you enough energy.

Take a healthy **lunch box** to work so that you always make a **good food choice** at lunchtime

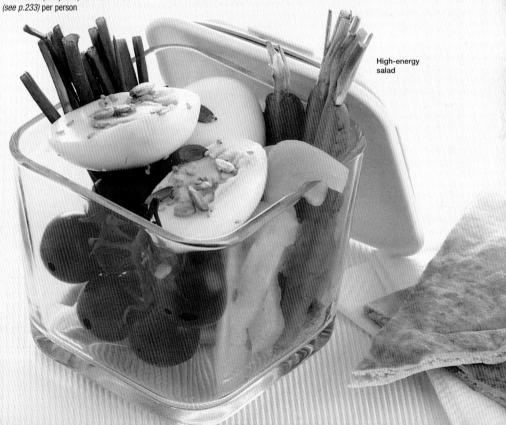

High-energy salad

Healthy soups

These soups, which range from a light, tasty broth to a hearty, filling soup, are low in fat and full of vitamins. Since they are all quick and easy to prepare, they are the perfect meal if you are pressed for time, or want something simple to eat. All recipes serve two.

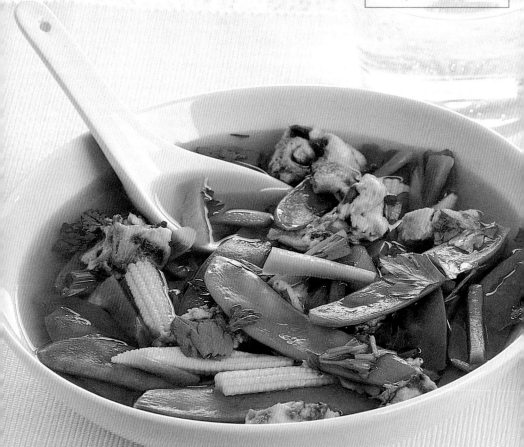

Japanese broth

Japanese broth

`ready in 15 minutes`

1.2 litres (2 pints) hot vegetable stock *(see p.296)*

100g (3½oz) carrots, cut into large matchstick pieces

100g (3½oz) baby sweetcorn, cut in half lengthways and across

100g (3½oz) mangetout

100g (3½oz) baby leeks (or spring onions), finely sliced

2cm (¾in) cube fresh ginger, finely grated

2 tablespoons rice wine

1 teaspoon soy sauce

1 teaspoon miso paste

Tabasco sauce to taste

A small handful fresh coriander, chopped

For the egg noodles:
2 eggs

2 tablespoons pumpkin seeds, coarsely ground

2 tablespoons water

Pour the hot stock into a saucepan, add the carrots and cook for 2 minutes. Add the corn, mangetout, leeks and grated ginger. Simmer for 10 minutes, then stir in the rice wine, soy sauce and miso paste.

To make the noodles, mix the eggs, seeds and water together and cook two thin, flat omelettes. Roll up each omelette and slice it across several times to make thin ribbons of egg.

Serve the hot soup in two bowls, topped with the egg ribbons and fresh coriander. Any leftover soup can be frozen for up to four weeks.

Pea & ginger soup

`ready in 15 minutes`

1 medium onion, finely chopped

¼ teaspoon cumin seeds

1 tablespoon olive oil

200g (7oz) frozen peas

1x400g (13oz) can butter beans, drained and rinsed

2cm (¾in) cube fresh ginger, finely grated

700ml (1¼ pints) chicken or vegetable stock *(see p.296)*

A small handful fresh coriander, chopped

A small handful fresh mint, chopped

Juice 1 lime

Freshly ground black pepper

2 tablespoons live natural low-fat yoghurt

3 spring onions, finely chopped

Heat the olive oil in a large saucepan, add the onion and cumin seeds and cook gently until the onion is soft but not coloured.

Add the peas, beans, ginger and stock, bring to the boil and lower the heat to a simmer. Add the fresh herbs and stir well. Simmer for about 5 minutes. Pour it all into a blender and zap until smooth.

Pour back into the saucepan and add the lime juice and black pepper.

Serve each portion with a swirl of yoghurt and the chopped spring onions sprinkled over the top.

You can also serve the soup chilled. Stir the yoghurt into the cold soup and garnish with the spring onions.

Salmon & sweet potato soup

`ready in 20 minutes`

2x150g (5oz) fillets salmon, skinned and cut into bite-sized pieces

Lemon juice to taste

Freshly ground black pepper

1 tablespoon olive oil

1 medium leek, trimmed and finely sliced

1 small bulb of Florence fennel, trimmed and finely sliced

200g (7oz) sweet potato, grated

75ml (3fl oz) dry white wine

600ml (1 pint) good fish stock (the better the stock, the better the soup)

2 tablespoons fresh dill, chopped (or 1 teaspoon dried dill)

2 tablespoons live natural low-fat yoghurt

Toss the salmon pieces in lemon juice and black pepper and set aside while you cook the vegetables.

Heat the oil in a wide-bottomed saucepan. Add the leek and fennel and soften for 5 minutes. Add the sweet potato, stir once and add the wine. Let it bubble for a couple of minutes, then stir in the stock and simmer for 15 minutes until the vegetables are cooked and the potatoes are collapsing into the liquid. Add the fish and chopped dill and simmer gently for 5 minutes until the fish is just cooked. Add seasoning to taste.

Ladle into two hot bowls and swirl the yoghurt into each serving.

Pestos for any meal

These are invaluable recipes, as they add flavour to any dish. Use a pesto as a sauce for grilled or baked fish, as a marinade or a dip, stir it into hot or cold quinoa for extra flavour or spread it over chicken breasts and cover with sliced tomatoes. All recipes serve two.

SERVING IDEAS

For lunch Serve the prawns with a few boiled new potatoes and a mixed leaf salad containing fresh coriander.

For dinner For a change, mash some feta cheese with your chosen pesto and spread the mixture on grilled chicken or fish as a topping.

Hemp seed & coriander pesto Ⓥ

`ready in` **2** `minutes`

2 tablespoons ground hemp seeds (buy coarsely ground seeds, or use a food blender or coffee/seed grinder)

3 tablespoons olive oil

A small handful fresh coriander (about five sprigs)

½ garlic clove

Freshly ground black pepper to taste

To make, see Hazelnut & dill pesto (*right*).

Walnut & basil pesto Ⓥ

`ready in` **2** `minutes`

30g (1oz) walnuts

A small handful basil (about 5 sprigs)

4 tablespoons olive oil

A drizzle walnut oil

Freshly ground black pepper to taste

To make, see Hazelnut & dill pesto (*right*).

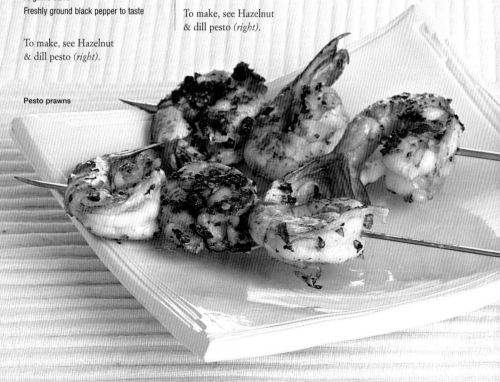

Pesto prawns

Pesto prawns

cook in **5** minutes

(marinade overnight)

8 large raw tiger prawns
3 tablespoons pesto of your choice

Put your chosen pesto in a shallow dish. Add the raw tiger prawns and coat them in the pesto. Leave to marinate for an hour or more.

Soak two wooden skewers in water and thread the tiger prawns onto the soaked skewers. Cook under a medium-hot grill for a couple of minutes on each side and serve.

The pesto prawns can also be left to cool once they have been cooked and eaten cold within 24 hours.

Hazelnut & dill pesto Ⓥ

ready in **2** minutes

30g (1oz) hazelnuts
A small handful fresh dill
(about 8 sprigs)
4 tablespoons olive oil
2 teaspoons lemon juice
Freshly ground black pepper to taste

The method for all pestos is very simple and the same for whichever mixture you choose.

Combine all the ingredients in a food processor and whizz together until you have a thick paste. Add more oil if the mixture is too stiff.

To make a smoother paste, zap the seeds (which are harder than the nuts) in a seed or coffee grinder for a few seconds before adding to the food processor.

Pesto dip Ⓥ

ready in **5** minutes

50ml (2fl oz) pesto of your choice
100ml (3½fl oz) reduced-fat fromage frais
Selection of raw vegetables such as carrots, peppers, broccoli and cauliflower

Mix your chosen pesto with the fromage frais and pour into a small bowl. Cut the fresh vegetables into thick fingers or chunks.

Use the pesto mix as a dipping sauce for the crudités.

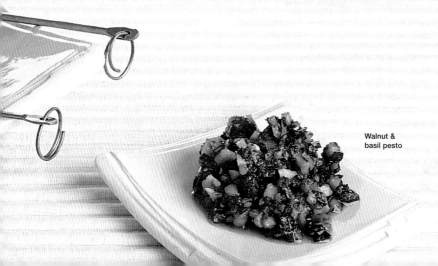

Walnut & basil pesto

Complete salads

These dishes are complete salads because they provide all the protein and complex carbohydrates you need for one meal; there's no need to prepare anything else to eat with them. Use ingredients that are as fresh as possible to give the best taste and flavour. All recipes serve two.

Sweet potato, feta & avocado salad **Ⓥ**

ready in 25 minutes

200g (7oz) sweet potato
1 tablespoon olive oil
1 tablespoon lemon juice
Freshly ground black pepper
1 bunch watercress
10 black olives, pitted
70g (2½oz) feta cheese
½ avocado, peeled

For the dressing:
2 tablespoons orange juice
2 tablespoons lemon juice
1 teaspoon soy sauce

Bake or boil the sweet potato in its skin until just cooked. Depending on its size and shape, this should take 15–20 minutes. Don't overcook the potato or you will end up with a mush. Peel while still warm and cut into 2.5cm (1in) cubes. Put in a bowl, toss with the oil and lemon juice, season with black pepper and leave to one side to cool.

Mix the dressing. Cut the stalks off the watercress, tear the top sprigs into two bowls and toss them in the dressing. Pile the sweet potato onto the leaves and add the olives. Chop the feta cheese and peeled avocado into the same sized chunks, pile on top of the sweet potato and serve.

You can also toast a couple of tablespoons of pinenuts and scatter them over each salad, or add a spoonful of a Food Doctor seed mix for added taste and crunch.

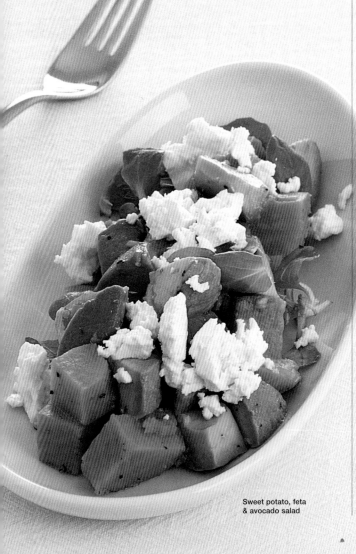

Sweet potato, feta
& avocado salad

Winter salad with cashews

ready in 10 minutes

75g (2½oz) peeled celeriac, coarsely grated

50g (2oz) raw unsalted cashew nuts

1 teaspoon caraway seeds

75g (2½oz) red cabbage, finely shredded

1 handful fresh parsley, coarsely chopped

1 tablespoon The Food Doctor Fennel and Caraway Seed Mix, or use ¼ teaspoon fennel seeds mixed with 1 tablespoon mixed pumpkin and sunflower seeds

For the dressing:
3 tablespoons live natural low-fat yoghurt

2 tablespoons lemon juice

1 garlic clove, crushed

Freshly ground black pepper

Put the celeriac in a bowl. Mix the dressing and add it to the bowl. Leave to one side.

Dry-roast the cashews in a dry frying pan and toss frequently to prevent burning. Repeat with the caraway seeds until they pop – it will take just a few seconds.

Combine the cashews and caraway seeds with the celeriac, mixing well. Gently stir in the red cabbage and the fresh parsley. Serve topped with the seed mix.

You can also serve the salad with grilled haloumi cheese on top.

Red rice salad ⓥ

50g (2oz) Camargue red rice

300ml (½ pint) weak stock

50g (2oz) yellow split peas or split mung beans

3 tablespoons The Food Doctor Rosemary & Garlic Seed Mix, or use 3 tablespoons mixed pumpkin, sesame, sunflower and linseeds with ½ teaspoon garlic, chopped

1 fat spring onion, finely sliced

½ large red pepper, chopped

½ courgette, cut into matchsticks

2 tablespoons fresh mixed herbs, chopped (parsley, coriander, mint, basil, rosemary, marjoram, etc.)

For the dressing:
50ml (2fl oz) olive oil

2 tablespoons lime juice

1 tablespoon soy sauce

Cook the rice in 150ml (¼ pint) stock for 25 minutes (it should be cooked but with a little bite). Drain off any liquid and put in a bowl.

Meanwhile, rinse the split peas and soak them in water for 10 minutes. Drain and simmer in the remaining stock for 10 minutes until they are soft but not collapsing. Tip into the bowl with the rice, add the dressing and allow to cool.

Once cold, add the rest of the ingredients. Mix well and serve.

For a change, use wild rice instead of red rice, but cook it until it explodes so that it is easy to eat. Or try stirring in a couple of tablespoons of sprouted seeds.

Chinese chicken salad

ready in 20 minutes

100g (3½oz) fine noodles (preferably buckwheat)

1 tablespoon sesame oil

150g (5oz) cold chicken meat, coarsely shredded

60g (2oz) beansprouts (either home-sprouted, or ready sprouted from a health food shop or supermarket)

2 spring onions, trimmed and finely sliced lengthways

½ red pepper, finely sliced

½ green pepper, finely sliced

1 tablespoon sesame seeds

For the dressing:
1 tablespoon soy sauce

2 tablespoons orange juice

1 tablespoon lemon juice

10cm (4in) cube fresh ginger, grated

1 teaspoon balsamic vinegar

1 tablespoon sesame oil

Mix all the ingredients for the dressing together in a jug or bowl.

Cook the noodles according to the instructions on the packet. Once cooked, drain, toss in the sesame oil and allow to cool.

While the noodles cook, prepare the rest of the ingredients and mix them together in a bowl. Pour over the dressing and allow to stand until the noodles are ready. Then toss in the drained, cooled noodles and serve with a crisp green salad.

Chicken & avocado salad

Quinoa is the base for this salad: it's gluten-free and has a low GI rating. Add the chicken and avocado, and this dish becomes a filling and healthy meal that is high in nutrients. Serves two.

| ready in **40** minutes |

150g (5oz) quinoa

220ml (7fl oz) vegetable or chicken stock *(see p.296)*

1 tablespoon olive oil

Juice 1 lemon

Approx 100g (3½oz) cold chicken, cut into bite-sized chunks

½ avocado

½ red pepper, roughly chopped

70g (2½oz) cucumber, roughly chopped

3 baby courgettes (approx 60g/2oz) cut into chunks

2–3 tablespoons mixed fresh herbs (mint, parsley, coriander and basil, depending wwon what is available), chopped

Put the quinoa into a medium-sized saucepan and pour in the stock. Bring to the boil and simmer the quinoa in the stock over a medium-low heat until the stock has all absorbed. This should take about 15–20 minutes, by which time the quinoa should be cooked. Stir in the olive oil and the lemon juice and set aside to cool.

Once cool, stir in the rest of the ingredients, divide between two plates and serve.

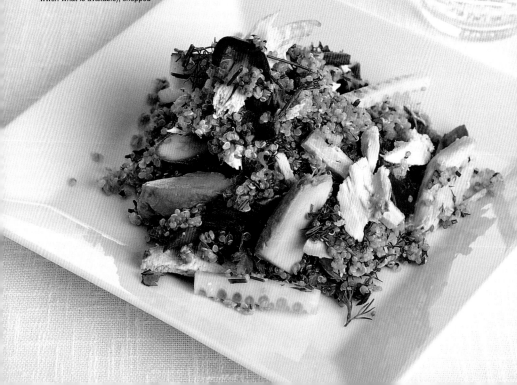

Remoulade & smoked meat

Remoulade is a French dish that is usually made with
mayonnaise. This recipe uses fromage frais instead,
which is low in fat and has a good protein content.
Remoulade also goes well with smoked mackerel.

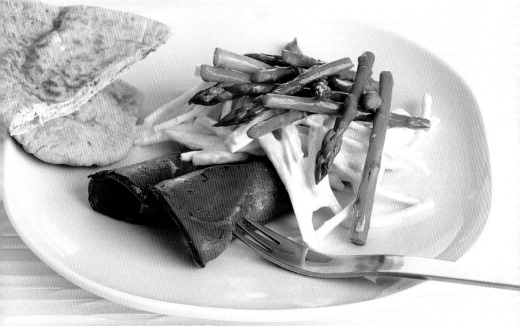

ready in 15 minutes

100ml (3½fl oz) live natural low-fat yoghurt
100ml (3½fl oz) reduced-fat fromage frais
2 tablespoons lemon juice
2 tablespoons Dijon mustard
Freshly ground black pepper
175g (6oz) celeriac, finely grated
12 spears asparagus
A drizzle of olive oil
A drizzle of lemon juice
4 slices smoked venison or smoked duck

Combine the yoghurt, fromage frais, lemon juice,
mustard, and black pepper in a bowl. Add the celeriac,
stir well and leave to stand for about 15 minutes for the
flavours to combine.

Meanwhile, steam the asparagus until just tender. This
should take approximately 10 minutes. Once cooked,
put the asparagus on a plate, drizzle with a little olive
oil and lemon juice while still hot and season with
freshly ground black pepper.

Divide the asparagus, the remoulade and the smoked
meat between two plates and serve. Serve with
wholemeal bread or flat bread as a light lunch for two.
This dish can also be used as a starter for four people.

Poached egg rosti ⓥ

This is the ideal easy meal to make when you don't have time to cook elaborate meals. If you are feeling hungry, cook two eggs per person and allow a little longer for the cooking time. Serves two.

ready in 25 minutes

300g (10oz) grated sweet potato
300g (10oz) grated celeriac
Zest and juice 1 lemon
1 tablespoon olive oil
2 tablespoons brown mustard seeds
A small bunch fresh dill, finely chopped
2 eggs

Mix the sweet potato and celeriac in a bowl with the lemon juice and zest. Heat the olive oil in a saucepan, add the mustard seeds and cook for a few seconds over a high heat until they pop. Pour the oil and seeds over the grated vegetables. Add the fresh dill and mix all the ingredients together.

Heat a little oil in a frying pan and add the vegetables, patting them down to form a cake. Cook over a medium-high heat for about 10 minutes to allow the underside to colour. Slip the pan under a high grill for another five minutes or so to brown the top.

Keep warm in a medium-hot oven while you poach the eggs *(see p.237)*. Serve the rosti with a poached egg placed on top of each portion.

SERVING IDEAS

For lunch Serve with a side salad and flat bread *(see p.298)*.

For dinner Crumble feta cheese over each egg and serve with a mixed salad.

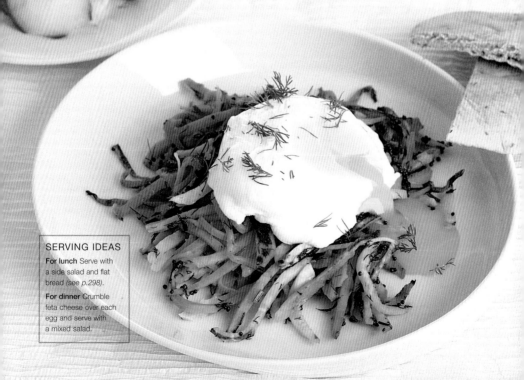

Cannellini bean stew with tomatoes Ⓥ

If you have time, you can cook dried cannellini beans for a slightly better texture. Soak them according to the instructions on the packet and cook them for approximately 1 hour. This recipe serves two.

ready in 15 minutes

1x400g (13oz) can cannellini beans or 200g (7oz) dried beans
8 cherry tomatoes, cut in half
1 teaspoon mixed herbs, dried
200ml (7fl oz) vegetable stock *(see p.296)*
Juice ½ lemon
1 teaspoon mustard
1 tablespoon olive oil
A small handful mixed fresh herbs, chopped, as a garnish

Put all the ingredients into a medium-sized pan, bring to the boil and simmer gently for 15 minutes. When the beans are cooked through, use a fork to gently break them up. Mix the stew well.

Divide the stew between two plates, scatter the chopped fresh herbs on top of each portion and serve.

SERVING IDEAS

For lunch For an instant protein to serve with this stew, use cold chicken pieces from the fridge, ready marinated tofu (available from delicatessens) or some smoked fish.

For dinner If you have time to cook, serve this as a side dish with Stuffed pork fillet *(see p.328)*, or grilled chicken or fish.

Use **canned tomatoes** from the **storecupboard** if you don't have any **fresh** tomatoes

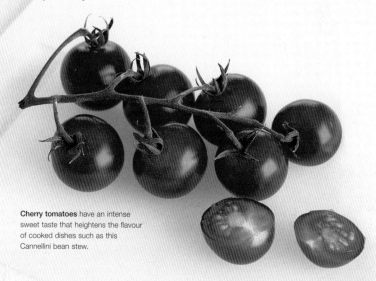

Cherry tomatoes have an intense sweet taste that heightens the flavour of cooked dishes such as this Cannellini bean stew.

Three ways with mushrooms

With their characteristic earthy flavour and meaty-tasting juices, mushrooms can sustain and even be enhanced by powerful flavours such as lemon, feta cheese and garlic. These recipes all serve two.

SERVING IDEAS

For lunch Serve the Greek mushroom & feta cheese salad with flat bread or wholemeal bread to soak up the juices.

For dinner Serve the Stuffed mushrooms with a mixed leaf salad or roasted tomatoes, or both. Serve the Mushroom bake with a crisp green salad.

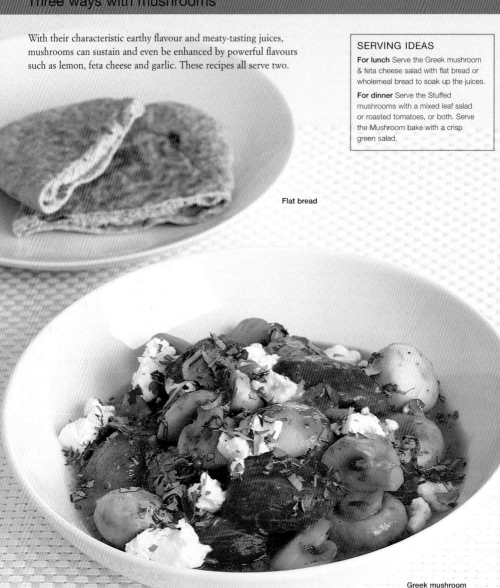

Flat bread

Greek mushroom & feta cheese salad

Greek mushroom & feta cheese salad

ready in **25** minutes

12 cherry tomatoes, skinned

8 baby onions or shallots (about the same size as the mushrooms; if bigger, cut in half)

2 tablespoons olive oil

200g (7oz) button mushrooms

100ml (3½fl oz) vegetable stock *(see p.296)*

50ml (2fl oz) white wine

1 bay leaf

2 teaspoons coriander seeds, whole

1 teaspoon black peppercorns, whole

1 tablespoon white wine vinegar

A small handful each fresh coriander and parsley, chopped

100g (3½oz) feta cheese, cubed

To skin the tomatoes, make a small slit in their skins, place in a bowl and pour over boiling water. Drain almost immediately and the skins should slip off. Leave to one side.

Heat the olive oil in a frying pan and gently brown the onions. Continue to cook over a low heat until they soften. Add the mushrooms and stir, then add the stock, white wine, bay leaf, coriander and peppercorns. Bring to the boil and simmer gently for 15 minutes until the onions are cooked. Add the tomatoes and vinegar, turn into a bowl and allow to cool. If you prefer, you can chill the mix in the fridge.

Serve with the feta gently folded into the mixture and the fresh herbs scattered on top.

Mushroom bake

ready in **20** minutes

1 medium aubergine

2 medium courgettes

A drizzle of olive oil

4 large portabello mushrooms

Freshly ground black pepper

2–3 medium tomatoes, sliced

200g (7oz) feta cheese, sliced

A squeeze of lemon juice

4 sprigs fresh rosemary

A handful fresh parsley, coriander and basil, chopped

Preheat the oven to 180°C/350°F/ Gas mark 4.

Thinly slice the aubergine and courgettes diagonally. Drizzle a little oil over them and brown on a griddle or under a grill.

Arrange the mushrooms in a lightly oiled ovenproof dish. Drizzle a little more olive oil over them and season with black pepper. Arrange 2–3 tomato slices over each mushroom, followed by slices of courgette and aubergine. Top with sliced feta and a squeeze of lemon juice. Tuck the rosemary around the mushrooms, cover with foil and bake for about 30 minutes until the mushrooms are soft.

Serve with the chopped herbs scattered over the top. This dish can also serve four as a starter.

Stuffed mushrooms

ready in **20** minutes

4 flat brown mushrooms, approx 50g (2oz) each

A drizzle of olive oil

Freshly ground black pepper

1 tablespoon olive oil

1 small onion, finely chopped

1 clove garlic, crushed or chopped

50g (2oz) fresh rye breadcrumbs

Zest 1 lemon

2 sprigs fresh sage, finely chopped

2 sprigs fresh thyme, finely chopped

2 tablespoons pinenuts, dry roasted

3 tablespoons The Food Doctor Sage & Thyme Seed Mix, lightly crushed, or use 3 tablespoons mixed pumpkin, sesame and sunflower seeds and ½ teaspoon each dried sage and thyme

60g (2½oz) feta cheese, crumbled

Preheat the oven to 180°C/350°F/ Gas mark 4.

Lightly oil a shallow ovenproof dish and lay the mushrooms side by side. Drizzle a little olive oil over each and season with black pepper. Cover loosely with foil and bake for 10–15 minutes.

Meanwhile, heat the oil in a frying pan over a low heat, add the onion and cook gently until soft. Add the garlic and bread and stir until the breadcrumbs turn brown and crisp. Add the lemon, sage, thyme, black pepper, pinenuts and seed mix. Mix well and stir in the feta.

Divide the stuffing evenly among the mushrooms, patting it down firmly. Pop under a grill to brown for a few minutes and serve.

Stir-fries

The secret of a successful stir-fry is the preparation – cooking is easy. These recipes are high on flavour and low on effort, so they may become firm favourites. All recipes serve two.

SERVING IDEAS

For lunch Serve the Coriander chicken stir-fry with brown or red rice, quinoa or socca. The Pork & spring vegetable stir-fry goes well with buckwheat noodles.
For dinner Omit the rice, quinoa, socca and buckwheat noodles and sprinkle on a tablespoon of toasted mixed seeds *(see pp.334–335).*

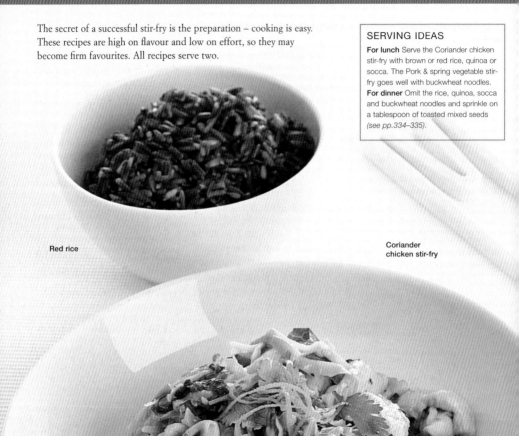

Red rice

Coriander
chicken stir-fry

Coriander chicken stir-fry

ready in **20** minutes

200g (7oz) chicken breast, finely sliced
1 teaspoon dry-roasted coriander seeds
100g (3½oz) green cabbage, finely sliced
2 tablespoons olive oil
4 tablespoons live natural low-fat yoghurt, flavoured with ½ teaspoon each ground cumin and ground chilli (to taste)

For the marinade:
1 teaspoon ground coriander
2 tablespoons fresh coriander, chopped (reserve a little for a garnish)
2 spring onions, finely sliced
2 teaspoons sesame seeds
3 tablespoons olive oil
Zest 1 orange (reserve a little for a garnish)
2 tablespoons orange juice
2 tablespoons lemon juice
Freshly ground black pepper

Combine the marinade ingredients in a bowl and mix. Add the chicken, stir well and leave to stand.

Heat a small saucepan over a medium-high heat, add the coriander seeds and dry-roast them for 30 seconds until they pop.

Just before cooking, add the roasted coriander seeds and shredded cabbage to the chicken.

Heat the oil in a wok and add the chicken mix. Cook over a medium-high heat until the chicken is cooked and the cabbage is wilting (add some water if it appears dry). Stir in the yoghurt and garnish with the orange zest and fresh coriander.

Mixed vegetable & bulgar wheat stir-fry

ready in **20** minutes

100g (3½oz) bulgar wheat
100ml (3½fl oz) boiling vegetable stock
100g (3½oz) asparagus stems
75ml (3fl oz) water
2 teaspoons Thai fry paste
1 teaspoon tamarind paste
1 tablespoon dry white wine
1 tablespoon rice wine vinegar
½ teaspoon chilli paste
100g (3½oz) broccoli in small florets
½ red pepper, cut into strips
½ yellow pepper, cut into strips
A drizzle of soy sauce
A drizzle of sesame oil
100g (3½oz) hot smoked fish, smoked tofu or feta cheese

Soak the bulgar wheat in the stock for 15 minutes, by which time it should be plump. Drain and squeeze through a fine sieve.

Heat lightly salted water in a saucepan, add the asparagus, bring to the boil and simmer for a minute or so. Drain and leave to one side.

Combine the water, Thai fry paste, tamarind paste, wine, vinegar and chilli paste in a small jug. Heat a wok, pour in the sauce and bring it to the boil. Toss in the broccoli and peppers, cook for 2 minutes, add the asparagus and stir for another minute. Stir in the bulgar wheat.

Serve with a drizzle of soy sauce and sesame oil, topped with the hot smoked fish, tofu or feta cheese.

Pork & spring vegetable stir-fry

ready in **20** minutes

150–200g (5–7oz) pork fillet
1 tablespoon olive oil
50ml (2fl oz) unsweetened apple juice 100g (3½oz) new baby carrots, cut lengthways
2 sticks celery, cut into short strips
50g (2oz) mangetout
1 fat or 2 thin spring onions, cut lengthways into 6cm (2½in) sticks
50g (2oz) broad beans
Freshly ground black pepper

For the marinade:
1 tablespoon soy sauce
2 tablespoons lemon juice
1 teaspoon fresh ginger, grated
1 tablespoon unsweetened apple juice

Trim any fat from the pork and cut it into short strips. Combine all the ingredients for the marinade, add the pork and allow to stand while you prepare the vegetables.

Heat the olive oil in a wok, lift the pork from the marinade and quickly brown the strips. Remove from the wok and put to one side. Pour the apple juice into the wok and add all the vegetables except the broad beans. Stir-fry for 5 minutes or so, return the pork to the wok and add the broad beans and the marinade. Continue to stir-fry for a further 5 minutes until the pork is cooked and the vegetables are *al dente*, then serve.

Smoked haddock tartare

It's important that you include fish in your diet at least twice a week: fish is both an ideal source of protein and rich in essential fats, which is vital for a healthy metabolism. This recipe is a fast and simple way to ensure that you get your quota. Serves two.

Use **unsmoked** haddock if **you prefer** a milder **flavour**

Yoghurt dressing

ready in **2** minutes

2 tablespoons live natural low-fat yoghurt
2 tablespoons reduced-fat fromage frais
1 tablespoon lemon juice
1 tablespoon olive oil

Combine all the ingredients in a small bowl or jug and mix together to a mayonnaise consistency.

Keep the dressing chilled in the fridge until the Smoked haddock tartare is ready to be served.

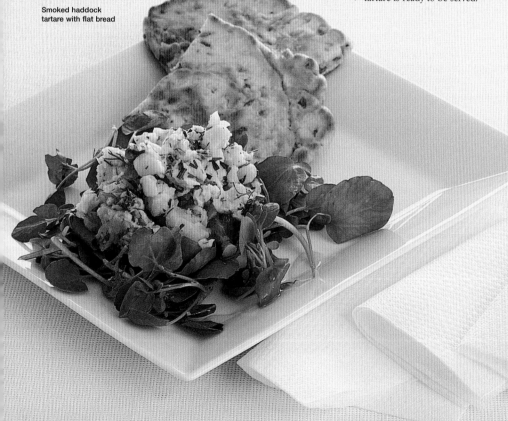

Smoked haddock tartare with flat bread

Smoked haddock tartare

| ready in **5** minutes |

200g (7oz) smoked haddock (undyed)
Juice and rind 1 lemon
½ teaspoon Dijon mustard
½ teaspoon capers, finely chopped
A small handful fresh dill, chopped
A small handful fresh chives, chopped
A large bunch fresh watercress, trimmed
and tossed in a drizzle each of olive oil and
fresh lemon juice

Carefully remove any skin and bones from the haddock. Using a large, sharp knife, cut the fish into thin strips, then chop the strips crosswise very finely to make tiny cubes. Don't be tempted to use a food processor to do this job, as it will leave the fish in a mushy pulp.

Combine the shredded fish with the lemon juice and rind, mustard, capers and the fresh herbs in a bowl and mix the ingredients well. Put the fish to one side while you make the flat breads (*see right*), or leave to marinate in the fridge for half an hour or so until you are ready to eat.

Once you have made enough flat breads, divide the fresh watercress between two plates and top each pile of watercress with half the haddock mix. Serve with the flat bread on the side and the yoghurt dressing in a small jug or bowl.

This makes a perfect light lunch for two people, or you can use it as a starter for four people.

Flat bread ⓥ

| ready in **10** minutes |

100g (3½oz) chick-pea flour
40ml (2fl oz) olive oil
200ml (7fl oz) water
A small handful fresh coriander, chopped
Zest of 1 lemon

Put the flour into a bowl, make a well in the middle and add the olive oil. Gradually pour in the water, mixing constantly with a whisk, until you have a batter about the consistency of double cream. (The batter shouldn't spread everywhere when poured into a pancake pan.) Add the coriander and lemon zest and stir well.

Heat a non-stick pancake pan until very hot, brush with olive oil and pour in about 100ml (4fl oz) of the batter. The batter should form a thick pancake about 20cm (8in) across. Lower the heat slightly and allow the flat bread to cook and brown before flipping it over and browning it on the other side. Lift out the flat bread, put it on a plate, cover with an upturned plate and keep in a warm oven while you use the rest of the mix.

This recipe should make at least four flat breads. Any excess flat breads can be kept covered in the fridge for up to two days or frozen for up to four weeks.

See page 298 for more flat bread recipes.

Yoghurt dressing

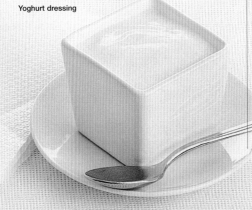

Pan-fried seafood

Seafood is a perfect ingredient to use when
preparing quick meals, as it only needs a few
minutes to cook through. Ensure that the seafood
you buy is as fresh as possible. Serves two people.

ready in **15** minutes

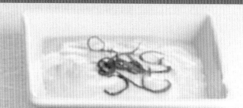

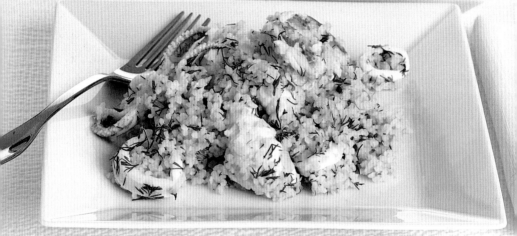

200g (7oz) mixed fish (raw prawns, prepared squid,
monkfish tail, white fish fillet), cut into bite-sized pieces

1 small cube of ginger, finely grated

Juice ½ lemon

Freshly ground black pepper

100g (3½oz) bulgar wheat, plus boiling water to cover

1 tablespoon olive oil

2 shallots, finely chopped

2 garlic cloves, crushed or finely chopped

A small bunch fresh dill, chopped

For the sauce:

6 tablespoons live natural low-fat yoghurt

Zest and juice 1 lime

Put the fish into a bowl. Toss them in the ginger and
lemon juice and add a grinding of black pepper. Leave
the fish to marinate for 5 minutes. Mix the sauce
ingredients together and decant into a small jug.

Put the bulgar wheat into another bowl and pour over
lightly salted boiling water until the bulgar wheat is just
covered. Leave to stand for 10 minutes, by which time
the bulgar wheat should be plump and soft.

Heat the oil in a frying pan, add the shallots and soften
over a low heat. Add the garlic and cook for a few
seconds. Lift the fish from the bowl, add it to the pan
and cook over a medium-high heat, tossing continually.
This shouldn't take more than a couple of minutes.
When cooked, drain and squeeze the bulgar wheat
through a sieve and add it and the marinating juices
to the pan. Add more lemon juice and black pepper
if needed and stir in the chopped dill. Serve with the
yoghurt and lime sauce on the side.

Hot griddled squid & salsa

The strong, sharp flavours of this salsa contrast well with the lightly spiced squid. Try to buy small or baby squid, as bigger squid can be too thick and become rubbery once cooked. Serves two.

ready in 20 minutes

300g (10oz) squid, cut into rings with the tendrils cut into 5–6cm (2–2½in) lengths

1 teaspoon fresh ginger, grated

Juice 1 lemon

Freshly ground black pepper

100g (4oz) bulgar wheat, plus boiling stock to cover

1 tablespoon olive oil

Rind ½ lemon

1 handful fresh parsley, finely chopped

A drizzle of olive oil

For the salsa:

A handful fresh mixed herbs such as mint, basil and parsley, chopped

1 large spring onion (or three small ones), finely chopped

1 fat garlic clove, crushed

Juice and rind 1 lime

Freshly ground black pepper

Put the squid in a bowl and combine with the ginger, lemon and black pepper. Leave for about 15 minutes.

Meanwhile, soak the bulgar wheat in the stock for 10 minutes, then drain through a sieve and squeeze out any excess stock. Stir in the olive oil, lemon rind and plenty of chopped parsley. Keep the bulgar wheat warm.

To make the salsa, mix the ingredients in a small bowl.

Use a slotted spoon to lift the squid from the marinade onto a lightly oiled, hot griddle over a high heat. Cook for 5–6 minutes, stirring occasionally to allow the squid to turn a golden colour. Serve immediately with the bulgar wheat, a mixed salad and the salsa on the side.

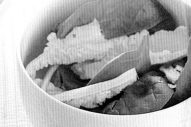

Fresh herb salsa

Mixed salad

Griddled squid with bulgar wheat

Coconut Thai fish

Fish is the finest of fast foods, and the more gently it is cooked the better. Heat the fish just until the flesh sets so that it retains its flavour and valuable nutrients. This recipe serves two.

ready in 15 minutes

100g (3½oz) corn or buckwheat noodles
2 teaspoons fresh lemongrass, chopped
2 teaspoons Thai fry paste
½ teaspoon ground turmeric
Juice and rind 1 lime
1 heaped teaspoon fresh ginger, grated
50g (2oz) fresh coconut, grated, or use creamed coconut
1 tablespoon olive oil
75g (2½oz) closed cap mushrooms, sliced
200ml (7fl oz) fish stock
200g (7oz) firm white fish fillet (haddock, hake, monkfish tail or halibut, according to what is available)
200g (7oz) pak choi, coarsely shredded
A small bunch fresh coriander or dill, chopped

Cook the noodles according to the instructions. Drain, toss with a little sesame oil and keep warm.

Combine the lemongrass, Thai fry paste, turmeric, lime, ginger and grated coconut in a bowl.

Heat the olive oil in a wok, add the spice mix from the bowl and stir for a minute to release the flavours. Add the mushrooms and stir for a few seconds. Pour in the fish stock, bring to the boil and add the shredded pak choi, stirring well. Add the fish almost immediately and simmer gently for a couple of minutes until the fish is just cooked, taking care not to break it up.

Add the noodles and mix gently. Divide between two plates, top with the coriander or dill and serve.

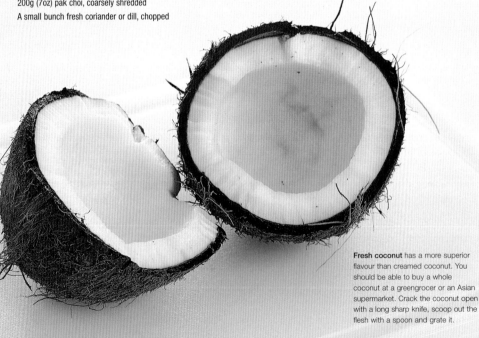

Fresh coconut has a more superior flavour than creamed coconut. You should be able to buy a whole coconut at a greengrocer or an Asian supermarket. Crack the coconut open with a long sharp knife, scoop out the flesh with a spoon and grate it.

Tuna carpaccio

This unusual way of preparing tuna means that the flavours are sealed in as the fish cooks and the flesh remains moist. Choose one of four crunchy toppings on pages 258–259 to suit your tastes. Serves two.

ready in 20 minutes

2x100g (3½oz) tuna steak
Enough crunchy topping
(see pp.258–259) to coat the steaks
A drizzle of olive oil

For the croutons:
2 thick slices rye bread
A drizzle of olive oil
1 garlic clove, crushed

Substitute **salmon** if you **prefer**, and ensure that it is as **fresh** as possible

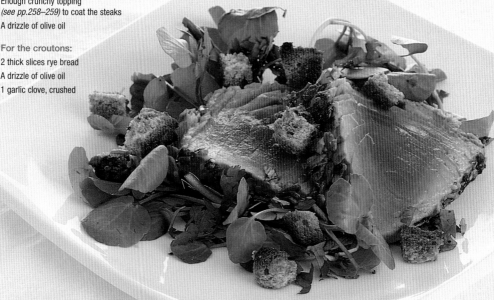

Spread the crunchy topping over the surface of a plate. Brush the tuna all over with olive oil and roll it in the crunchy topping, pressing down lightly to coat it well. Then wrap the tuna tightly in aluminium foil.

Heat a large cast-iron pan, or a stainless steel frying pan with a heavy base, over a very high heat until really hot. Put the wrapped tuna in the pan and press down gently so that it makes good contact with the hot surface. Cook for 3 minutes or so, turning regularly. Remove from the heat and leave to cool in the foil. The tuna should be cooked on the outside and pink on the inside.

Preheat the oven to 180°C/350°F/Gas mark 4.

To make the croutons, brush both sides of the bread slices well with olive oil and crushed garlic. Cut the bread into cubes, place on a baking sheet and bake in the oven for about 20 minutes, turning once, until the croutons are well browned and crunchy.

Once the tuna is cold, slice each steak thinly and arrange the slices on a bed of fresh salad leaves and herbs. Scatter the croutons over the top and serve.

Sautéed dishes

The term "sauté" comes from the French word *sauter*, "to jump". By lightly frying food at a high temperature it literally jumps in the pan and remains tender because it cooks so quickly. This is a great way to cook poultry to prevent it becoming tough. All recipes serve two.

SERVING IDEAS

For lunch Serve any of the three dishes with brown or red rice or flat bread *(see p.298)* if you are feeling hungry.

For dinner Serve the Sautéed pigeon and Spicy chicken with Refried yellow peas *(see p.288)*, steamed green beans or a mixed salad. The Spicy chicken sauce cools down the fiery chicken and should be added according to taste.

Spicy chicken sauce

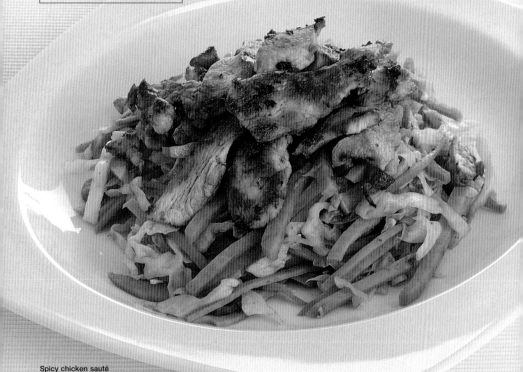

Spicy chicken sauté

Spicy chicken sauté

ready in **10** minutes

2 chicken breasts (approx 100g/3½oz each), cut into strips
2 tablespoons olive oil
2 teaspoons tamarind paste
50ml (2fl oz) water
150g (5oz) spring cabbage, finely shredded
150g (5oz) sweet potato, grated
Freshly ground black pepper

For the sauce:
2 tablespoons reduced-fat fromage frais
2 tablespoons live natural low-fat yoghurt
Juice and rind 1 lime
¼ teaspoon ground cumin

For the marinade:
¼–½ teaspoon hot chilli powder (depending on taste)
1 small cube fresh ginger, grated
1 teaspoon soy sauce
Juice ½ lime

Mix the marinade ingredients, add the chicken and leave to one side while you prepare the vegetables.

Heat the oil in a frying pan over a medium heat, add the chicken strips and sauté quickly until they are cooked and have turned golden.

Combine the tamarind paste and water and pour into a wok. Bring to the boil and toss in the vegetables. Stir-fry until the cabbage has just wilted and the vegetables are hot.

Mix the sauce ingredients and pour into a jug or bowl. Pile the chicken onto the vegetables and serve.

Sautéed chicken livers

ready in **5** minutes

150g (5oz) chicken livers
1 tablespoon olive oil
1 tablespoon lemon juice
½ teaspoon balsamic vinegar
A small handful fresh parsley, chopped
Freshly ground black pepper
2 generous handfuls mixed leaves with fresh herbs
2 flat breads *(see p.298)*
French dressing to taste

Rinse and clean any stringy or discoloured bits from the chicken livers and pat the livers dry.

Before cooking the livers, which take 2 minutes, make the flat breads if you don't have any ready made in the fridge or freezer.

Heat the olive oil in a frying pan over a medium heat, toss in the chicken livers and brown them for 2 minutes, turning frequently. Remove them from the heat when their outsides are browned and their insides are still pink, or their texture becomes grainy and dry.

Sprinkle the lemon juice, vinegar and parsley over the livers, season with black pepper and stir the ingredients together.

Put one flat bread on each plate and pile the mixed leaves on top. Drizzle with French dressing, top with the chicken livers and serve.

Sautéed pigeon breasts

ready in **20** minutes

2 tablespoons olive oil
200g (7oz) red onions, chopped
1 garlic clove, finely chopped or crushed
100g (3½oz) mushrooms, sliced
4 pigeon breasts
2 teaspoons mushroom ketchup (or sauce)
1 tablespoon orange juice
75ml (3fl oz) dry white wine
Freshly ground black pepper
A small handful fresh parsley, chopped

Heat a tablespoon of olive oil in a frying pan over a low heat, add the onions and soften, then add more olive oil and cook the mushrooms and garlic until the mushrooms are soft and beginning to brown. Transfer to a warmed serving dish using a slotted spoon.

Turn the heat up and brown the pigeon breasts on both sides. Add the mushroom ketchup, juice and wine and stir. Turn the heat down, cover and simmer for 5 minutes until the pigeon breasts are cooked, but still pink in the middle.

Make four three-quarter length slices in each breast, creating a fan shape. Divide the mushroom and onion mix between two plates and top with two pigeon breasts each. Add black pepper and a tablespoon of lemon juice to the sauce in the pan, simmer for a couple of seconds and pour over the breasts. Scatter with parsley and serve.

Meat escalopes

You need to cook with paper-thin pieces of veal or turkey for these recipes. Place the meat between two sheets of greaseproof paper and bang it out with a wooden rolling pin or the back of a large wooden spoon. This also helps to tenderize the meat. Each recipe serves two.

Veal escalope with brown mushrooms

ready in **10** minutes

2 veal escalopes (approx 100g/3½oz each)
1 garlic clove, crushed
Freshly ground black pepper
Juice 1 lemon
2 tablespoons olive oil
1 small onion, chopped
100g (3½oz) brown mushrooms, sliced
50ml (2fl oz) dry white wine
2 tablespoons live natural low-fat yoghurt
A handful fresh parsley, chopped

Lay the meat in a shallow dish, rub the garlic and black pepper into both sides of each escalope and sprinkle with lemon juice. Leave to one side to marinate while you prepare the rest of the dish.

Heat the oil in a shallow pan over a low heat, add the onion and sauté for a few minutes until it begins to soften. Add the mushrooms to the pan and cook gently until they take on colour. Lift out the onions and mushrooms with a slotted spoon and keep them warm in an oven set at a low temperature.

Turn the heat up, lift the escalopes from the marinade and put them in the pan. Brown each side over a medium-high heat – this should take about 2 minutes. Once they have taken on a golden colour, lift them from the pan and put them into a warmed dish. Put the dish into the warm oven.

Pour the wine into the pan and let it bubble for a few seconds. Stir in the marinade, mix the sauce well and bring it to boiling point. Remove the pan from the heat and stir in the yoghurt. Put the pan back over a very low heat, bring to just below boiling point and stir well to combine all the flavours. Stir in the mushroom and onion mix and heat through.

Pour the sauce over the escalopes, scatter with plenty of chopped parsley and serve.

Turkey escalope with shiitake mushrooms

ready in **20** minutes

2 escalopes turkey (approx 100g/3½oz each fillet)
1 garlic clove, crushed
Freshly ground black pepper
Juice 1 lemon
1 small onion, chopped
100g (3½oz) shiitake mushrooms, sliced
2 tablespoons olive oil
50ml (2fl oz) dry white wine
2 tablespoons live natural low-fat yoghurt
A handful fresh dill, chopped

Prepare this recipe by following the same method as for the Veal escalope with mushrooms (*see left*).

Shiitake mushrooms give a stronger flavour than brown mushrooms, and are known to be a good immune booster.

If fresh shiitake mushrooms are unavailable, buy a packet of dried mushrooms: soak 20g (¾oz) in enough boiling water to just cover for 20 minutes. Add the mushroom stock to the frying pan at the same time that you pour in the wine.

Scatter with fresh dill and serve.

Escalopes may sound complicated, but are **easy** to **prepare** and always **popular**

Freshly grated
carrot

SERVING IDEAS

For lunch Serve with a mixed salad and a small portion of quinoa if you are feeling hungry.

For dinner Serve with some steamed broccoli and a freshly grated carrot side salad or a spoonful of Refried split yellow peas (see p.288).

Veal escalope
with mushrooms

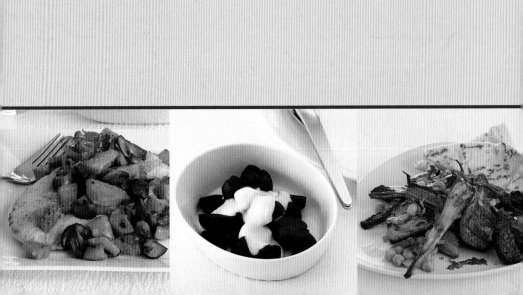

Slow cook

Make use of time spent at home by trying out these tempting recipes.
They are all the more delicious for being cooked slowly.

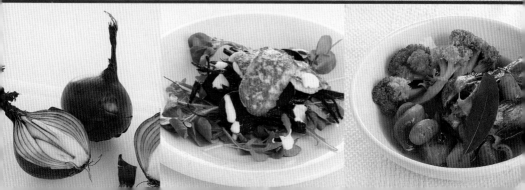

Beetroot & butter bean soup ⓥ

Fresh beetroot is full of minerals such as magnesium, iron and folic acid, while the butter beans provide necessary fibre. This soup freezes beautifully for two to three months. Serves two.

2 tablespoons olive oil
1 red onion, chopped
400g (13oz) beetroot, peeled and diced
800ml (1½ pints) vegetable stock *(see p.296)*
1x400g (13oz) can butter beans, rinsed and drained
Juice and zest 1 orange
Juice 1 lemon
Freshly ground black pepper
2 tablespoons live natural low-fat yoghurt

Heat the olive oil in a saucepan over a low heat, soften the onion for 3–4 minutes, then add the beetroot pieces and stir well for a couple of minutes.

Add the hot stock, bring to the boil and simmer for 30–40 minutes until the beetroot is tender. (This will depend on how old the beetroot is.)

Add the butter beans and orange juice and zest and cook for about 10 minutes. Pour the soup into a blender and whizz until smooth. Return to the pan to reheat, add the lemon juice to taste and season with plenty of black pepper.

Serve hot with a tablespoon of yoghurt swirled into each portion of soup.

> **SERVING IDEAS**
>
> **For lunch** Serve each portion with a slice of wholemeal or rye bread.
>
> **For dinner** Add a palmful of mixed pumpkin, sunflower and sesame seeds to each bowl of soup.

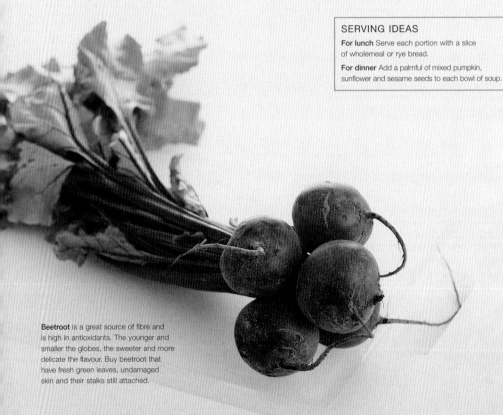

Beetroot is a great source of fibre and is high in antioxidants. The younger and smaller the globes, the sweeter and more delicate the flavour. Buy beetroot that have fresh green leaves, undamaged skin and their stalks still attached.

Roast beetroot with haloumi ⓥ

Slowly roasting beetroot sweetens and enriches its flavour. Haloumi cheese can turn slightly rubbery if it is left to cool for too long, so cook it just before you are ready to eat. Serves two.

SERVING IDEAS

For lunch Serve as a light lunch with wholemeal, rye or flat bread (see p.298).

For dinner Serve as a side dish with Fritatta (see p.291).

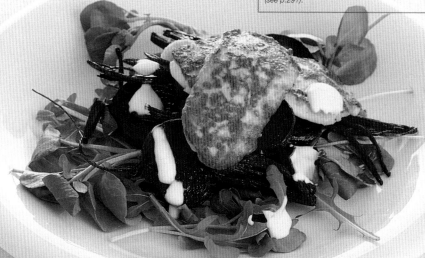

8 small beetroot, preferably organic (approx. 500g/1lb 2oz)

4 tablespoons olive oil

3 sprigs fresh rosemary or 1 teaspoon dried rosemary

4 garlic cloves, unpeeled (just cut off the tip)

1 heaped teaspoon horseradish sauce

Juice 1 lemon

Freshly ground black pepper

200g (7oz) light haloumi cheese

2 handfuls mixed green leaves, including watercress and rocket

French dressing to taste

Preheat the oven to 200°C/400°F/Gas mark 6.

Scrub the beetroot well. Trim off any leaves and cut each beetroot in half. Put a tablespoon of olive oil in a roasting tray and toss the beetroot in the oil. Scatter the garlic and rosemary around the beetroot, cover the pan loosely with foil and bake for 20–25 minutes.

Remove the foil, turn the beetroot over and bake uncovered for a further 20–25 minutes.

Depending on their size, the beetroot should be cooked, but not mushy. Lift them from the tray and keep warm. Pick out any rosemary twigs, remove the garlic cloves and squeeze the soft centres out of their outer skins and back into the pan. Add the horseradish, remaining olive oil, lemon juice and black pepper and stir well. Keep to one side while the haloumi cooks.

Arrange the washed leaves on a serving plate. Slice the haloumi into thin slices and cook them either in a medium-hot lightly oiled griddle pan or on a rack in the hot oven. Brown the slices (about 3 minutes on each side in the pan, but a little longer in the oven).

Arrange the beetroot on the leaves and the haloumi on top. Drizzle with a little French dressing and serve.

Savoury squashes

With their golden flesh and soft, slightly sweet taste, squashes are rich in nutrients and complex carbohydrates. Winter varieties, such as acorn or butternut squashes, are not restricted to a particular season because they store well, so you should be able to buy them quite easily. All recipes serve two.

SERVING IDEAS

For lunch Serve the Baked squash with a green leaf side salad.

For dinner Serve any of the squash recipes with meat or fish as a vegetable accompaniment. Alternatively, heat a tin of lentils and stir it into the Baked squash to make a hearty stew.

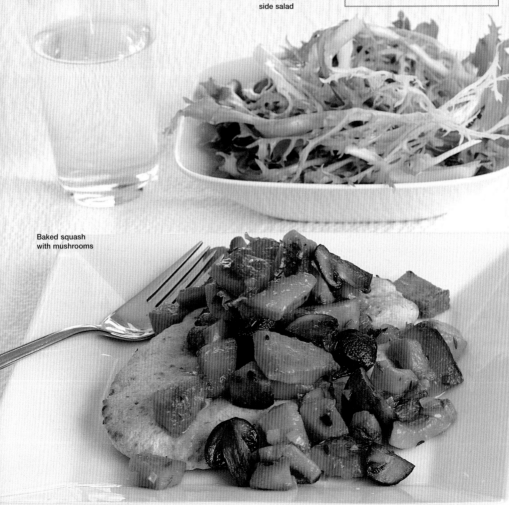

Green leaf
side salad

Baked squash
with mushrooms

Baked squash with mushrooms

1 small squash (approx 400g/13oz)

50g (2oz) brown or exotic mushrooms, sliced

2 whole garlic cloves

1 teaspoon cumin seeds, coarsely crushed

1 small onion, finely chopped

1 tablespoon olive oil

Juice 1 lemon

A handful fresh mixed herbs (coriander, parsley, chives, etc.), chopped

50g (2oz) crumbled feta cheese

Preheat the oven to 200°C/400°F/Gas mark 6.

Peel and cut the squash into 5cm (2in) cubes. Wipe and slice the mushrooms. Rub the loose skin off the garlic cloves, but don't peel them, just cut off their tips. Put all these ingredients in a bowl together with the cumin seeds, onion and olive oil and toss well.

Lightly oil a shallow baking dish, tip the squash mix into it and spread the ingredients out. Cover the dish with aluminium foil and bake until the squash is soft (about 30 minutes).

Remove the garlic cloves, squeeze the cooked flesh from their skins and stir it into the squash mix. Drizzle the bake with fresh lemon juice, scatter the chopped fresh herbs and crumbled feta cheese on top and serve.

Stuffed squash

2 small acorn squashes

1 tablespoon olive oil

Freshly ground black pepper

1 leek (approx 100g/3½oz), finely sliced

½ teaspoon caraway seeds

100g (3½oz) brown risotto rice

250ml (8fl oz) light vegetable stock

4 tablespoons The Food Doctor Original Seed Mix, or toast 4 tablespoons of your own seeds (see p.335)

50g (2oz) hard goat's cheese, grated

Preheat the oven to 200°C/400°F/Gas mark 6.

Cut the bulbous end off each squash (use the leftover flesh for other squash recipes), leaving two ends of squash each weighing 250–300g (8–10oz).

Scoop out the seeds, then use a sharp knife and a spoon to cut out as much flesh as you can, leaving the skin intact. Drizzle olive oil inside each hollowed out squash, season with black pepper and put them on a baking tray in the oven for 30 minutes to soften the skin and remaining flesh.

Soften the leek in the oil in a large saucepan over a low heat. Add the squash and caraway seeds and stir for a few seconds. Add the rice and stir to combine the flavours. Pour in the stock and simmer until the rice is plump and *al dente*. Add the mixed seeds and black pepper.

Put the mixture into the softened squash shells, sprinkle the goats' cheese on top, slide under a hot grill for 5 minutes and serve.

Squash with quinoa

100g (3½oz) quinoa, plus 250ml (8fl oz) light vegetable stock

1 courgette (approx 100g/3½oz), sliced into 5mm (¼in) rings

1 tablespoon olive oil

1 small onion, finely sliced

100g (3½oz) firm-fleshed squash, cut into 2cm (¾in) cubes

Juice ½ lemon

Freshly ground black pepper

75ml (3fl oz) vegetable stock

12 cherry tomatoes, cut in half

A small handful fresh tarragon, chopped

Simmer the quinoa in the stock in a saucepan without a lid. After 25 minutes the quinoa should be cooked and all the stock absorbed.

Brush a ridged griddle pan with olive oil and, once hot, brown the courgette slices on both sides. (If you don't have a griddle, cook the courgette slices with the squash.)

Heat the oil in a wok or large frying pan with a lid and soften the onion. Add the squash and the lemon juice and stir for a few seconds. Add the black pepper and the stock, cover and simmer for about 10 minutes. Then add the tomatoes and courgettes and stir well. Lastly, add the quinoa and tarragon. When the quinoa is heated through, serve.

This dish can also be eaten cold with a drizzle of olive oil and balsamic vinegar drizzled on top. Alternatively, add a spoonful of Yellow pepper sauce (see p.297).

Roasted root vegetables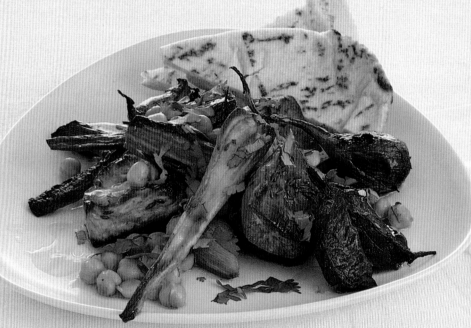

Cook these vegetables in a wide, shallow casserole or baking tray so that they roast evenly and turn crisp at the edges. The larger the vegetable chunks, the longer they will take to cook. Serves two.

> **SERVING IDEAS**
>
> **For lunch** Serve with flat bread for a light lunch.
>
> **For dinner** Serve as a side dish with the Citrus-baked chicken dish on page 282.

100g (3½oz) leeks, sliced diagonally
100g (3½oz) parsnips
150g (5oz) sweet potato
150g (5oz) celeriac
200g (7oz) red onion, thinly sliced end to end
100g (3½oz) carrot
100g (3½oz) beetroot
4 whole garlic cloves, with skin intact
1 teaspoon caraway seeds
4 tablespoons olive oil
Freshly ground black pepper
1x400g (13oz) can chick-peas, rinsed and drained
A drizzle of lemon juice and olive oil

Preheat the oven to 175°C/340°F/Gas mark 4.

Cut all the root vegetables except the onion and leek into even-sized chunks. Put all the vegetables into a large baking tray or casserole dish together with the garlic and caraway seeds. Toss the vegetables in the olive oil to coat them and season with black pepper.

Roast for about an hour, turning occasionally to prevent burning. When the vegetables are almost cooked, fold in the rinsed and drained chick-peas and return to the oven for about 10 minutes.

Before serving, drizzle with a little more olive oil and lemon juice to taste and serve.

Gratin of celeriac, red onion & asparagus ⓥ

Celeriac tastes quite similar to mashed potato when cooked. Combined with the caramelized onions and tangy feta cheese, it makes a delicious main meal or side dish. Quantities are for two.

300g (11oz) celeriac
2 large red onions, quartered and finely sliced
3 tablespoons olive oil
½ teaspoon ground cinnamon
½ teaspoon balsamic vinegar
1 tablespoon fresh lemon juice
12 thin asparagus shoots, with the tough end broken off
Crumbled feta cheese to garnish
A drizzle of olive oil
Freshly ground black pepper

SERVING IDEAS

For lunch Serve with a mixed leaf salad and wholemeal bread.

For dinner Serve with a poached egg on top of each portion, or with grilled fish or meat.

Preheat the oven to 180°C/350°F/Gas mark 4.

Peel the celeriac and cut it into slices about 1cm (½in) thick. Line the bottom of a small flan dish with overlapping layers of the celeriac. Drizzle with olive oil and season with black pepper and cook in the oven for 40 minutes or so.

Heat the oil in a frying pan over a low heat and soften the onions. Add the cinnamon, vinegar and lemon juice and continue cooking slowly to caramelize them. Don't let the onion slices become hard, so add more olive oil to the pan if the contents begin dries up.

Drop the asparagus into boiling water and cook for about 5 minutes, until just *al dente.*

Cover the celeriac with the caramelized onions and press down. Arrange the asparagus on top and crumble feta over the top. Put the dish under a hot grill for about 5 minutes until the feta cheese starts to brown.

Divide between two plates and serve. If you have individual gratin dishes, you could prepare and cook each helping separately.

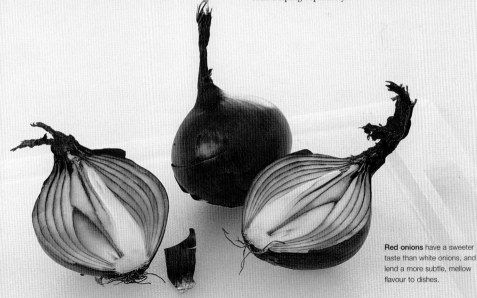

Red onions have a sweeter taste than white onions, and lend a more subtle, mellow flavour to dishes.

Red rice dishes

Red rice, also known as Camargue red rice, has a pleasant nutty flavour and a wine-coloured appearance when cooked. It has a medium GI rating and takes less time to cook than brown rice, so it's a useful addition to your storecupboard. Both recipes serve two.

Chicken & red rice with roast tomatoes

75g (2½oz) red rice
4 small chicken thigh fillets, skinned
Juice 1 lemon
1–2 tablespoons dried oregano
Freshly ground black pepper
2 tablespoons olive oil
1 small onion, chopped
2 garlic cloves, finely chopped
4 teaspoons freshly grated ginger
1 tablespoon dry white wine
300ml (½ pint) chicken or vegetable stock (see p.296)
1 teaspoon whole coriander seeds
4 medium tomatoes, cut in quarters
A drizzle of olive oil
Fresh sprigs of marjoram or coriander

Put the red rice in a saucepan and cover with cold water to soak while you prepare the chicken thighs.

Lay the chicken thighs out flat, make a couple of diagonal incisions into (not through) the outer flesh and rub in half the lemon juice, oregano and black pepper. Turn the thighs over and rub in the remaining juice and herbs. Leave for at least 15 minutes.

Heat a tablespoon of olive oil in a frying pan and soften the onion over a low heat. Add the garlic and ginger and heat gently for a few seconds. Add the chicken pieces (and more oil if necessary) and gently brown the chicken on both sides. Pour in the white wine and let it bubble, then add the stock, the drained rice and coriander seeds. Bring to the boil, turn the heat down and cover. Simmer very gently for about 30–35 minutes until the rice is plump and soft. Most of the stock should be absorbed by this time.

About 15 minutes before the end of the cooking time, preheat the oven to 180°C/350°F/Gas mark 4.

Put the quartered tomatoes in a small baking dish, drizzle with oil and season with freshly ground black pepper. Toss the tomatoes in the oil to cover them well and roast for 10–15 minutes.

Before serving the chicken and rice, top each portion with some of the tomatoes and torn herbs.

Thai fried rice

125g (4oz) red rice
250ml (8fl oz) light vegetable stock
2 tablespoons olive oil
100g (3½oz) pork fillet, cut into strips
1 small onion, chopped
½ green pepper, finely sliced
½ teaspoon ground cumin
¼ teaspoon chilli paste
2 lime leaves, crushed
1 garlic clove, crushed or chopped
Juice 1 lime
100g (3½oz) cooked prawns
75ml (3fl oz) dry white wine or unsweetened apple juice
Freshly ground black pepper
A small handful fresh coriander, chopped

Cook the rice in the stock for about 30–35 minutes. Drain and reserve.

Heat a tablespoon of olive oil in a wok. Add the pork and cook over a high heat, turning frequently, until the meat is lightly browned (about 5–10 minutes). Lift out the meat and keep it warm.

Add more oil to the wok if necessary and cook the onion and pepper over a low heat until soft. Add the cumin, chilli, lime leaves, garlic and lime juice and stir together for a minute or so. Add the prawns and stir well, then return the pork to the pan, add the wine or apple juice and stir to combine the flavours. Add the rice and season with freshly ground black pepper to taste. Serve garnished with coriander leaves.

These dishes include **complex carbohydrates** so they must be served with some **protein**

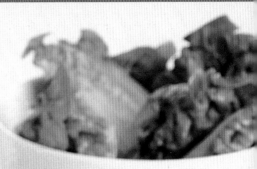

SERVING IDEAS

For lunch Both dishes just need a crisp green leaf side salad.

For dinner Serve with some steamed green vegetables if you want a change from a salad. You could also add a tablespoon of live natural low-fat yoghurt or toasted seeds (see p.335).

Crisp green
leaf side salad

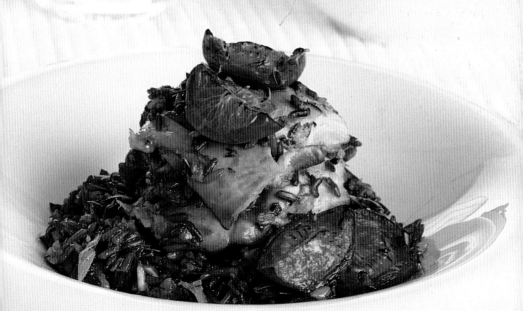

Chicken & red rice
with tomatoes

Citrus-baked chicken

This is a simple way to liven up a simple chicken dish. The strong citrus flavours give the chicken a sharp, slightly sweet taste. Keep any left-over meat in the fridge to eat cold the next day. Serves two.

4 skinned joints of chicken (leg and thigh joined together)
1 tablespoon olive oil
1 large onion, finely sliced

For the marinade:
Juice and zest 1 lemon
Juice and zest 1 lime
Juice and zest 1 orange
Zest ½ grapefruit
1 tablespoon soy sauce
50ml (2fl oz) olive oil
3 or 4 sprigs fresh basil, shredded

Combine all the marinade ingredients in a bowl. Make a couple of slits across the top of the chicken flesh and leave the joints to marinate for a couple of hours, or even overnight.

Preheat the oven to 175°C/340°F/Gas mark 4.

Heat a tablespoon of olive oil in a frying pan over a low heat and soften the onion. Add 2 tablespoons of the marinade and allow the onion to caramelize. Arrange the onion slices in the base of a shallow ovenproof dish.

Gently brown the chicken joints on both sides in the frying pan, then lay them on top of the onion, add 2 tablespoons of the marinade, cover and cook in the oven for about half an hour. The chicken should be tender with the juices running clear when pierced with a sharp knife. Lift onto two plates and serve.

> ### SERVING IDEAS
> **For lunch** Serve with bulgar wheat and a salad.
>
> **For dinner** The strong citrus flavours of this dish go well with the slightly sweet Roast Vegetable side dish on page 278.

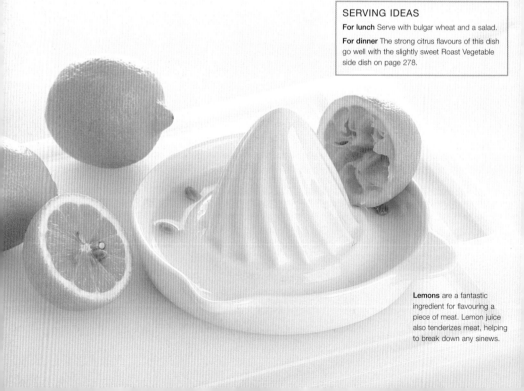

Lemons are a fantastic ingredient for flavouring a piece of meat. Lemon juice also tenderizes meat, helping to break down any sinews.

Lamb shank with garlic & rosemary

This dish must be cooked slowly to release all the flavours and reduce the liquid to a rich, dark gravy. You can, if you wish, double the cooking time for a very slow-baked dish. Serves two.

2x175g (6oz) lamb shanks (or 1 lamb shank
approx 350g/11½oz)
2 large sprigs rosemary, each broken into 3 or 4 pieces
1 large garlic clove, peeled and cut into thin sticks
1 tablespoon olive oil
8 shallots, peeled (or 1 medium onion, cut into 6)
1 medium/large carrot, cleaned and cut into chunks
250ml (8fl oz) dry white wine
1 bay leaf
2–3 sprigs fresh thyme
3–4 sprigs fresh marjoram
Freshly ground black pepper
250ml (8fl oz) stock

Prepare the lamb shanks by making 6 or 7 small slits in each shank and stuffing the garlic sticks and rosemary sprigs into them. Wrap in kitchen foil and leave overnight to absorb the flavours.

Preheat the oven to 150°C/300°F/Gas mark 2 to slow-cook for 3½ hours, or 140°C/275°F/Gas mark 1 to cook very slowly for 7 hours.

Heat the oil in a small casserole over a high heat and brown the lamb shanks all over. Tip in the shallots, carrot chunks and white wine and allow to bubble for a few seconds. Tuck in the bay leaf, thyme and marjoram and season with a good grinding of black pepper. Add stock just until the liquid doesn't quite cover the shanks and put the casserole, tightly covered, in the oven.

When the lamb is ready, remove any skin or fat and serve with the stewed vegetables and juices spooned over the top. This dish only needs some steamed broccoli or kale served with it.

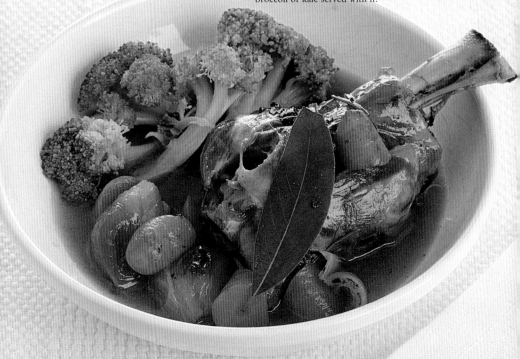

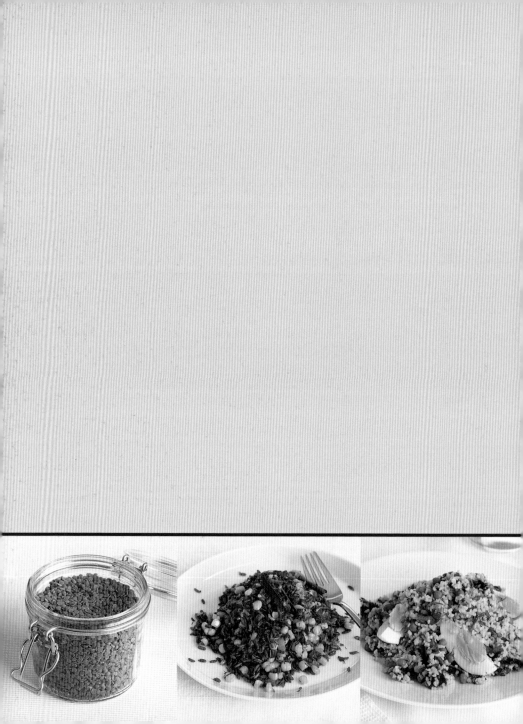

So there's nothing in the fridge

Of course there is. These recipes use basic proteins and carbohydrates from the fridge and storecupboard to make tasty meals.

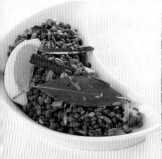
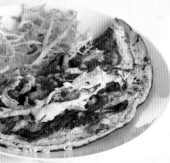
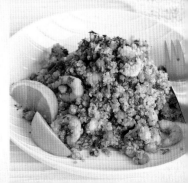

Quinoa & prawn salad

Keep your freezer stocked with frozen peas and cooked prawns for recipes such as this. The prawns must be thoroughly defrosted before you eat them, but they shouldn't take long to thaw. Serves two.

ready in 15 minutes

SERVING IDEAS

For lunch or dinner Depending on what is in the fridge, serve with a green salad or chopped tomatoes and scatter some chopped fresh herbs (if you have any) over each portion to give some extra flavour.

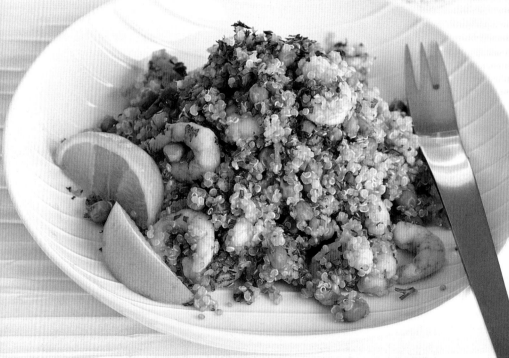

100g (3½oz) quinoa
200ml (7fl oz) stock
1 tablespoon olive oil
Juice ½ lemon
50g (2oz) frozen prawns, thawed and drained
50g (2oz) frozen peas, cooked and cooled
A small handful mixed fresh herbs, chopped

Simmer the quinoa in the stock until the stock has absorbed, by which time the quinoa should be soft and plump. Allow the quinoa to cool.

Stir in the olive oil, some lemon juice (if you have any), the prawns and the cooled peas, mix well, add the fresh mixed herbs and serve.

Sardine salad

Sardines are rich in omega-3 fats – one of the essential fats that the body needs in order to function properly. They are also a good source of protein and supply calcium. Serves two.

ready in 25 minutes

8 dried mushrooms
4 strips of roast pepper from a jar
6 sun-dried tomatoes
A drizzle of olive oil and lemon juice
1 can sardines in oil, drained

Soak the mushrooms in warm water for 20 minutes. Then drain them and chop them coarsely.

Chop the peppers and sun-dried tomatoes. Combine with the mushrooms, olive oil and lemon juice (if you have any) to taste. Fold in the sardines, break them up coarsely with a fork and serve.

SERVING IDEAS

For lunch or dinner Serve on flat bread *(see p.298)* or on wholemeal toast. Top with any chopped fresh herbs you may have.

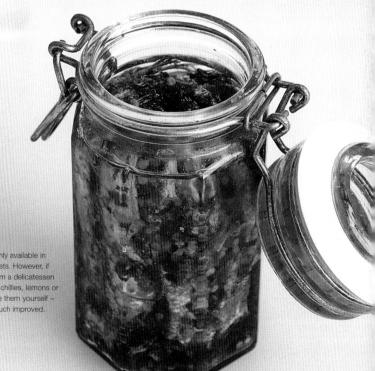

Sardines are commonly available in cans from supermarkets. However, if you can buy them from a delicatessen marinated in olive oil, chillies, lemons or peppers – or marinate them yourself – their flavour will be much improved.

Lentil & bean dishes

Pulses such as chick-peas and lentils are an ideal source of complete protein. Keep a selection of tinned and dried lentils and beans in your storecupboard for recipes such as these – and use your imagination as to what you can find to serve with them. All recipes serve two.

Baked beans

ready in **15** minutes

1 tablespoon olive oil
1 small onion, chopped
1 garlic clove, crushed or finely chopped
1 stick celery, chopped (or use 1 teaspoon celery seed)
1x400g (13oz) can haricot beans, drained and rinsed
1x250g (8oz) can chopped tomatoes
4 teaspoons soy sauce
50ml (2fl oz) unsweetened apple juice
Freshly ground black pepper

Heat the olive oil in a saucepan and soften the onion over a low heat. Add the garlic and the chopped celery (or celery seed) and cook for another minute or two. Tip in the beans, tomatoes, soy sauce and apple juice, and season with black pepper to taste. Stir well and simmer over a reasonably high heat for about 10 minutes until well thickened, then serve.

Chilli chick-peas

ready in **10** minutes

1 tablespoon olive oil
1 small onion, finely chopped
1 tablespoon tomato paste
1 teaspoon curry powder
¼ teaspoon chilli powder
1x400g (13oz) can chick-peas, rinsed and drained
4 sun-dried tomatoes, cut into strips

Heat the oil in a saucepan and soften the onion over a low heat. Stir in the tomato paste, curry powder and chilli powder and mix well for a few seconds. Stir in the chick-peas and sundried tomatoes and heat the ingredients together until the chick-peas are hot. This is meant to be a dry dish, but add a tablespoon of water to prevent sticking if necessary.

Serve with a squeeze of lemon juice and fresh herbs if you have some.

Refried split yellow peas

ready in **20** minutes

100g (3½oz) dried split yellow peas (or split mung beans)
150ml (¼ pint) weak vegetable stock
2 tablespoons olive oil
1 small onion, chopped
1 teaspoon cumin seeds, dry roasted
Squeeze of lemon juice

Soak the peas or beans for about 10 minutes, or at least rinse very well. Put them in a saucepan, add the stock and simmer until soft but not mushy, which should take 10–15 minutes. Drain and set aside.

Heat the olive oil in a saucepan and soften the onion over a low heat until it turns brown at the edges – this will bring out the sweet flavour of the onion. Add the cumin seeds, stirring for a few seconds. Tip the peas into the mix and stir over a medium heat for 2 minutes so that the peas take on the flavours of the onions and seeds.

Just before serving, stir in a squeeze of lemon juice to taste.

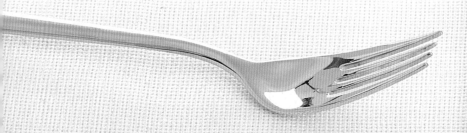

Lemony lentils

ready in 25 minutes

100g (3½oz) puy lentils
1 small onion, finely chopped
¼ unwaxed lemon, finely chopped
1 bay leaf
2 garlic cloves
1 small piece of cinnamon
1 small piece of star anise,
about 2 "petals"
400ml (¾ pint) water
1 teaspoon soy sauce
2 wedges lemon, to serve

Put all the ingredients except the soy sauce into a saucepan, bring to the boil and simmer gently for about 25 minutes until the lentils are soft but not collapsing. If the mixture looks too watery, raise the temperature slightly and boil away some of the liquid.

Add the soy sauce, stir and serve with a wedge of fresh lemon.

Lemony lentils

SERVING IDEAS
For lunch Serve the Baked beans on toast with a poached egg.

For dinner Serve the Chilli chick-peas with a mixed salad. Serve the Refried split yellow peas with a hard-boiled egg, and the Lemony lentils with 2 tablespoons of mixed seeds.

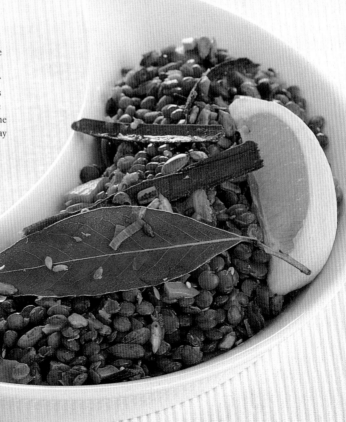

Lentil stew ⓥ

Try this storecupboard supper when the fridge holds nothing tempting to eat. Use dried lentils, which only take 10 minutes to cook, or grab a can of lentils instead. Serves two.

25g (¾oz) dried mushrooms
1 small onion, finely chopped
1 tablespoon olive oil
¼ teaspoon cumin seeds
¼ teaspoon turmeric
100g (3½oz) red lentils or 1x200g (7oz) can unsweetened lentils
300ml (½ pint) stock
100g (3½oz) frozen peas

Cover the mushrooms with warm water and soak for about 20 minutes. Then drain and slice them, removing the stems if they seem tough.

Soften the onion in the oil in a medium-sized saucepan over a low heat. Add the spices and cook for a few seconds, then add the lentils and stock and simmer, with the pan covered, for 5 minutes. Add the peas and sliced mushrooms and cook for a further 5 minutes. By this time the stock should be almost absorbed and the lentils soft and starting to collapse. If you use canned lentils, add them with the peas and use just 100ml (3½ fl oz) of stock.

If you have any fresh herbs such as parsley or coriander, chop a good handful into the lentil stew and serve.

> ### SERVING IDEAS
>
> **For lunch or dinner** You could scatter your favourite Food Doctor seed mix on top of the stew, or use a mixture of pumpkins, linseeds and sunflower seeds.
> If you have the right ingredients in the fridge, make a side salad to serve with the stew.

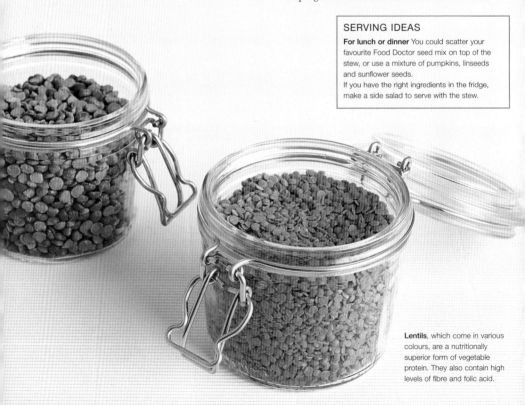

Lentils, which come in various colours, are a nutritionally superior form of vegetable protein. They also contain high levels of fibre and folic acid.

Simple fritatta

This quick and easy dish is so versatile that you can add any fillings you find: canned vegetables or pulses, frozen prawns or peas, roast peppers or artichokes from a jar or sundried tomatoes. Serves two.

| ready in **5** minutes |

4 eggs

3 tablespoons live natural low-fat yoghurt

1 teaspoon Dijon mustard

Freshly ground black pepper

1 onion, chopped

1 tablespoon olive oil

Fresh herbs (if you have any)

SERVING IDEAS

For lunch or dinner If you have any leftover Roasted root vegetables *(see p.278)*, serve those with the fritatta, or add a handful of fresh herbs. Alternatively, serve with flat bread *(see p.298)*.

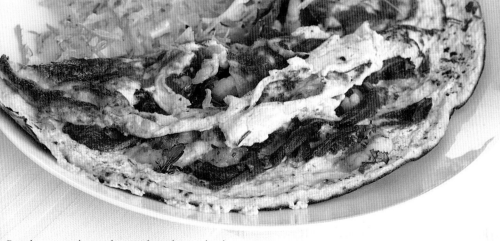

Beat the eggs, yoghurt and mustard together in a bowl and season with freshly ground black pepper.

Soften the onion in the olive oil in an omelette pan over a low heat. Pour in the egg mixture. Scatter in whatever filling you have to hand and cook gently to set and brown the bottom. Slip under a warm grill to brown the top and then serve.

Egg pilau v

Pilau is usually made with rice, but this recipe uses bulgar wheat, which has a lower GI rating than rice. If you don't have any eggs in the fridge, try using tofu or even leftover cold chicken pieces. Serves two.

ready in 15 minutes

100g (3½oz) bulgar wheat,
plus enough hot stock to cover

2 tablespoons olive oil

3 teaspoons Dijon mustard

Lemon juice to taste

8 sun-dried tomatoes

2–3 hard-boiled eggs

SERVING IDEAS

For lunch or dinner Add a handful of chopped fresh parsley and some frozen peas, if you have them, to add colour and flavour to the egg pilau.

Cover the bulgar wheat with boiling stock and leave it to stand for 10 minutes until soft. Drain and squeeze the grains through a fine sieve. Then stir in the olive oil, mustard and some lemon juice if you have any.

Drain the pieces of sundried tomato from a jar, slice them and toss them into the bulgar wheat. Pile the mixture onto two plates, arrange the quartered whard-boiled eggs on top and serve.

Spicy red rice & corn ⓥ

Red rice is a superior-quality unmilled short-grain rice, so it's slightly sticky when cooked. If you don't have red rice though, you can use brown. Buy cans of sweetcorn without sugar or salt. Serves two.

1 tablespoon olive oil
2 whole cloves
2 cardamom pods (split)
1 small stick cinnamon
1 small onion, finely chopped
100g (3½oz) red rice
300ml (½ pint) stock
1 small can sweetcorn, drained and rinsed
Chopped fresh herbs (if you have any)

Heat the oil in a saucepan over a medium heat and add the spices. Cook for a couple of minutes before adding the onion. Soften the onion over a low heat and allow it to take a little colour, then add the rice and stir into the oil for a few seconds. Add the stock, bring to the boil and simmer gently for 35 minutes until the rice is cooked, but not soggy, and the stock is absorbed. Stir in the sweetcorn, cook over a low heat for 5 minutes to combine the flavours and serve with a garnish of herbs.

> ## SERVING IDEAS
> **For lunch or dinner** Lightly steam some vegetables or prepare a side salad to serve with the rice and sweetcorn if you have any suitable ingredients in the fridge.

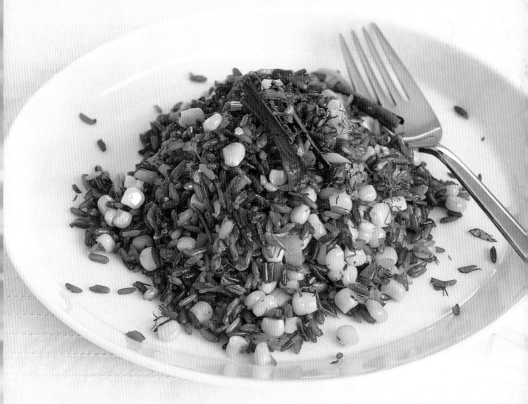

Stocks & sauces

Many of the recipes in this book require stocks or sauces. If you cook your own stocks – and freeze them in small portions – you'll find that they'll give your food a delicious depth of flavour. The sauces can also be frozen for up to three months or kept in the fridge for three days.

Chicken stock

1 chicken carcass, left over from pot-roasting *(see p.317)*, or ask your butcher for 500g–1kg (1–2lb) chicken bits for stock
1 large carrot, scraped and chopped
1 large stick celery
1 large onion
3 sprigs fresh parsley
6 whole peppercorns
A sparse teaspoon sea salt or Lo salt

Remove any remaining meat from the chicken carcass and use for the Chinese chicken salad on page 251, or the Chicken & avocado salad on page 252.

Put the all the bones and skin of the chicken into a large saucepan and add the remaining ingredients (including any onions and lemons that may be left over from roasting). Cover with cold water and bring to the boil. Lower the heat and simmer for at least 2 hours. Then turn off the heat and allow to cool.

Strain the stock and discard all the vegetables and bones. Allow the liquid to stand, then scoop any excess fat off the top of the stock with a spoon or ladle. Return the liquid to the saucepan and boil for about 10 minutes to give the stock a stronger taste.

Use the stock for any recipes in this book requiring bouillon or stock, or use to make a delicious and simple Chicken soup *(see p.301)*.

Vegetable stock Ⓥ

2 medium carrots, trimmed and cut into chunks
3 sticks celery, cut into chunks
1 medium onion, quartered
½ small cabbage, coarsely shredded
2 garlic cloves, peeled and coarsely chopped
2 sprigs parsley
6 peppercorns
2 tablespoons soy sauce
2 litres (3½ pints) water

Put all the ingredients into a large saucepan, bring to the boil and simmer over a low heat for an hour and a half. Strain the liquid, adjust the seasoning and use.

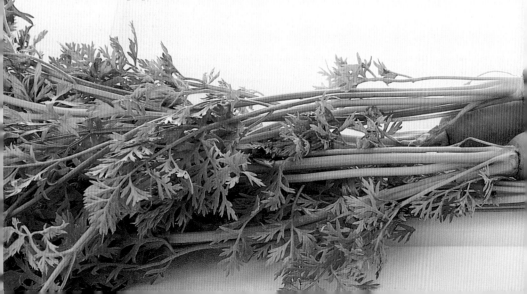

Rich tomato sauce

2 tablespoons olive oil
1 medium onion, finely chopped
1 medium carrot, finely chopped
1 stick celery, finely chopped
2 garlic cloves, chopped or crushed
2x400g (13oz) cans chopped tomatoes
1 teaspoon tamarind paste
750ml (1¼ pints) dry white wine
2 teaspoons dried mixed herbs
Freshly ground black pepper
2 tablespoons fresh parsley, chopped

Heat the oil in a large saucepan and add the onion, carrot and celery. Soften for about 10 minutes over a low heat, then add the garlic. Raise the heat and cook for a further 5 minutes to intensify the flavours.

Add the tomatoes and tamarind paste, stir well and cook for a further 5 minutes.

Pour in the white wine and allow to bubble for a couple of minutes. Stir in the dried herbs and season with freshly ground black pepper.

Lower the heat, cover the pan and simmer gently for 20 minutes, stirring occasionally.

Once cooked, stir in the fresh parsley. The sauce should be quite thick and rich.

Use the sauce as the base for a balanced soup (just add stock and a can of cannellini or barlotti beans). It can also be blended to make a smoother soup, or served with chunky vegetables. Use as a sauce for the Stuffed gem squash *(see p.316)*, or to accompany the Mixed nut & haloumi roast *(see p.299)*.

Yellow pepper sauce

1 large yellow pepper
2 tablespoon olive oil
Juice ½ lemon
½ teaspoon soy sauce
A small handful chives, chopped
Freshly ground black pepper
A splash Tabasco sauce

Preheat the oven to 200°C/400°F/Gas mark 6.

Cut the pepper in half lengthways, deseed it and cut each half into three thick strips. Put on a baking tray and drizzle with the olive oil. Put in a hot oven and bake for 30 minutes, turning once.

Tip the peppers and any juices into a food processor together with the rest of the ingredients. Whizz to make a smooth, thick sauce.

For a quicker version, buy a jar of marinated roast peppers, drain and use instead. Serve the sauce with Squash with quinoa *(see p.277)* and Baked trout *(see p.315)*.

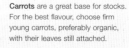

Carrots are a great base for stocks. For the best flavour, choose firm young carrots, preferably organic, with their leaves still attached.

Flat breads ⓥ

These yeast-free breads are a cross between a pitta bread and a pancake. The quantities listed are enough for two people, but you can make more and keep them for up to four weeks in the freezer.

Fennel & caraway buckwheat bread

| ready in **10** minutes |

100g (3½oz) buckwheat flour

3 tablespoons The Food Doctor Fennel & Caraway Seed Mix, finely ground, or grind 1 tablespoon each pumpkin, sunflower and sesame seeds, ½ teaspoon caraway seeds and ½ teaspoon fennel seeds

40ml (2fl oz) olive oil

200ml (7fl oz) water

Chilli & garlic gram bread

| ready in **10** minutes |

100g (3½oz) chick-pea flour

3 tablespoons The Food Doctor Garlic & Chilli Seed Mix, finely ground, or grind 1 teaspoon chilli flakes, 1 garlic clove, crushed, 1 tablespoon each pumpkin, sunflower and sesame seeds

40ml (2fl oz) olive oil

200ml (7fl oz) water

To make either, put the flour and ground seeds in a bowl, make a well in the middle and add the olive oil. Gradually pour in the water, mixing with a whisk, until you have a thick batter the consistency of double cream. (The batter needs to be poured into a pancake pan without spreading everywhere.)

Heat a pancake pan until very hot, brush with olive oil and pour in approximately 100ml (4fl oz) of the batter. This should make a thick pancake about 20cm (8in) across. Lower the heat slightly and allow the flat bread to brown before turning and browning the other side. Lift out, cover and keep warm while you finish cooking the rest of the batter.

If you want to add extra flavour to these breads, add some chopped fresh mixed herbs to the batter.

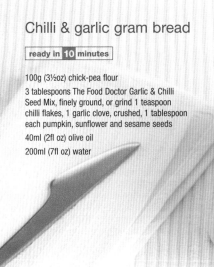
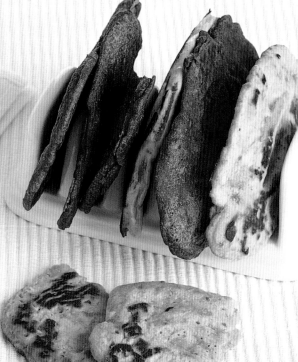

Mixed nut & haloumi roast ⓥ

The high nut content of this dish makes it rich in omega-6 fats, which are vital for good health. You can prepare the raw ingredients in advance and cook the dish later. It's also good served cold. Serves two.

Choose nuts that are raw and unsalted for your cooking. Ideal choices are almonds, walnuts, a few Brazil nuts, cashew nuts, pinenuts and hazelnuts.

ready in **10** minutes

150g (5oz) raw unsalted mixed nuts
1 small onion, peeled and quartered
75g (2½oz) mushrooms, quartered
50g (2oz) oat flakes or quinoa flakes
1 tablespoon sesame seeds
2 heaped tablespoons mixed dried herbs
2 tablespoons fresh parsley, chopped
1 large egg, lightly beaten with a fork
1 tablespoon mustard (or 1 teaspoon powdered mustard)
Juice 1 lemon
Freshly ground black pepper
150g (5oz) haloumi cheese, sliced approx 3 mm (⅛in) thick

Preheat the oven to 180°C/350°F/Gas mark 4.

Put the nuts, onion and mushrooms into a food processor and whizz together until the nuts are coarsely chopped. Tip the contents into a bowl and add the oat flakes or quinoa, sesame seeds, dried herbs and fresh parsley, stirring well. Add the beaten egg, mustard and lemon juice and season with black pepper.

Lightly oil a 14cm x 20cm (5½ x 8in) oblong loaf tin. Press half the mixture into the bottom of the tin, lay the haloumi slices over the nut mix, cover with the rest of the mix and press down gently. Cover the loaf tin with foil and bake for 45 minutes.

When the dish is ready to be eaten, heat up some Rich tomato sauce *(see p.297)*, cut the nut roast into slices and serve it with the sauce and some steamed broccoli.

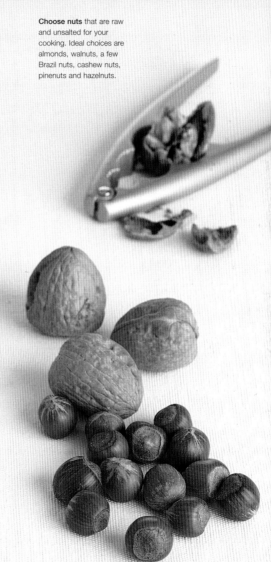

Chicken dishes for every occasion

With its high protein content and versatility, chicken is an ideal lean meat to use for cooking healthy meals. These recipes use cheaper cuts of chicken meat to make deliciously tasty dishes that you can serve for a variety of occasions. Each recipe serves two.

Three-grain
wheatfree bread

Sliced chicken terrine,
with caperberries and
chopped tomatoes

Chicken terrine

500g (1lb) chicken thigh fillets
(which are moister than breast meat)

Rind 1 lemon

2 large spring onions, cut into chunks

2 teaspoons soy sauce

2 teaspoons grated nutmeg

2 teaspoons olive oil

4 tablespoons reduced-fat fromage frais

Freshly ground black pepper

2 good handfuls mixed fresh herbs
(including a little fresh sage), chopped

2 tablespoons olive oil

2 garlic cloves, crushed

400g (13oz) spinach, cut into shreds

Preheat the oven to
150°C/300°F/Gas mark 2.

Put the chicken, lemon rind and
spring onions into a food processor
and blitz until they are well minced.

Combine the mince, soy sauce,
nutmeg, olive oil and fromage frais
in a bowl. Season with black pepper
and fresh herbs. Leave to stand
while you prepare the spinach.

Heat the oil in a wok, add the garlic
and soften over a medium heat. Add
the spinach. When it wilts, drain.

Lightly oil a terrine, add the mince
and spinach in layers, cover with
foil and bake for 1 hour until the
juices are clear. Drain the juices and
grill for 5 minutes to brown. Cover
with a layer of foil and press down
the mix using weights or cans.
Leave to cool, draining off any
more juice.

Can be kept in the fridge for 3–4
days, or frozen for 4 weeks.

Chicken liver paté

2 tablespoons olive oil

120g (4oz) brown mushrooms, chopped

250g (8oz) chicken livers (organic livers are best) with any stringy or discoloured bits cut off

3–4 large sprigs fresh parsley, chopped

3 sprigs fresh thyme, chopped (or ½ teaspoon dried thyme)

1 teaspoon red wine vinegar

½ teaspoon balsamic vinegar

1 teaspoon soy sauce

1 teaspoon mustard

1 teaspoon lemon juice

Freshly ground black pepper

Heat a tablespoon of olive oil in a frying pan and cook the mushrooms over a medium heat, browning them just a little to bring out the flavour. Tip the cooked mushrooms into a food processor or blender.

Heat the rest of the olive oil in the pan, gently sauté the livers for about 2 minutes on each side (don't overcook them: they should be just pink inside). Remove with a slotted spoon and add to the mushrooms, together with the parsley and thyme.

Add the vinegars, soy sauce, mustard lemon juice and black pepper to the juices in the pan and simmer for 2 seconds. Add to the blender.

Whizz the ingredients for a few seconds. Scrape into a pot and cover.

Store in the fridge for up to three days, or freeze for up to a month if the livers were not previously frozen.

Spring chicken

4 small chicken thighs

1 tablespoon olive oil

12 shallots

50g (2oz) small brown mushrooms

10 cherry tomatoes

3 stems celery, cut into short sticks

100g (3½oz) baby carrots

100g (3½oz) broad beans

50ml (2fl oz) dry white wine

200ml (7fl oz) chicken stock *(see p.296)*

Preheat the oven to 150°C/300°F/Gas mark 2.

Skin the chicken thighs and cut away any fat. Put them in an ovenproof casserole. Heat the oil in a frying pan over a high heat and brown each of the vegetables in turn, adding them to the chicken as you go (except the broad beans). Pour the wine into the hot pan, let it bubble for a couple of seconds and add to the casserole. Add the stock, the black pepper and the fresh herbs and cover tightly.

Cook for 1¼ hours, stirring a couple of times. Add the broad beans 15 minutes before the end of the cooking time. The meat should be well cooked and coming away from the bone.

This stew can be refrigerated and reheated the next day or frozen for up to one month.

Simple chicken soup

60g (2oz) brown Basmati rice

50g (2oz) reserved cold chicken meat

1 litre (1¾pints) chicken stock, plus extra to cook the rice

1 tablespoon lemon juice

1 generous tablespoon fresh parsley, chopped

Freshly ground black pepper

Cook the rice according to the instructions on the packet using the extra chicken stock (rather than water). This should take about 20 minutes to cook.

Meanwhile, shred the cold chicken into smallish pieces. Put the stock into a bowl and add the chicken pieces. Once the rice has cooked, add it and any remaining fluid to the stock, together with the lemon juice. Stir in the parsley and season with black pepper.

This will make approximately 1 litre (1¾pints) of soup that can be refrigerated for two days, or frozen for up to four weeks. When you come to eat the soup, heat it until just simmering and serve.

Moroccan beef

This delicious dish is full of warm, spicy flavours and beefy juices. It can be refrigerated and reheated the next day – or double-up the quantities and freeze the portions for up to four weeks. Serves two.

400–500g (13oz–1lb) very lean beef, trimmed and cubed

½ teaspoon each ground cinnamon, ground coriander, ground ginger and ground cumin

2 tablespoons olive oil

1 onion, chopped

2 garlic cloves, finely chopped or crushed

1x400g (13oz) can chopped tomatoes

16 prunes

150g (5oz) broad beans (shelled weight)

A small handful fresh coriander, chopped

2 tablespoons The Food Doctor Original Seed Mix, or 2 tablespoons toasted sesame seeds *(see p.335)*

Preheat the oven to 160°C/320°F/Gas mark 3.

Put the beef in a bowl and toss in the ground spices to coat the meat. Leave for a few minutes, then heat a tablespoon of the olive oil in a pan and gently brown the beef in small amounts at a time over a high heat. Once browned, lift the beef out of the pan and into a casserole dish.

Heat the remaining oil in the pan and add the onion, softening it over a low heat. Once the onion is softened, add the garlic. Cook together for a minute or so, then pour in the tomatoes and stir the ingredients together. Pour the mixture over the beef pieces and stir in the prunes. Cook in the oven for 30 minutes.

After half an hour, remove the casserole from the oven and add the beans. Stir them in and add a little stock if necessary. Replace the dish in the oven and cook for a further 30 minutes.

When you come to serve the stew, stir in the fresh coriander, sprinkle the seeds on top and eat with bulgar wheat or brown rice and a green salad.

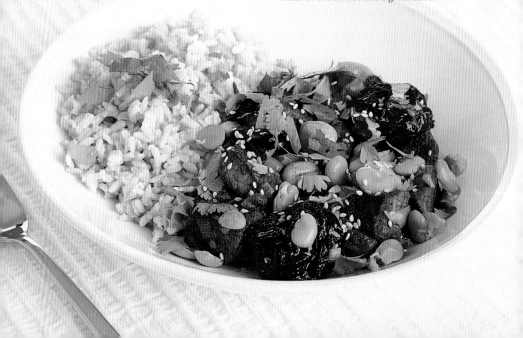

bazant

Normandy pheasant

Pheasant is a rich-tasting but lean meat, so it's a good choice of protein. A hen pheasant is an ideal size to serve two. The dish can be refrigerated and eaten hot the next day, or frozen for up to one month.

1 prepared jointed pheasant (or 2 pheasant breasts)
½ tablespoon cider vinegar
1 tablespoon unsweetened apple juice
1 garlic clove
1 tablespoon olive oil
1 small onion, finely sliced
1 medium-sized cooking apple, peeled, cored and sliced
½ tablespoon calvados or brandy (optional)
50ml (2fl oz) stock

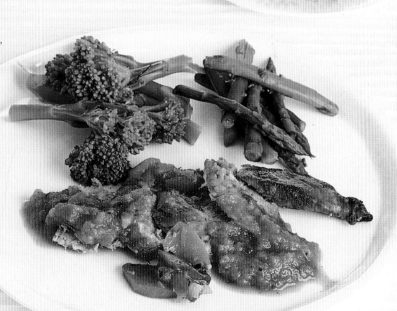

Put the pheasant in a bowl together with the vinegar, apple juice and garlic and marinate it for at least 15 minutes, or preferably an hour.

Heat the olive oil in a saucepan, lift the pheasant from the marinade (which you should reserve) and gently brown the outside of the bird. Once browned, lift the pheasant from the pan and keep it to one side.

Heat the remaining oil in the pan and add the onion. When it starts to soften, add the apple slices. Cook together for 5–10 minutes until the apple starts to soften too, and then replace the pheasant. Pour over

the calvados or brandy and set alight, shaking the pan around while the spirit burns off. Then add the marinade and the stock to the pan and season with a good grinding of freshly ground black pepper.

Bring to the boil, lower the heat and cook over a very gentle heat for approximately 45 minutes, by which time the meat should be tender.

Lightly steam some green vegetables or arrange a salad of crisp mixed leaves when you are ready to serve the dish. If you are eating the pheasant for lunch, you can also add a portion of brown rice or bulgar wheat.

Stews & casseroles

Whether you want to take the strain out of cooking on the night of a special dinner, or stock the freezer with balanced nutritious meals, all these recipes are adaptable enough to be cooked, chilled and reheated the next day or frozen for up to one month. Each recipe serves four.

Pork and beans

400g (13oz) lean pork (leg or fillet) cut into cubes

2 tablespoons olive oil

1 large onion, finely chopped

2 garlic cloves, finely chopped or crushed

1x400g (13oz) can chopped tomatoes

1x400g (13oz) can haricot beans, drained and rinsed

1 green pepper, deseeded and chopped

100ml (3½fl oz) apple juice

2 teaspoons soy sauce

3 sprigs fresh sage, chopped

Freshly ground black pepper

Preheat the oven to 160°C/320°F/Gas mark 3.

Heat the oil in a frying pan, and sauté the meat over a high heat, a few cubes at a time, until lightly browned. Remove from the pan and put into a casserole.

Add the onion to the pan and soften over a low heat. Toss in the garlic and cook for 2 minutes more. Tip into the casserole.

Add the tomatoes, beans, green pepper, apple juice, soy sauce and sage to the casserole and season with black pepper. Mix well.

Cover the casserole and cook in the oven for about 45 minutes or until the meat is tender.

Beef goulash

400–500g (13oz–1lb) very lean beef, trimmed and cubed

2 teaspoons paprika (smoked paprika gives a lovely flavour)

2 teaspoons caraway seeds

2 tablespoons olive oil

1 onion, finely sliced

1x400g (13oz) can tomatoes

150g (5oz) sweet potato, peeled and cubed

150g (5oz) celeriac, peeled and cubed

1 bay leaf

200ml (7fl oz) stock

2 tablespoons live natural low-fat yoghurt

Preheat the oven to 160°C/320°F/Gas mark 3.

Put the beef, paprika and caraway seeds in a bowl and toss together.

Heat a tablespoon of oil in a frying pan over a high heat and brown the beef, a few cubes at a time. Lift out and put in a casserole.

Heat the remaining oil in the pan and soften the onion over a low heat. Stir in the tomatoes, sweet potato and celeriac. Add to the beef with the stock and bay leaf.

Cook for 1 hour in the oven. Stir a couple of times and check if the stock level needs topping up.

Add the yoghurt just before serving.

Chick-pea stew

2 medium courgettes

2 tablespoons olive oil

1 medium onion, finely sliced

2 garlic cloves, crushed or finely chopped

2 large sticks celery, sliced

1x400g (13oz) can chick-peas, drained and rinsed

1x400g (13oz) can tomatoes

75g (2½oz) green beans, topped and tailed and cut in half

1 bay leaf

Freshly ground black pepper

2 tablespoons The Food Doctor Chilli Seed Mix, coarsely ground, or use ¼ teaspoon chilli flakes and 2 tablespoons mixed pumpkin and sunflower seeds

A large handful fresh parsley or coriander, chopped

Preheat the oven to 180°C/350°F/Gas mark 4.

Cut the courgettes in half and slice them lengthways into fairly thick slices. Brush each slice with olive oil and brown under a medium-hot grill or on a ridged griddle pan.

Heat a tablespoon of olive oil in a frying pan and soften the onions. Add the garlic and celery and cook together for a minute or so. Add the chick-peas, tomatoes, beans, courgettes, bay leaf and black pepper. Cook for 2 minutes, then put all the ingredients in an ovenproof casserole and cook for 30 minutes.

Add the seeds and herbs just before you are ready to serve the stew.

Venison stew

2 tablespoons chick-pea flour

400–500g (13oz–1lb) stewing venison, trimmed and cubed

2 tablespoons olive oil

12 shallots

1 tablespoon red wine

300ml (½ pint) stock

½ teaspoon ground nutmeg

2 whole cloves

1 small stick cinnamon

A pinch cayenne

Freshly ground black pepper

8 juniper berries, lightly crushed

A handful fresh parsley, chopped

Preheat the oven to 160°C/320°F/Gas mark 3.

Sprinkle the chick-pea flour onto a plate and lightly coat the cubes of meat in the flour.

Heat a tablespoon of olive oil in a frying pan and, once the pan is hot, lightly brown the venison, a few cubes at a time. Lift out the browned pieces of meat and put them into a casserole dish.

Heat the remaining oil and lightly brown the shallots over a medium heat. Lift them out and add them to the venison in the casserole.

Pour the red wine and the stock into the frying pan and stir well to mix them in with the pan juices. Bring to the boil and then pour into the casserole.

Add the spices and juniper berries to the stew, combine well, and cook in the oven for about 1½ hours, by which time the meat should be tender and nearly breaking up.

When you come to serve the stew, scatter the fresh parsley over the top of the dish.

Venison stew

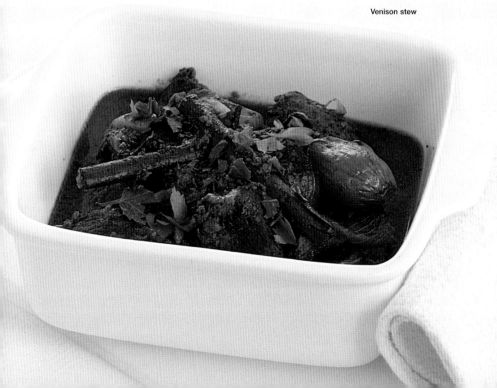

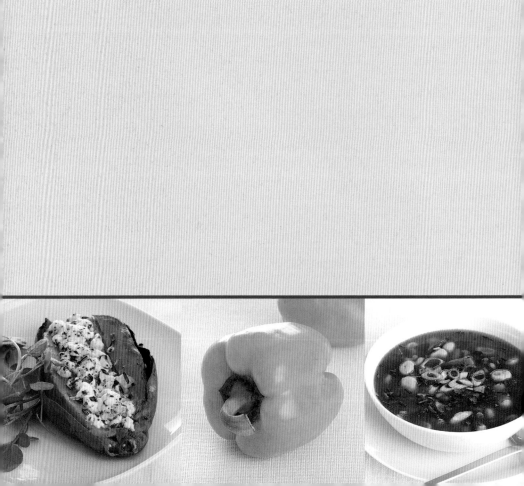

Family Food

These healthy recipes are designed to be enjoyed by the whole family.

Adapt any ingredients to suit your family's tastes.

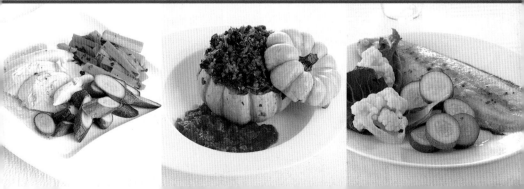

Beef carpaccio

Carpaccio, an Italian hors d'oeuvre consisting of paper-thin sliced meat or fish, is usually served raw. This lightly cooked version served with croutons means that the whole family should enjoy eating it.

100g (3½oz) beef fillet per person

1 tablespoon ground The Food Doctor Garlic & Chilli Seed Mix per person, or use 1 teaspoon chilli flakes, 1 crushed garlic clove and 1 tablespoon mixed pumpkin and sunflower seeds per person

1 tablespoon olive oil

For the croutons:
1 slice of rye bread per person

1 tablespoon olive oil

Brush the beef all over with olive oil and then roll the meat in the ground seeds, pressing them well into the meat. Wrap the beef fillets tightly in aluminium foil.

Place a large cast iron pan over a very high heat until really hot. Put the wrapped beef into the pan and press it down lightly so that it makes good contact with the hot surface. Cook for a minute, turning a couple of times. The beef should be cooked on the outside and very pink on the inside when you remove it from the heat. Put the beef, still wrapped in the foil, in the fridge and leave it to cool.

Preheat the oven to 180°C/350°F/Gas mark 4.

Cut a thick slice of rye bread per person and brush both sides well with olive oil and crushed garlic. Cut the bread into cubes, place on a baking sheet and bake for approximately 20 minutes, turning once. They should be well browned and crunchy.

Wait until the beef is very cold before serving it because it will be easier to slice. Slice each fillet as thinly as possible using a long, very sharp knife.

SERVING IDEAS
For lunch or dinner
Serve the thinly sliced beef on a bed of fresh salad leaves and mixed herbs, with some of the rye bread croutons scattered over the top.

Three-bean soup ⓥ

This robust soup is a great way of getting the family to eat more pulses (such as flageolet beans), which are inexpensive, are high in protein and fibre and carry a low GI rating. This recipe serves four.

ready in **15** minutes

1 tablespoon olive oil

2 shallots, finely sliced

1 garlic clove, finely chopped

100g (3½oz) green beans, topped and tailed and cut in three

1 litre (1¾ pints) hot vegetable stock *(see p.296)*

200ml (7fl oz) tomato passata (cooked tomato concentrate)

100g (3½oz) broad beans (weight after shelling – or use frozen)

1x400g (13oz) can flageolet beans

Juice 1 lemon

Freshly ground black pepper

2 tablespoons mustard

2 spring onions, finely chopped

2 tablespoons fresh parsley, chopped

Heat the oil in a large saucepan, add the shallots and soften them over a low heat. Add the garlic and green beans and stir together for a minute. Pour in the hot stock and passata and simmer for 5 minutes until the green beans are nearly tender. Add the broad beans, the flageolet beans and lemon juice and season with freshly ground black pepper. Simmer for a further 5 minutes.

Stir in the mustard and serve immediately, topped with the spring onions and chopped parsley.

> ### SERVING IDEAS
>
> **For lunch** Serve each portion of soup with a fresh wholemeal roll.
>
> **For dinner** Add a tablespoon of live natural low-fat yoghurt to each bowl of soup and sprinkle a generous tablespoon of toasted mixed seeds on top *(see p.335).*

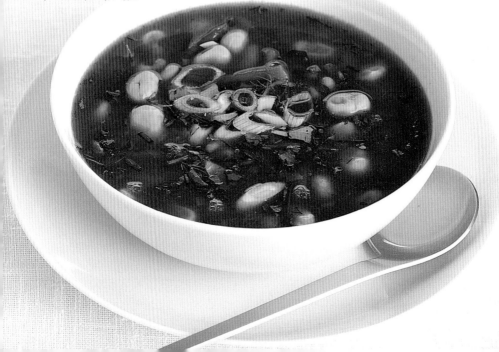

Smoked fish & sweet potato cakes

Sweet potato may not seem an obvious ingredient for a fishcake recipe, but it packs a lot of nutrition into a single meal and is especially easy to digest. This recipe serves four.

4 sweet potatoes (150–200g/5–7oz each)
4 tablespoons lemon juice
400g (13oz) hot smoked fish (trout, mackerel or salmon)
2 teaspoons fish sauce
8 tablespoons fresh parsley, finely chopped
A little olive oil
4 lemon wedges

Boil the sweet potato whole in very lightly salted water until soft for about 25 minutes. Remove from the water, peel and mash in a bowl together with the lemon juice. Flake in the fish, the fish sauce and the parsley and stir gently to combine the ingredients.

Divide the mixture into 16 small cakes. Heat a little oil in a non-stick frying pan and brown the cakes on both sides, turning only once. Serve with a wedge of lemon at the side of each plate.

This meal can also serve eight as a starter.

The **tang** of smoked fish combines **beautifully** with the **milder flavour** of sweet potato to make a **delicious** main course

> **SERVING IDEAS**
>
> **For lunch** This meal is quite filling and should only need a mixed salad, but if you are feeling hungry add a serving of quinoa.
>
> **For dinner** Serve with a large salad of mixed leaves and some sliced tomato on the side.

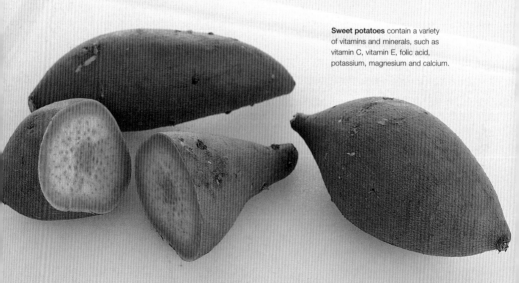

Sweet potatoes contain a variety of vitamins and minerals, such as vitamin C, vitamin E, folic acid, potassium, magnesium and calcium.

Moroccan chicken

With its warm, fragrant, slightly sweet flavours,
Moroccan food brings out the best in chicken.
Use chicken breasts for this recipe, as they won't
dry out. This recipe serves four.

ready in **25** minutes

4 chicken breasts (approximately 100g/3½oz each)
4 tablespoons olive oil
2 onions, chopped
2 garlic cloves, chopped or crushed
2x400g (13oz) cans chopped tomatoes
2 teaspoons fresh ginger, grated
2 cinnamon sticks
4 tablespoons orange juice
2 tablespoons lemon juice
300ml (½ pint) chicken stock *(see p.296)*
4 tablespoons fresh coriander, chopped

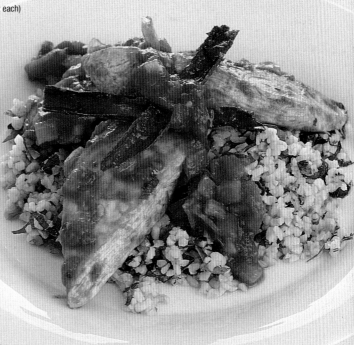

Cut each chicken breast diagonally into three strips.
Heat 2 tablespoons of olive oil in a saucepan with a lid
and gently brown the chicken breasts on both sides.
Lift from the pan and put to one side.

Heat the rest of the olive oil in the same pan, add the
onions and soften over a low heat. Add the garlic,
tomatoes, ginger, cinnamon and orange and lemon juice

and simmer together for about 5 minutes. Replace
the chicken breasts, add the stock and combine well.

Bring to the boil and simmer very gently for about
10 minutes. Stir in the fresh coriander and serve on a
bed of brown rice, quinoa or bulgar wheat with a salad
of mixed leaves.

Baked sweet potato with feta ⓥ

This is one of those meals that cooks itself and only needs minimal preparation before serving. Unlike ordinary potatoes, it doesn't matter if sweet potatoes are slightly al dente in the middle. Serves four.

4 sweet potatoes (150–200g/5–7oz each)

300g (11oz) feta cheese

2 plump spring onions

2 tablespoons olive oil

2 tablespoons orange juice

Freshly ground black pepper

2 rounded teaspoons caraway seeds (or fennel or cumin could be used instead)

A good handful fresh parsley, chopped

Preheat the oven to 180°C/350°F/Gas mark 4.

Spear each potato with a metal kebab skewer to speed up the cooking time: the skewer will conduct the heat to the centre of the potato.

Cook the potatoes in the oven for about 40 minutes (depending on their size).

While the potatoes are cooking, chop or crumble the feta cheese into a small bowl. Finely chop the spring onions and toss them in with the feta cheese. Add the olive oil, orange juice and black pepper. Roast the seeds in small pan over a medium high heat to give a more intense, toasted flavour and stir them in with the feta. Leave to marinate while the potatoes are cooking.

When the sweet potatoes are cooked, remove from the skewer, cut them open and drizzle over a little olive oil. Scatter the feta mix on top, sprinkle with the chopped parsley and serve.

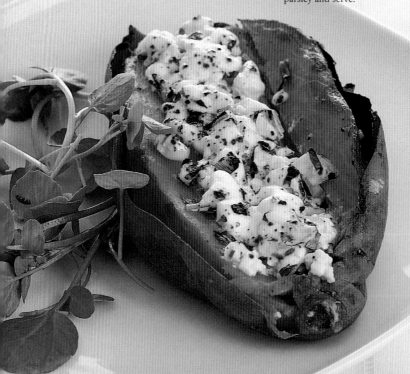

SERVING IDEAS

For lunch or dinner
This dish should make a filling lunch or dinner, so serve it with a simple crisp green salad. You can add some toasted seeds *(see p.335)* for extra protein or, if everyone is feeling very hungry, grill a few mini chicken breasts to serve with this dish.

Roast vegetable quinoa pilau 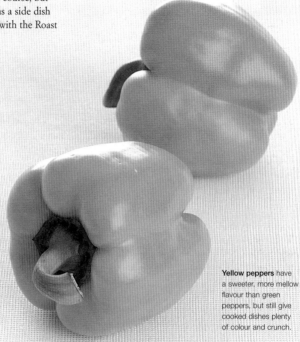

This recipe makes a tasty vegetarian main course, but
you can halve the quantities and serve it as a side dish
to accompany simply grilled meat or fish with the Roast
pepper sauce on page 297. Serves four.

8 tablespoons olive oil
1 medium onion, finely chopped
2 garlic cloves, crushed or finely chopped
400g (14oz) quinoa, rinsed and drained
500ml (17fl oz) stock
20 baby plum tomatoes (approx 300g/10oz)
Freshly ground black pepper
12 baby courgettes (approx 350g/11½oz)
1 large yellow pepper
2 medium red onions, finely sliced
A few squeezes of lemon juice
1 teaspoon balsamic vinegar
½ teaspoon cinnamon powder
2 tablespoons fresh mint, chopped

Yellow peppers have
a sweeter, more mellow
flavour than green
peppers, but still give
cooked dishes plenty
of colour and crunch.

Heat 2 tablespoons of olive oil in a large saucepan.
Soften the onion over a low heat, add the garlic and
stir. Add the drained quinoa, stir for a minute, then
add the stock. Bring to the boil and simmer gently.
It will take approx 20 minutes for the quinoa to cook,
by which time all the stock should be absorbed.

Preheat the oven to 180°C/350°F/Gas mark 4.

Cut the tomatoes in half, put them on a small baking
tray, toss in 2 tablespoons of olive oil and season with
a good grinding of black pepper. Roast in the oven for
about 15 minutes until soft, with the juices running.
When cooked, drizzle with the vinegar.

Slice the courgettes lengthways – about four slices to
each small courgette – and slice the pepper into thin
strips. Heat 2 tablespoons of olive oil in a griddle pan
or frying pan, add the courgettes and pepper and cook
over a medium heat for about 15 minutes, turning once,
until brown on both sides.

Heat the final 2 tablespoons of olive oil in a frying pan,
add the red onion and cook over a low heat for about
10 minutes, turning frequently, until it starts turning
brown. Sprinkle with the cinnamon and cook for
another couple of minutes.

Put the quinoa in a warmed bowl and toss with the
tomatoes, courgettes and pepper, lemon juice, vinegar
and a little olive oil. Top with the cinnamon, onions and
the chopped mint. You can, if you wish, crumble some
feta cheese on top too. Serve with a mixed leaf salad.

Spinach bake ⓥ

This all-in-one dish is easy to make and tastes delicious. The combination of iron-rich spinach, nutritious eggs and mixed seeds makes this a balanced yet satisfying meal. Serves four.

SERVING IDEAS

For lunch If you have any flat breads in the freezer, serve them with the Spinach bake, or make some fresh flat breads (see p.298).

For dinner Scatter some chopped fresh parsley on top of the dish for extra flavour.

2 or 3 large tomatoes (about 400g/13oz), sliced

1 medium onion, finely sliced

4 tablespoons olive oil

2 teaspoons balsamic vinegar

Freshly ground black pepper

2 garlic cloves, chopped

300g (10oz) spinach, washed and coarsely shredded

4 eggs

2 tablespoons live natural low-fat yoghurt

2 tablespoons ground The Food Doctor Chilli and Garlic Seed Mix, or grind 1 teaspoon chilli flakes, 1 crushed garlic clove and 2 tablespoons mixed pumpkin and sunflower seeds

Crumbled feta cheese as a garnish

Preheat the oven to 200°C/400°F/Gas mark 6.

Put the tomatoes, onion, 2 tablespoons of olive oil and the vinegar in a roasting tin, season with freshly ground black pepper and roast until the onion is soft – about 45 minutes. Shake the tin occasionally to prevent burning. When cooked, roughly mash the vegetables together.

Heat a tablespoon of olive oil in a large saucepan, add the garlic and cook over a low heat for a minute. Add the spinach and cook until it has wilted.

Beat the eggs, yoghurt, ground seeds and black pepper together and make three flat omelettes.

Lightly oil a deep, round baking dish roughly the same size as the omelettes. Place one omelette in the bottom, cover with a third of the spinach and half the tomatoes and repeat. Top with the third omelette and the rest of the spinach. Scatter feta cheese on top, put in the oven for 10 minutes or under a grill to brown and serve.

Baked trout with fresh herbs

Trout is quite a delicate-tasting fish and only needs a few simple ingredients to bring out its flavour. Buy the freshest fish you can find on the day that you want to eat this dish. Serves four.

ready in 20 minutes

4 small trout, approx 150g (5oz) each without head

Juice 1 lemon

Freshly ground black pepper

4 small handfuls fresh herbs (use whatever is in season: dill, fennel, basil, parsley, chives, marjoram, mint or lemon balm)

75ml (5fl oz) dry white wine

> ### SERVING IDEAS
> **For lunch or dinner**
> Serve each fish with a mixed leaf salad with added fresh herbs and hot, mashed chick-peas. Try serving some Yellow pepper sauce on the side *(see p.297).*

Preheat the oven to 150°C/300°F/Gas mark 2.

If you prefer, ask your fishmonger to gut the trout and remove its head. You could use two larger fish between four, but add an extra 5 minutes or so to the cooking time.

Rinse the fish to remove loose scales and wash the insides. Pat dry with kitchen paper and place in an oiled shallow ovenproof dish. Season the inside of the fish with lemon juice and black pepper and tuck a small handful of mixed fresh herbs into each cavity. Sprinkle the white wine over each fish, season with black pepper, cover the dish with foil and put in the oven to bake.

Small fish should only take 15 minutes to bake – the flesh should be just cooked but still nice and moist.

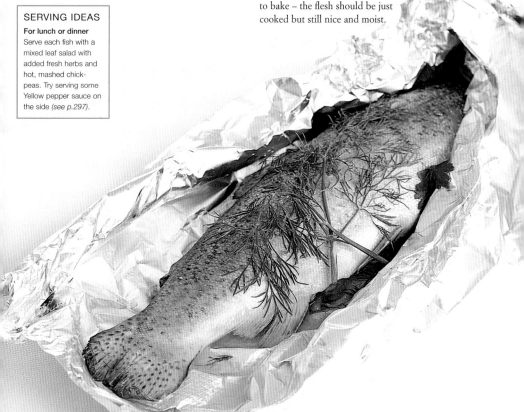

Stuffed gem squash

The easiest way to cut a squash in half is to use a very sharp knife and apply pressure with the heel of your free hand to back of the blade – or carefully hit the knife with a rolling pin. Serves four.

4 gem squashes
50g (2oz) bulgar wheat
250ml (8fl oz) light stock
2 tablespoons olive oil
1 medium onion, finely chopped
2 garlic cloves, finely chopped
250g (8oz) steak mince, as lean as possible
1 tablespoon smoked paprika
3–4 good sprigs fresh parsley, chopped
Freshly ground black pepper
300ml (½ pint) Rich tomato sauce *(see p.297)*

Cut each squash in half across its middle and scrape out the seeds. Put the squashes in a steamer to cook for 10 minutes until they are beginning to soften, but are not thoroughly cooked through.

Put the bulgar wheat in a bowl and pour in the boiling stock. Soak for 10 minutes, then squeeze the bulgar wheat through a fine sieve to remove excess moisture.

Preheat the oven to 170°/325°F/Gas mark 3.

Heat the oil in a saucepan and soften the onion and garlic over a low heat. Turn up the heat a little, add the steak mince, break it up with a fork and stir until it is well browned. Stir in the paprika, then the bulgar wheat and parsley and season with freshly ground black pepper.

Put the squashes into a shallow baking dish and pack some of the stuffing into each squash, piling it up if necessary. Cover with foil and cook for half an hour, by which time the flesh of the squash should be soft.

Serve with the Rich tomato sauce and some Roasted root vegetables *(see p.278)*.

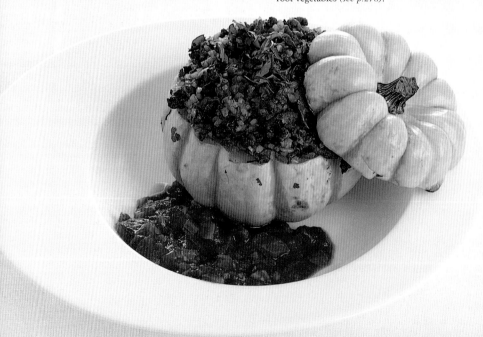

Pot-roast chicken

It's worth cooking a large chicken, as you can use the leftover cuts of meat for other recipes: Chicken & avocado salad *(see p.252)*, Chinese chicken salad *(see p.251)* and Chicken soup *(see p.301)*. Serves four.

1 chicken, about 2kg (4½lb)
1 medium onion
½ lemon
A few sprigs fresh thyme
Freshly ground black pepper
2 tablespoons olive oil
100ml (3½fl oz) white wine
A small handful fresh parsley, chopped

SERVING IDEAS

For lunch Serve with some Roasted root vegetables *(see p.278)* and a small helping of plain red or brown rice.

For dinner Lightly steamed carrots and courgettes are all you need to serve with this satisfying dish.

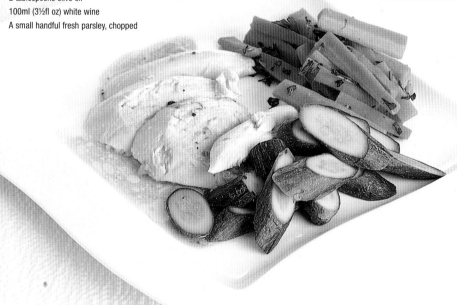

Preheat the oven to 180°C/350°F/Gas mark 4.

Check that the cavity of the chicken is clear and then stuff it with the onion and lemon. Tuck sprigs of fresh thyme inside the chicken and under the wings and legs. Drizzle the olive oil over the bird and season with black pepper. Put the chicken in either a deep casserole with a lid or a high dome-covered baking dish. Pour white wine around the bird, cover and cook for 45 minutes. Remove the lid and return to the oven for a further ten minutes to brown the bird. Set the bird aside while you tip the juices from the pan and the chicken cavity into a small pan and skim off any fat.

Remove the skin, carve the bird and serve with a little sauce poured over the meat.

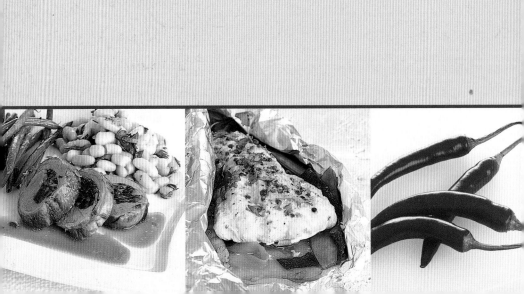

Food for friends

When you follow my principles, cooking for friends doesn't mean you have to compromise, as you will see from these impressive dishes.

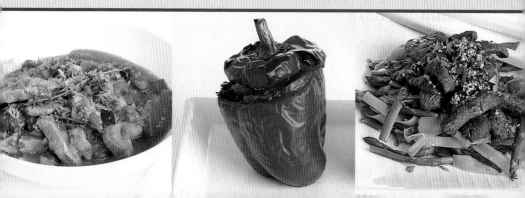

Moroccan stuffed peppers ⓥ

Buy a mix of different coloured peppers to give
a more vibrant effect when you serve this dish.
It can be served as a vegetarian main course
for four people or as a starter for eight.

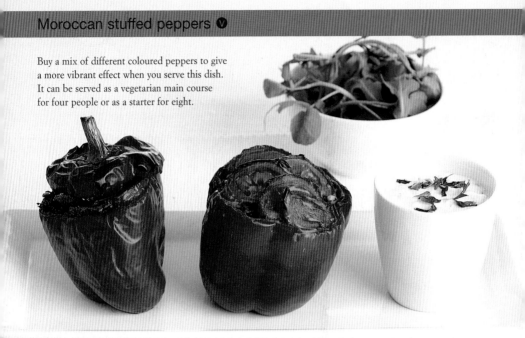

250g (9oz) red rice
3 tablespoons olive oil
400g (13oz) onions, finely chopped
400ml (¾pint) light stock
20g (1oz) currants
A small handful each mint, parsley and dill, finely chopped
25g (¾oz) pinenuts
8 peppers
1 large tomato (optional), sliced
50ml (2fl oz) water
1 tablespoon lemon juice
1 teaspoon olive oil

For the sauce:
3 tablespoons live natural low-fat yoghurt
3 tablespoons fat-reduced fromage frais
Juice ½ lemon
A couple of sprigs of fresh mint, finely chopped

Soak the red rice in cold water until needed.

Heat the oil in a large saucepan and soften the onion
over a low heat until it turns golden. Add the rice, stock
and currants and simmer for 30 minutes. Stir in the
chopped herbs and stir well.

Preheat the oven to 180°C/350°F/Gas mark 4.

Add the pinenuts to the rice mix. Cut the stalk ends off
the peppers and scoop out the seeds and any pith. Fill
each pepper with the rice and top with a slice of tomato
(or you can put the cut end of pepper back on top).

Place the peppers upright in a baking dish positioned
fairly tightly together to support each other. Mix the
water, lemon juice and olive oil and pour it around the
base of the peppers. Cover with foil or a lid. Bake for
an hour until the peppers are soft, but not collapsing.

Mix the yoghurt, fromage frais, lemon juice and mint
together and serve separately in a small pot. Serve the
peppers with a watercress salad.

Chilli fish with stir-fried vegetables

Use any type of firm white fish for this recipe to match the fiery flavours of the chilli sauce. Sea bass, orange roughy or halibut are all good choices. Quantities for this recipe make enough for four.

4 white fish fillets, approx 75–100g (2½–3½oz) each
Freshly ground black pepper
850ml (1½ pints) fish stock

For the sauce:
4 tablespoons white wine
4 spring onions, finely chopped
4 garlic cloves, peeled whole
1 teaspoon chilli paste
1 teaspoon rice vinegar

For the stir-fry:
4 tablespoons olive oil
4 teaspoons caraway seeds
4 teaspoons brown mustard seeds
300g (10oz) sweet potato, grated
200g (7oz) bean sprouts

First, make the sauce: combine all the ingredients except the chilli paste and vinegar in a small pan, bring to the boil and simmer gently for about 15 minutes until the garlic is soft. Mash the garlic with a fork and stir in the chilli paste and vinegar.

Preheat the oven to 160°C/320°F/Gas mark 3.

Place the fish fillets in a shallow dish and season with a good grinding of black pepper. Pour over the sauce, cover the dish with foil and bake for 10–15 minutes until the fish is just cooked.

Meanwhile, heat the oil in a wok, add the seeds and cook them until they pop. Throw in the sweet potato and bean sprouts and stir fry for 3–4 minutes until the vegetables are piping hot.

Pile the fish onto the stir-fried vegetables and serve with the chilli sauce spooned over the top.

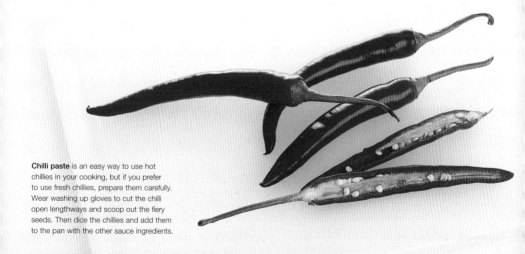

Chilli paste is an easy way to use hot chillies in your cooking, but if you prefer to use fresh chillies, prepare them carefully. Wear washing up gloves to cut the chilli open lengthways and scoop out the fiery seeds. Then dice the chillies and add them to the pan with the other sauce ingredients.

Fish parcels with ribbon vegetables

This is a very quick and easy dish to serve for friends, and it looks impressive too. Keep the foil for each portion opened slightly when you serve it to prevent the fish cooking further. Serves four.

ready in 20 minutes

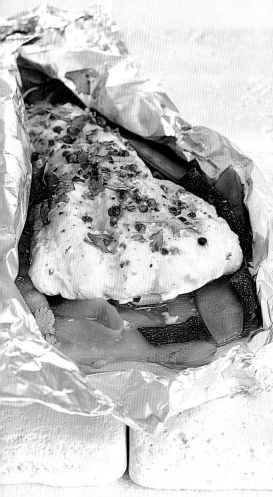

4 skinless white fish fillets, about 100g (3½oz) each

100g (3½z) leeks

100g (3½oz) courgettes

200g (7oz) sweet potato

100g (3½oz) mangetout

100ml (3½fl oz) water

Juice 1 lemon

1 teaspoon fresh grated ginger

1 teaspoon soy sauce

4 tablespoons finely ground The Food Doctor Fennel and Caraway Seed Mix, or grind ½ teaspoon fennel seeds, ½ teaspoon caraway seeds and 2 tablespoons mixed pumpkin and sunflower seeds

Freshly ground black pepper

A large handful fresh coriander, finely chopped

1 lemon, quartered

Preheat the oven to 175°C/340°F/Gas mark 4.

Cut the leeks finely lengthways into short strips, toss into boiling water for a couple of minutes to soften and then drain. Using a vegetable peeler, peel the courgettes and sweet potato into wide ribbons. Heat the water, half the lemon juice, ginger and soy sauce in a wok. Toss in the vegetables and stir fry for a minute or two.

Place the fish on a plate, drizzle each fillet with lemon juice and season with freshly ground black pepper. Coat each fillet in the ground seeds.

Cut four sheets of foil, large enough to wrap up each fish fillet, and lightly oil the surface of the foil. Lay a quarter of the vegetables on each sheet of foil and place a fillet on top. Carefully join the two long sides of foil and fold up the ends to make a loose parcel. Place the parcels on a baking sheet. Bake for 10–15 minutes, depending on the size of the fillet. The fish should be just cooked when you take it out of the oven.

Serve immediately in the parcel with the soy sauce from the wok and fresh coriander sprinkled on top. Add a wedge of fresh lemon at the side. This dish would go well with red rice or bulgar wheat.

Spicy fish stew

The better the fish stock, the tastier this stew is. Ask your fishmonger for offcuts and make a stock based on the chicken stock recipe on page 296, or buy a good-quality fish stock. Serves four.

400g (13oz) mixed fish fillets (tuna, salmon, sea trout, cod, coley, scallops or prawns)

Lemon juice to taste

Freshly ground black pepper

2 tablespoons olive oil

1 medium onion, finely chopped

1 stick celery, chopped

3 small courgettes (approx 200g/7oz), cut into thick chunks

1 garlic clove, finely chopped or crushed

1 bay leaf and 1 sprig thyme

½ teaspoon ground cumin seeds

1x200g (7oz) can chopped tomatoes

1 tablespoon tomato paste

2 teaspoons toasted sesame seed oil

75ml (3fl oz) white wine

150ml (¼ pint) fish stock

2 tablespoons fresh coriander, chopped

2 tablespoons The Food Doctor Chilli & Garlic Seed Mix, coarsely ground, or grind 1 teaspoon chilli flakes, 1 garlic clove and 2 tablespoons mixed pumpkin and sunflower seeds

Remove any skin from the fish fillets and cut them into large, bite-sized chunks. Put the pieces in a bowl, squeeze lemon juice over them, season with black pepper and leave to one side.

Heat the oil in a casserole and soften the onion and celery over a low heat. Add the courgettes and garlic and cook over a medium-high heat until the onion and celery start to take colour. Add the herbs and cumin seeds, tomatoes and paste and the sesame oil. Simmer for a couple of minutes and then pour in the white wine. Allow to bubble hard for a further minute or two. Pour in the stock, bring the stew to boiling point and simmer for about 15 minutes.

At this point, the stew can be cooled and kept in the fridge for up to 24 hours if you are preparing the dish in advance.

When you are ready to serve the stew, ensure that it is boiling before adding the fish pieces, then lower the heat and cook gently for 10–15 minutes. Just before serving, stir in the fresh coriander and ground seeds.

Serve in a bowl with a simple green salad and flat bread (*see p.298*) to mop up the juices.

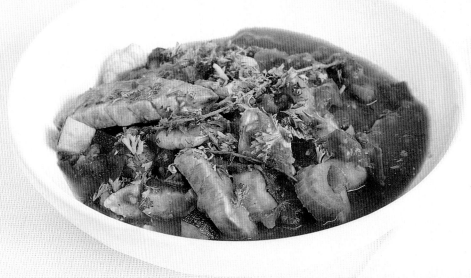

Spiced duck breast

Indian five-spice powder is different to Chinese five-spice, and is available from any Asian store. This recipe serves four.

4 duck breasts

3 tablespoons ground Indian five-spice powder

1 teaspoon fresh ginger, grated

100ml (3½fl oz) live natural low-fat yoghurt

200g (7oz) bulgar wheat or quinoa, plus enough boiling stock to just cover the bulgar wheat

2 tablespoons olive oil

Rind 1 lemon, finely chopped

A small bunch fresh coriander, chopped

Juice and finely chopped rind ½ orange

3–4 sprigs fresh mint, chopped

Remove any skin and all the fat from each duck breast. Combine the five spice, ginger and yoghurt in a bowl and leave the duck breasts to marinate for at least half an hour, but preferably for a couple of hours.

Meanwhile, soak the bulgar wheat in boiling stock for 10 minutes, then drain. Stir in the olive oil, lemon rind and chopped coriander and keep warm. If using quinoa, simmer it gently in about 500ml (approx ¾ pint) of stock until the liquid has been absorbed and the quinoa is tender (add a little more stock if it boils away too fast). Add the olive oil, rind and coriander to the quinoa and keep the dish warm.

Warm a griddle over a medium-high heat and brush or spray it with olive oil. Wipe most of the marinade off the duck breasts and cook them on the griddle for 3–4 minutes on each side so that they are brown on the outside and still pink inside. Mix the orange and mint with the marinade, warm gently and serve separately.

A watercress side salad goes well with this dish.

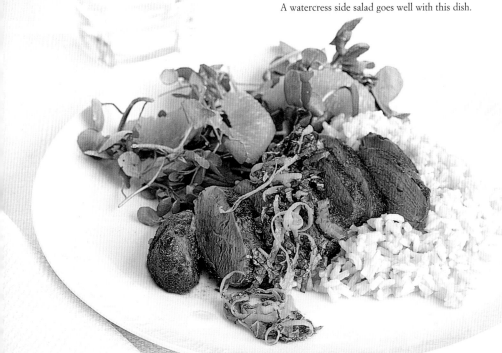

Moroccan rabbit stew

You should be able to get rabbit from your butcher, or buy boned rabbit in most supermarkets, but if you can't, buy chicken thighs instead as their flesh is not dissimilar. This recipe serves four or more.

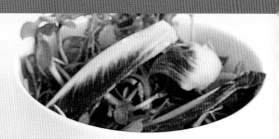

500g (1lb) tomatoes peeled and chopped, or 1x400g (13oz) can chopped tomatoes

1 rabbit, jointed, or 8 chicken thighs, skinned

4 tablespoons olive oil

3 medium onions, peeled and roughly chopped

1 garlic clove, chopped or crushed

1 whole cardamom pod, cracked

½ teaspoon allspice (or nutmeg if allspice is not available)

1 teaspoon cinnamon powder

40ml (2fl oz) red wine vinegar

50ml (2fl oz) unsweetened apple juice

Freshly ground black pepper

Approx 500ml (¾ pint) water

3 tablespoons fresh coriander or parsley, chopped

SERVING IDEAS

For lunch Serve with plain brown rice or bulgar wheat and a green salad.

For dinner Arrange a large mixed leaf salad or lightly steam a good quantity of vegetables to serve with the stew.

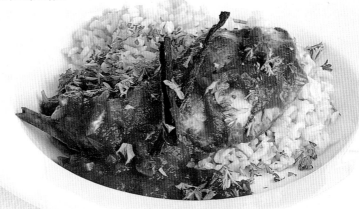

To peel the tomatoes, cover with boiling water and allow to stand for 5 minutes until the skins split. Drain and peel off the skins.

Heat the oil in a large casserole and brown the rabbit pieces, then lift them out and put them to one side. Tip the onions into the casserole and cook over a gentle heat until golden brown. Add the garlic and stir well.

Add the tomatoes, cardamom, allspice, cinnamon, vinegar, apple juice and rabbit pieces to the casserole, season with freshly ground black pepper and stir well. Pour in the water until it just covers the ingredients and bring to the boil. Turn the heat down low and simmer gently for an hour. Remove the lid, raise the heat slightly and simmer for half an hour to reduce the liquid.

Stir in the coriander or parsley and serve.

Calves' liver with coriander

You can also make this recipe using lambs' liver or venison liver, but if you use either of these alternatives, soak them in milk for half an hour before cooking to improve their flavour. Serves four.

ready in **10** minutes

400g (13oz) calves' liver
2 tablespoons chick-pea flour
2 tablespoons ground coriander
4 tablespoons olive oil
2 medium onions, chopped
100ml (3½fl oz) white wine
1 teaspoon soy sauce
200ml (7fl oz) very light hot stock
Juice and zest 2 large oranges
A large handful fresh coriander, chopped

Clean any stringy bits from the liver and cut into wide strips. Mix the flour and ground coriander in a shallow bowl and roll the pieces of liver in the flour.

Heat a tablespoon of olive oil and very quickly brown the liver – just a few seconds on each side. Lift the pieces from the pan and keep warm.

Heat the remainder of the oil and cook the onion until it starts to take colour. Meanwhile, stir the white wine and soy sauce into the hot stock. Then lift the onion from the pan and keep warm with the liver.

Pour the stock into the pan and bring it to the boil. Allow it to bubble, scraping up any residues in the pan. Add the orange juice and zest and return the liver and onion to the pan. Simmer very gently for 1 minute. Remove from heat, stir in the fresh coriander and serve with rosti *(see p.254)*.

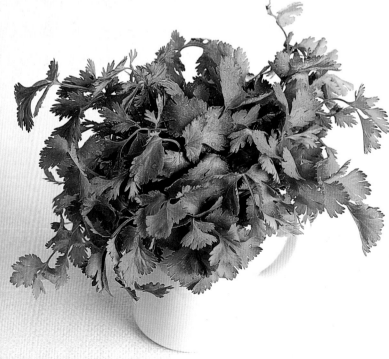

Coriander is a strong, pungently flavoured fresh herb that can lift any dish. To store coriander, put it in a jar of water, cover the leaves with a plastic bag and keep in the fridge, changing the water every two days and picking out any wilted leaves.

Chinese five-spice lamb

Once you have marinated the lamb, this is a quick and impressive-looking dish to make for friends. Lean pork or beef would make a good alternative to lamb. Quantities listed are enough for four.

4 teaspoons Chinese five-spice paste

2 shallots, finely grated

2 tablespoons olive oil

Juice 1 lemon

2 teaspoons soy sauce

400g (13oz) lean lamb, cut into fairly large strips

Freshly ground black pepper

Juice 1 grapefruit

100ml (3½fl oz) water

200g (7oz) carrots

12 spears thin asparagus

4 small spring onions

300g (10oz) mangetout

2 tablespoons toasted sesame seeds *(see p.335)*

A small bunch fresh coriander, chopped

A drizzle of sesame oil

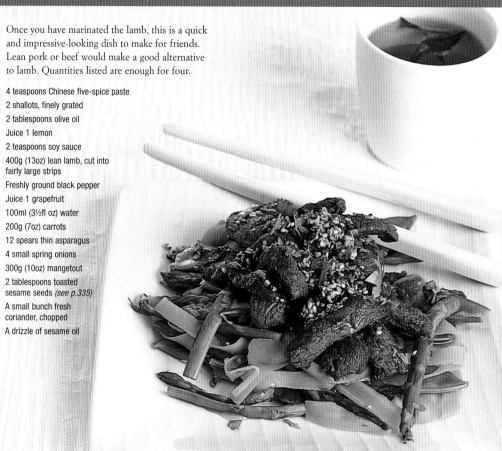

Put the spice, shallots, olive oil, lemon juice and soy in a bowl. Add the lamb, mix thoroughly, season with black pepper, and marinate for half an hour, or longer.

Clean the carrots and slice them into ribbons using a potato peeler (if they are very small, just cut them in half). Snap the tough ends off the asparagus and halve them. Cut the spring onions into thin strips. Bring a pan of water to the boil and simmer the asparagus for a couple of minutes to slightly soften them.

Heat the grapefruit juice and water in a wok over a high heat, add all the vegetables and boil quite fast until the juice has evaporated and the vegetables are just tender.

Cook the strips of lamb quickly on a hot griddle, or under a hot grill, turning frequently until well browned.

Serve the lamb on the vegetables, topped with toasted sesame seeds, the chopped coriander and a drizzle of sesame oil.

Stuffed pork fillet

The preparation time for this recipe takes about 20 minutes, so this task can be done ahead of time and the uncooked dish refrigerated for 24 hours if it's more convenient for you to do so. Serves four.

1x400–500g (13oz–1lb 2oz) pork fillet

Freshly ground black pepper

3 tablespoons lemon juice

2 tablespoons olive oil

1 medium onion, chopped

75g (3oz) mushrooms, chopped

1 dozen pitted black olives, coarsely chopped

1 tablespoon fresh parsley, chopped

1 tablespoon fresh sage, chopped

Zest 1 lemon

50ml (2fl oz) vegetable stock
(see p.296)

(see p.296)

> ### SERVING IDEAS
> **For lunch or dinner**
> Serve with cannellini beans (soaked and cooked according to the instructions on the packet) scattered with fresh parsley and steamed green beans.

Cut five pieces of fine cooking string, each about 40cm (16in) long, and tie a slip knot with a tail at one end of each piece.

Lay the fillet on a board, slice halfway through the meat lengthways and fold the fillet out flat. Gently flatten the fillet by banging it with a rolling pin. Work the strings underneath the fillet so that they are evenly spaced with a piece near each end. Season with freshly ground black pepper and sprinkle with a tablespoon of lemon juice. Leave to one side while you make the stuffing.

Heat a tablespoon of oil in a pan and soften the onion over a low heat. Add the mushrooms, olives, herbs and lemon zest and season with a good grinding of pepper. Cook for 5 minutes, then spoon the mix down the centre of the fillet. Gently squeeze the sides together and hold in place with the string (pull one end through the slip knot and tighten). Start at the ends and work towards the middle, securing the knots as you go.

Preheat the oven to 180°C/350°F/Gas mark 4.

Heat a tablespoon of oil in a frying pan over a high heat. Brown the meat all over and then place it in a shallow ovenproof dish. Pour the stock and lemon juice over the meat, cover with a lid or cooking foil and cook for half an hour before serving.

Osso bucco

This dish looks most impressive served on the bone, although the meat should fall away easily from the bone when you come to distribute it onto your guests' plates. Serves four.

1 slice of shin of veal, cut though the bone, weighing approx 500–600g (1lb–1lb 4oz) and about 8cm (3in) thick

2 tablespoons olive oil

400ml (¾ pint) Rich tomato sauce *(see p.297)*

150ml (¼ pint) dry white wine

For the gremolata:

2 tablespoons fresh parsley, chopped

1 teaspoon lemon zest, finely chopped

1 garlic clove, chopped

Preheat the oven to 180°C/350°F/Gas mark 4.

Heat the oil in a large saucepan over a high heat and brown the meat. Transfer to a casserole dish. Pour the wine into the pan and let it bubble for 30 seconds, then add the tomato sauce and bring to the boil. Pour this over the veal and transfer the dish to the oven to cook for about 45 minutes.

Mix the gremolata ingredients together just before serving and sprinkle a little over each portion.

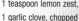

> ## SERVING IDEAS
>
> **For lunch** Serve with steamed vegetables such as broccoli, flat bread *(see p.298)* and the sauce in a jug.
>
> **For dinner** Serve with the sauce in a jug and a large mixed leaf salad.

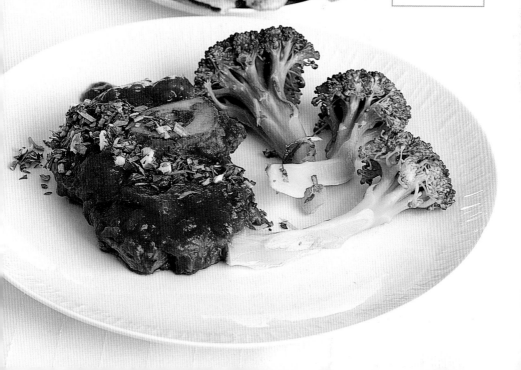

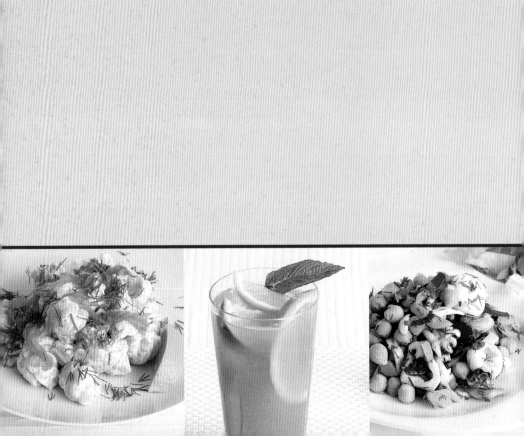

Lazy
weekends

You don't have to be a slave to the kitchen all the time. These dishes are perfect for a lazy weekend and won't take much time to make.

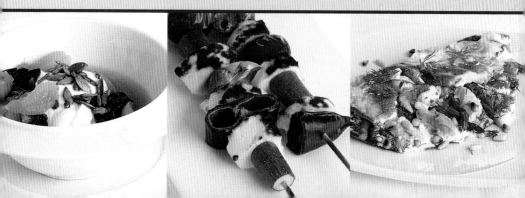

Apple tonics

Make these delicious drinks to give you a boost at any time of day. Apples have beneficial effects on the digestive system and help to remove toxins, while ingredients such as lemon balm clear the mind and calm the nerves – perfect for a relaxing weekend. Serves two.

Love apple livener ⓥ

ready in **1** minute

200ml (7fl oz) tomato passata (cooked tomato concentrate)
200ml (7fl oz) unsweetened apple juice
1 teaspoon fresh ginger, grated
Pinch of cayenne pepper
Freshly squeezed lime juice to taste
2 slices lime

Mix the tomato passata and apple juice together. Add the ginger, cayenne and lime juice. Serve chilled with slices of lime.

Carrot & apple fizz ⓥ

ready in **1** minute

200ml (7fl oz) chilled carrot juice
200ml (7fl oz) unsweetened apple juice
400ml (¾ pint) sparkling water
Slices fresh lemon, lime and orange
A sprig lemon balm

Mix the chilled carrot juice and apple juice together and dilute with the sparkling water. Add the slices of lemon, lime and orange and the sprig of lemon balm and serve.

Apple zing ⓥ

ready in **10** minutes

200ml (7fl oz) boiling water
1 ginger tea bag
Juice 1 lemon
200ml (7fl oz) unsweetened apple juice
2 slices lemon

Pour the boiling water over the tea bag. Add the lemon juice and allow to cool. Mix in the apple juice and pour into glasses filled with ice cubes. Add a slice of lemon to each glass and serve.

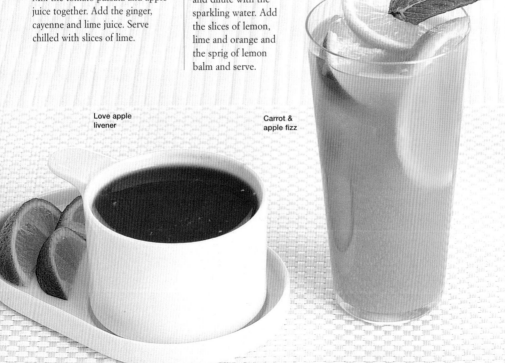

Love apple livener

Carrot & apple fizz

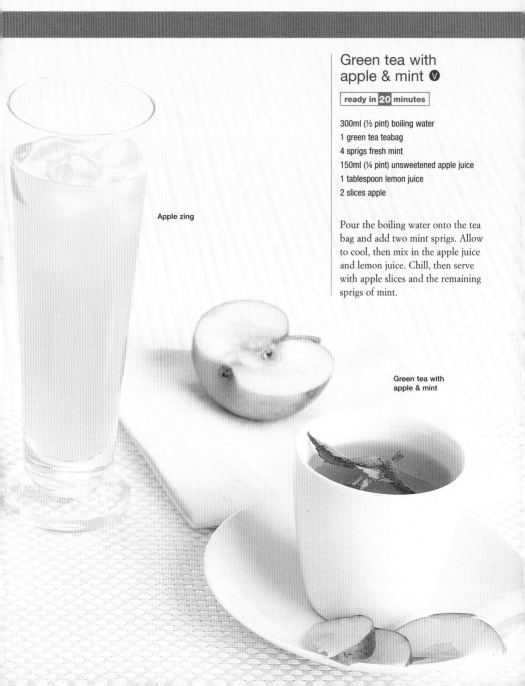

Green tea with apple & mint ⓥ

ready in **20** minutes

300ml (½ pint) boiling water
1 green tea teabag
4 sprigs fresh mint
150ml (¼ pint) unsweetened apple juice
1 tablespoon lemon juice
2 slices apple

Pour the boiling water onto the tea bag and add two mint sprigs. Allow to cool, then mix in the apple juice and lemon juice. Chill, then serve with apple slices and the remaining sprigs of mint.

Apple zing

Green tea with apple & mint

Jasmine fruit compote with toasted seeds

You need to soak the dried fruit the night before you make this recipe, but it's so quick and easy to do that it won't feel like a chore. Vary the fresh fruits according to the season (such as raspberries, strawberries or blueberries), and use mint tea if you prefer. Serves two.

Jasmine fruit compote 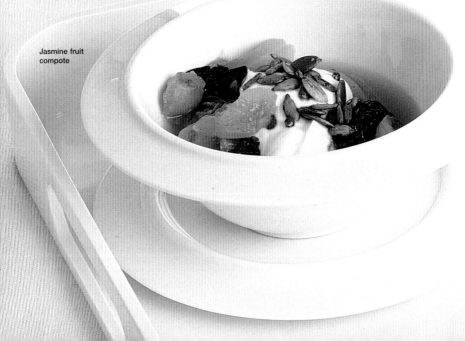 🅥

ready in	**5**	minutes

150ml (5fl oz) green tea with jasmine
8 organic dried apricots, cut in half
6 dried prunes, cut in half
50ml (2fl oz) apple juice
½ crisp apple, cored and sliced
½ crisp pear, cored and sliced

Prepare by making the tea the night before. Allow to cool, add the dried fruit and steep overnight.

When you are ready to eat the compote, strain the tea off the fruit and stir the apple juice into it. Mix the fresh fruit with the soaked fruit in a bowl and pour over the juice. Top with a good dollop of the Fromage frais and yoghurt cream and a couple of tablespoons of toasted seeds *(see right)*.

You could also use the toasted Breakfast crunch, described on page 232, as an alternative topping.

Fromage frais & yoghurt cream 🅥

ready in	**2**	minutes

This is a delicious topping or base. Fromage frais has a better fat profile than crème fraiche.

2 tablespoons reduced-fat fromage frais
2 tablespoons live natural low-fat yoghurt

Beat the two ingredients together to make a soft, thick cream. You can also use this spread on flat bread *(see p.298)* with fruit on top.

Jasmine fruit
compote

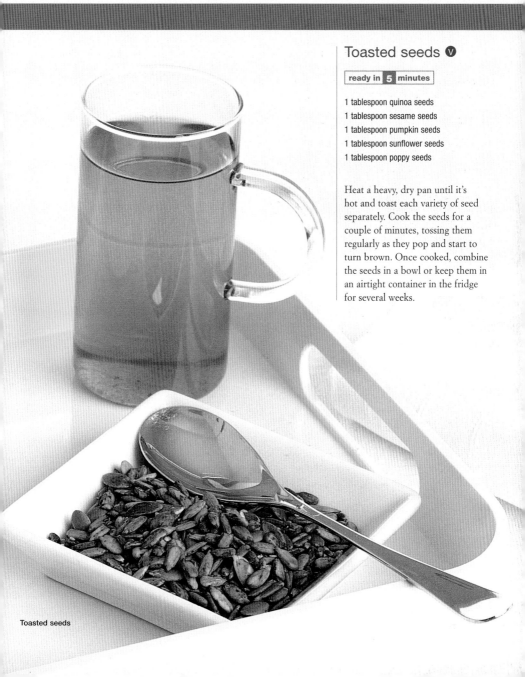

Toasted seeds Ⓥ

ready in **5** minutes

1 tablespoon quinoa seeds
1 tablespoon sesame seeds
1 tablespoon pumpkin seeds
1 tablespoon sunflower seeds
1 tablespoon poppy seeds

Heat a heavy, dry pan until it's hot and toast each variety of seed separately. Cook the seeds for a couple of minutes, tossing them regularly as they pop and start to turn brown. Once cooked, combine the seeds in a bowl or keep them in an airtight container in the fridge for several weeks.

Toasted seeds

Haloumi brochettes with spicy salsa V

This recipe makes a great barbecue dish or a quick evening meal. You can, if you wish, substitute the haloumi with fish, such as tuna, sword fish, monk fish or scallops. Quantities are enough for two.

ready in 15 minutes

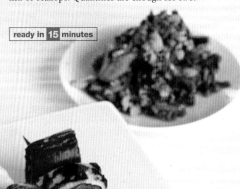

4 thick slices of light haloumi cheese, approx 40g (1½oz) each

1 small courgette (approx 50g/2oz)

4 cherry tomatoes

8 small mushrooms (crimini mushrooms are small and firm and have a good flavour)

8 chunks red pepper

A drizzle olive oil

Cut the haloumi cheese into chunks. Soak four – or more, if you need them – wooden skewers in water, then thread the vegetables and cheese alternately onto the skewers: use something substantial such as a mushroom or courgette at either end, and position the tomato in the middle between the chunks of cheese.

Brush each brochette with a little olive oil and brown on a heated griddle, under a grill or on the barbecue. Turn frequently for even cooking and then serve.

Spicy salsa

35ml (1½fl oz) olive oil

½ tablespoon ground The Food Doctor Chilli Seed Mix, or grind ¼ teaspoon chilli flakes and ½ tablespoon sunflower seeds

½ spring onion, sliced

1 small chunk sweet red pepper

Juice ½ lime

2 teaspoons soy sauce

2 teaspoons orange juice

A sprig each fresh parsley, mint, coriander and basil

Put all the ingredients in a blender and blitz for a few seconds. The result should be coarse and chunky, not completely smooth. Pour the salsa into a bowl and serve with the brochettes.

SERVING IDEAS

For lunch Serve with the salsa and flat bread.

For dinner Arrange a large mixed salad to serve with the Haloumi brochettes and the salsa sauce.

Butter bean colcannon

Colcannon is usually made with mashed potato, but since mashed potato has a high GI rating, this recipe uses butter beans instead. The ham is optional if you want to make this a vegetarian dish. Serves two.

ready in **20** minutes

1x400g (13oz) can butter beans, drained and rinsed

Vegetable stock *(see p.296)* to cover the beans

2 teaspoons Dijon mustard

1 tablespoon reduced-fat fromage frais

2 good sprigs fresh parsley, chopped

2 tablespoons olive oil

100g (3½oz) onion, finely sliced

100g (3½oz) green cabbage, shredded

1 garlic clove, crushed

25ml (1fl oz) water

¼ teaspoon soy sauce

80g (3oz) lean ham, shredded

Put the beans in a saucepan and barely cover them with stock. Bring to boil and simmer for 5–10 minutes until the stock has reduced to about 25ml (1fl oz). Mash the beans with a potato masher, then mix in the mustard, fromage frais and parsley. Leave to one side in a bowl.

Heat a tablespoon of olive oil in a frying pan and soften the onion over a low heat. Add the cabbage and garlic and stir well. Add the water and soy sauce, turn the heat up and simmer, covered, for about 10 minutes until the cabbage is soft. Stir occasionally to prevent any ingredients sticking.

Tip the onion mix into the bowl of mashed beans and mix well. Then stir in the ham.

Heat the remaining oil in a non-stick frying pan and add the mash. Flatten it down to fill the pan and cook over a medium heat to brown the under side. Slip under a hot grill to brown the top before serving.

SERVING IDEAS

For lunch or dinner This dish is filling enough to serve on its own, or if you are hungry you could cook one poached egg per person and serve them on top of the colcannon.

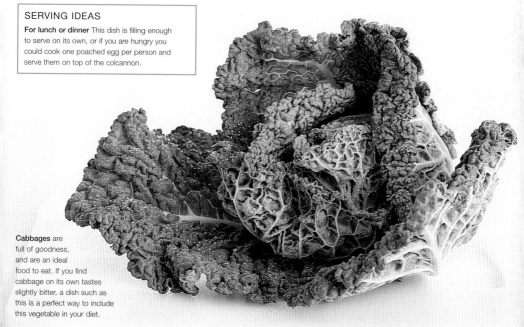

Cabbages are full of goodness, and are an ideal food to eat. If you find cabbage on its own tastes slightly bitter, a dish such as this is a perfect way to include this vegetable in your diet.

Easy toppings

This range of toppings can be spread on The Food Doctor High Bran and Seed Bagels, Mixed Cereal Puffed Crackers, flat breads or wraps, eaten wwith scrambled eggs, or even served together in small dishes like a mini tapas selection. All recipes serve two.

Roast tomatoes

ready in **15** minutes

8–10 cherry tomatoes
1 tablespoon olive oil
Freshly ground black pepper
Crumbled feta cheese as a garnish

Preheat the oven to 180°C/350°F/Gas mark 4.

Put the tomatoes in a small roasting pan and toss in the black pepper and olive oil. Roast for 15 minutes or until soft and serve with the crumbled feta cheese.

Soft herring roes

ready in **5** minutes

4–6 herring roes
1 tablespoon olive oil
Freshly ground black pepper
Fresh lemon juice to taste

Rinse the roes and remove any discoloured bits. Heat the olive oil in a pan and gently sauté the roes until they are turning golden and curling into a ball. Season with black pepper and a little lemon juice and serve.

Sautéed mushrooms Ⓥ

ready in **10** minutes

200g (7oz) flat or exotic mushrooms
2 tablespoons olive oil
Freshly ground black pepper
Fresh lemon juice to taste
2 tablespoons fresh herbs, chopped

If the mushrooms are large, slice them finely; if small, leave whole or cut them in half. Heat the olive oil in a pan and sauté the mushrooms over a medium heat until they start to collapse and turn brown. Season with black pepper and lemon juice and add whatever fresh herbs you have in the fridge.

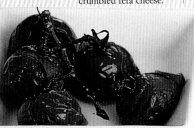

Roast tomatoes

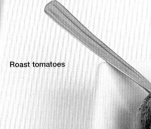

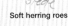
Soft herring roes

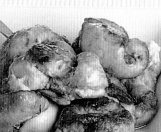

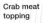
Crab meat topping

Crab meat topping

ready in **10** minutes

25ml (1fl oz) reduced-fat fromage frais
25ml (1fl oz) live natural low-fat yoghurt
2 spring onions, finely chopped
½ teaspoon Dijon mustard
Zest and juice 1 lime
1 teaspoon fresh ginger, grated
A small handful fresh coriander, chopped
A few drops Tabasco sauce
Freshly ground black pepper
200g (7oz) crab meat
½ teaspoon Thai fish sauce
1 little gem lettuce,
finely shredded
2 wedges fresh lemon

Put the fromage frais and yoghurt into a bowl and add the spring onions, mustard, lime juice and zest, ginger, coriander, Tabasco, black pepper and fish sauce. Mix well. Gently fold in the crab meat.

Put the shredded lettuce on top of two flat breads or wraps and spoon half the crab meat mix over each. Serve with a wedge of fresh lemon on each plate.

Lean ham

ready in **1** minute

Choose a lean ham baked on the bone in your local delicatessen or supermarket and have the slices cut very thinly. Arrange the slices of ham on a plate and serve.

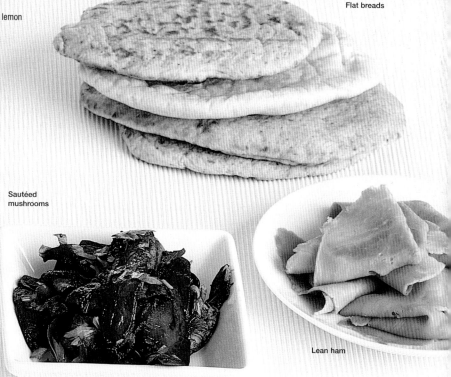

Flat breads

Sautéed
mushrooms

Lean ham

Smart salads for relaxed occasions

The great thing about these salads is that not only do they look impressive and taste delicious, they are quick and easy to make using a can of chick-peas as a base ingredient. The quantities listed serve two, but can easily be increased to serve four or six people.

Warm chick-pea & seafood salad

ready in **10** minutes

2 tablespoons olive oil
1 garlic clove, crushed
1 teaspoon harissa paste
150g (5oz) can chick-peas
150g (5oz) cooked mixed seafood salad, available from most supermarkets
Juice 1 lemon
A good handful each fresh parsley and dill, coarsely chopped

Heat a tablespoon of olive oil in a pan over a low heat, add the garlic and allow it to take a little colour. Then add the harissa paste.

Drain and rinse the chick-peas and toss them in the hot oil for a couple of minutes. Allow them to get hot and begin to turn golden. Add the seafood salad and lemon juice and heat everything together gently.

Tip the contents of the pan into a salad bowl. Stir the fresh parsley and dill into the warm salad.

Serve with flat bread *(see p.298)* and a mixed leaf salad.

Artichoke, chick-pea & spinach salad Ⓥ

ready in **5** minutes

150g (5oz) can chick-peas
100g (3½oz) artichokes marinated in oil (from a delicatessen or a jar)
½ red onion, finely chopped
A large handful baby spinach leaves
A small handful pitted black olives

For the dressing:
Juice ½ lemon
Freshly ground black pepper
3 tablespoons olive oil

Drain and rinse the chick-peas and tip them into a salad bowl. Drain and quarter the artichokes and combine them and the onion in the bowl with the chick-peas. Add the spinach leaves and olives.

To make the dressing, whisk the lemon juice, black pepper and olive oil together. Pour the dressing over the salad and toss the ingredients well to mix. Serve with some flat breads *(see p.298)*.

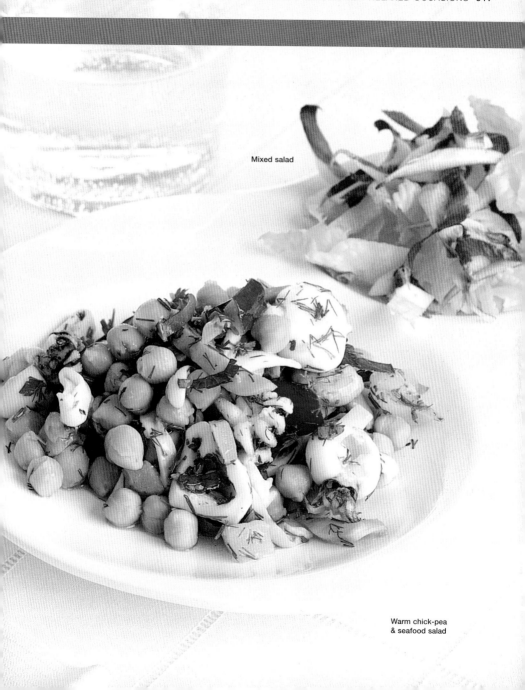

Mixed salad

Warm chick-pea
& seafood salad

Barbecue skewers

The beauty of these skewers is that even if you don't own a barbecue, you can use a medium-hot griddle or grill, pile the cooked skewers onto a plate and serve them outside. All recipes serve two; increase the quantities if you invite guests.

Skewers are **easy** to **prepare** and **quick** to **cook** so they are **ideal** for a **lazy weekend** meal or snack

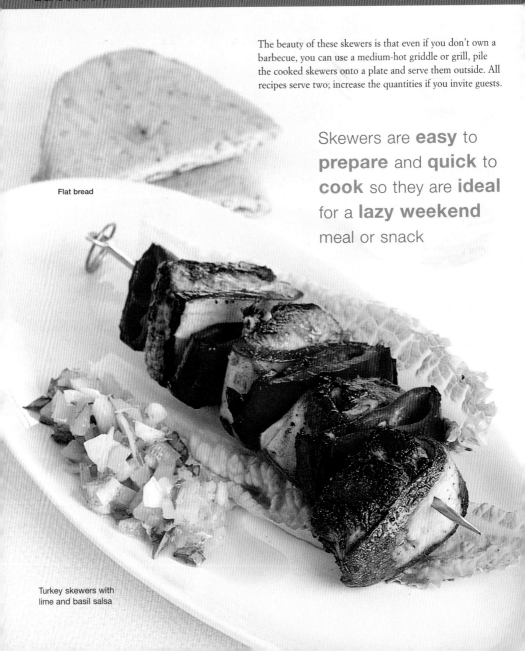

Flat bread

Turkey skewers with lime and basil salsa

Turkey skewers with lime & basil salsa

150–200g (5–7oz) boneless turkey

2 medium courgettes, cut into lengthways slices 7mm (¼in) thick

2 large red peppers, cut into 20 chunks

For the marinade:
2 teaspoons Chinese five-spice paste

Juice and zest 1 lime

2–3cm (¾in–1¼in) fresh ginger, grated

2 garlic cloves, crushed

1 tablespoon olive oil

2 teaspoons sesame oil

Freshly ground black pepper

For the salsa:
A small handful fresh basil, chopped

1 small green onion

½ yellow pepper

Freshly ground black pepper

1 garlic clove

2 tablespoons olive oil

Juice and zest ½ lime

Mix the marinade in a bowl, cut the turkey into 16 even-sized chunks and add to the marinade. Leave for at least half an hour in the fridge.

Blitz the salsa ingredients in a food processor for a few seconds.

To thread the skewers, partly wrap a piece of meat in a courgette slice, then alternately thread the peppers and wrapped meat onto four soaked wooden skewers. Cook on a griddle or barbecue for 15 minutes over a medium heat. Serve with the salsa, a green salad and flat bread.

Swordfish skewers with salsa

ready in 20 minutes

200g (7oz) swordfish steak, skinned

2 small courgettes, cut into thick slices

For the marinade:
Juice 1 lime

2 tablespoons olive oil

1 garlic clove, crushed or topped

2cm (¾in) fresh ginger, grated

Freshly grated black pepper

Soy sauce to taste

For the salsa:
50g (2oz) red onion, chopped

50g (2oz) cucumber, chopped

Cut the fish into 12 chunks. Mix the marinade in a bowl, add the fish and leave to marinate for at least 15 minutes.

Soak four wooden skewers in water, then alternately thread five slices of courgette and three pieces of fish on to each skewer (conserve the marinade). Cook on a barbecue or griddle over a medium heat to brown the courgettes and just cook the fish (overcooking the fish will leave it tough).

Tip the marinade into a food processor, add the onion and cucumber and blitz for a couple of seconds. Turn out into a small bowl and serve with the skewers and a little soy sauce.

Mediterranean chicken skewers

4 chicken thighs, each trimmed of fat and cut into three pieces

8 shallots or pickling onions

8 cherry tomatoes

100ml (3½fl oz) vegetable stock (see p.296)

For the marinade:
2 tablespoons olive oil

3 tablespoons lemon juice or white wine vinegar

1 teaspoon tomato paste

1 garlic clove, finely chopped

Freshly ground black pepper

A few sprigs fresh thyme, finely chopped (or ½ teaspoon dried thyme)

Combine the marinade ingredients in a bowl, add the chicken pieces and leave to marinate for at least 15 minutes, or longer if possible.

Put the shallots in a small saucepan, pour in the stock, bring to the boil and simmer for 5 minutes. Drain and set aside.

Soak four wooden skewers in water, then alternately thread two shallots, three chicken pieces and two baby tomatoes on each skewer, starting and ending with the shallots.

Grill on a barbecue or griddle over a medium heat until the chicken pieces are cooked through.

Serve with some Rich tomato sauce or Yellow pepper sauce (see p.297).

Weekend brunch rice dishes

A rice dish such as kedgeree is a classic brunch meal that is normally made with refined white rice. By substituting the white rice for brown or red rice, you can create "slow-burning" low-GI rice dishes that will supply you with steady energy levels for longer. All recipes serve two.

Orange rice with tofu

1 tablespoon olive oil
1 small onion, finely chopped
100g (3½oz) acorn squash, peeled and cut into 2cm (¾ in) cubes
3 cardamom pods
Rind 1 orange (carefully peel the rind off the orange in large pieces so they can be lifted out before serving)
250ml (8fl oz) vegetable stock *(see p.296)*
100g (3½oz) red rice or brown Italian rice
150g (5oz) marinated tofu, cubed, or 3 hard-boiled eggs, roughly chopped
A small handful fresh mint or coriander, chopped
Freshly ground black pepper

Heat the oil in a medium-sized saucepan over a low heat and cook the onion, squash and cardamom pods until the onion has softened.

Add the orange rind and the stock to the pan and bring to a simmer. Add the rice, cover and simmer gently for 25 minutes. Remove the lid, stir in the tofu and cook for a further 5 minutes.

Add the mint or coriander, season with black pepper and add the chopped eggs if you are not using tofu. Remove the orange rind and cardamom pods and serve.

Coconut rice pilau V

1 tablespoon olive oil
1 small onion, finely chopped
150g (5oz) brown Italian rice (short grain)
300ml (½ pint) vegetable stock *(see p.296)*
60g (2oz) creamed coconut
1 teaspoon ground turmeric
Freshly ground black pepper
A small bunch parsley, finely chopped
Juice ½ lemon
3 hard-boiled eggs

Soften the onion in the olive oil over a low heat. Add the rice and stir for a few seconds. Pour in the hot stock and bring to a simmer. Add the coconut and stir until dissolved. Simmer for 20–25 minutes until the rice is cooked.

Stir in the turmeric, black pepper to taste, parsley and lemon juice. The liquid should be almost absorbed but with some creamy juice still left. If the rice has absorbed the liquid too quickly, add another 50ml (2fl oz) hot stock.

Divide between two plates with the hard-boiled eggs cut into quarters and arranged around the rice. Garnish with some more chopped fresh parsley and serve.

Red rice kedgeree

1 flat teaspoon cumin seeds
450ml (¾ pint) boiling water
150g (5oz) red rice
200g (7oz) smoked haddock, undyed
1 tablespoon olive oil
A little grated nutmeg
½ teaspoon ground turmeric
1 tablespoon lemon juice
Freshly ground black pepper
2 tablespoons fresh parsley, chopped
2 tablespoons live natural low-fat yoghurt
2 poached eggs *(see p.237)*

For the poaching flavouring:
1 lemon slice
1 sprig fresh parsley
1 bay leaf
4 black peppercorns

Dry roast the cumin seeds in a large hot pan for a few seconds until they pop. Pour the boiling water into the pan, add the rice and simmer for 25 minutes.

Put the poaching flavourings and fish in a saucepan. Add cold water until the fish is just covered. Bring to the boil over a medium heat. Turn off the heat and leave for 10 minutes. Drain. Flake the fish, remove any skin or bones and put in a bowl.

Combine the olive oil, nutmeg, turmeric, lemon juice and black pepper. Drain the rice and combine with the fish and parsley in an ovenproof dish. Serve with the two poached eggs and yoghurt poured over the top.

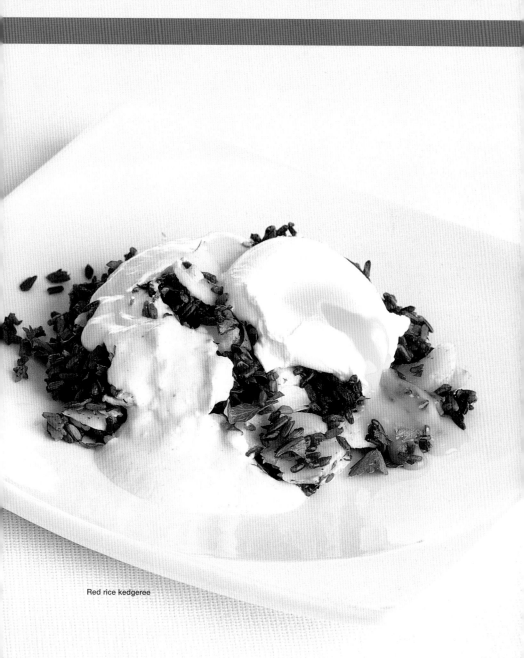

Red rice kedgeree

Squash and feta rosti ⓥ

This rosti is a great vegetarian option. It tastes just as good cold so make a little extra and save some for the next morning's snack. Serves two.

ready in 20 minutes

2 tablespoons olive oil

1 onion (approx. 100g/3½oz), finely chopped

½ teaspoon caraway seeds

2.5cm (1in) piece fresh root ginger, peeled and grated

325g (11oz) firm squash, such as butternut, peeled, deseeded and coarsely grated

100g (3½oz) feta cheese, crumbled

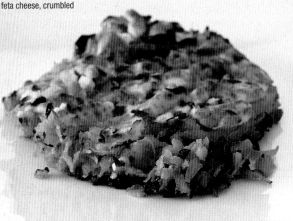

Heat the oil in a small non-stick frying pan, add the onion and caraway seeds and cook until the onion is softened and golden. Add the ginger and grated squash and stir-fry gently for 3–4 minutes to combine the ingredients and soften the squash.

Add the feta and mix well. Pat down the mixture in the pan and draw it in from the sides, to make a cake. Leave over a medium-high heat for about 5 minutes, to firm and brown the base.

Put the pan under a hot grill for a further 5 minutes to brown the top. Cut in half and serve.

SERVING IDEAS

For lunch Serve with a piece of toasted rye or wholemeal bread.

For dinner Serve with a large mixed salad. Add a little extra feta to increase the protein quota too.

Herby scrambled eggs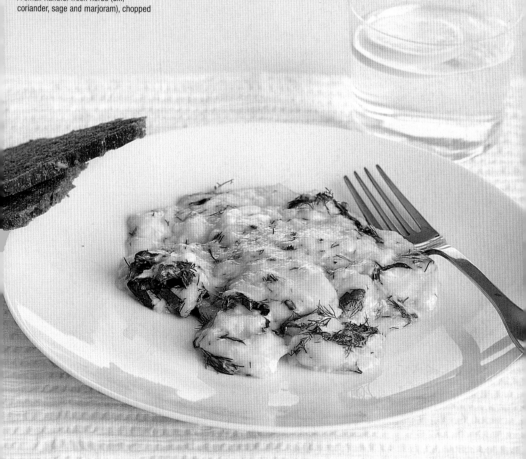

Although this is such a simple recipe, it's important that you don't overcook the eggs. Aim for a soft, creamy consistency; if the eggs become watery or rubbery, they've been cooked too long. Serves two.

ready in 5 minutes

4 small eggs

A drizzle of olive oil

A pinch of ground turmeric

Freshly ground black pepper

A small handful fresh herbs (dill, coriander, sage and marjoram), chopped

Break the eggs into a bowl, season with black pepper and a pinch of turmeric and whisk together.

Heat a little olive oil (or, for a treat, use unsalted butter) in a heavy, non-stick pan over a medium heat. Pour in the egg mixture and move the eggs slowly around the pan. Cook until the eggs set into soft flakes. Once cooked, stir in plenty of chopped fresh herbs and serve immediately with wholemeal toast or rye bread.

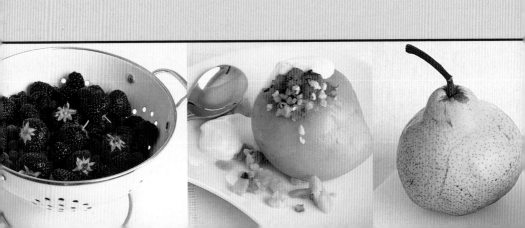

Occasional desserts

Eating sweet food perpetuates the feeling of wanting more, so don't have these delicious desserts too often.

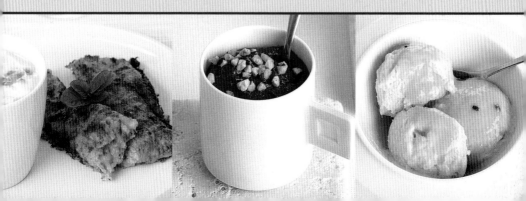

Poached pears ❤

It doesn't matter too much whether the pears you use for this recipe are slightly hard: poaching the fruit will soften their flesh and bring out more of their flavour. Serves two.

2 pears
250ml (8fl oz) jasmine tea
1 tablespoon unsweetened apple juice
½ small stick cinnamon
1 clove
2 mint leaves
½ teaspoon arrowroot powder
2 tablespoons live natural low-fat yoghurt or reduced-fat fromage frais

Peel the pears, removing the black part of the core that shows and leaving the stalk intact. Put the pears in a saucepan large enough to hold them both and add the jasmine tea, apple juice, spices and mint leaves. Simmer for 10–15 minutes, by which time the pears should be soft but still holding their shape.

Lift the pears from the pan and put them into a serving dish. Rapidly boil the fluid in the pan, reducing it to about 200ml (7fl oz).

Mix the arrowroot in a small cup with 2 tablespoons of cold water. Add a little of the tea mix from the pan and stir well. Pour this mix back into the pan and stir well over a low heat. Simmer for a couple of minutes, stirring all the time until the mixture has thickened to a syrupy consistency. Pour the sauce over the pears and chill in the fridge.

Serve with a tablespoon of natural yoghurt or fromage frais and some sauce poured over each pear.

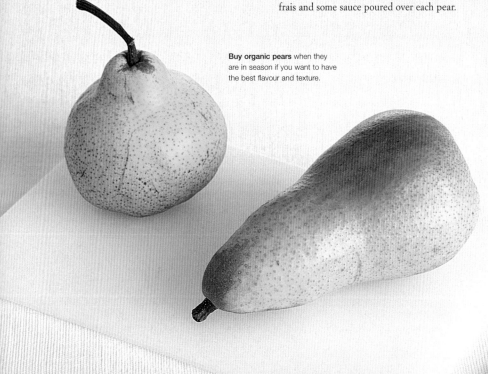

Buy organic pears when they are in season if you want to have the best flavour and texture.

About the Author

Ian Marber MBANT Dip ION

Nutrition consultant, author, broadcaster and health journalist

Ian studied at the Institute for Optimum Nutrition, and now heads The Food Doctor clinic at Notting Hill, London. He contributes regularly to many of Britain's leading magazines and newspapers and appears regularly on TV and radio shows. He has also made a 15-part series for the Discovery Health channel. He is currently studying for a master's degree in nutrition therapy.

Undiagnosed food sensitivities in his twenties led to Ian becoming interested in nutrition. His condition was later identified as coeliac disease, a life-long intolerance to gluten. He is now an acknowledged expert on nutrition and digestion, and many of his clients are referred to his clinic by doctors and gastroenterologists.

Ian advises on all aspects of nutrition, in particular on the impact that correct food choices can have on health. He is known to give motivational, positive and practical advice that can make a real difference to your well-being.

Ian's first book, *The Food Doctor – Healing Foods for Mind and Body*, co-written with Vicki Edgson in 1999, has sold more than 1 million copies and been translated into nine languages. Ian subsequently wrote *The Food Doctor in the City* and *In Bed* with *The Food Doctor. In 2003, The Food Doctor Diet* became an instant bestseller and was tested on Channel 4's *Richard and Judy* by three volunteers, who each lost a dress size in only three weeks. Richard and Judy tested Ian's subsequent book, *The Food Doctor Everyday Diet* on six new volunteers over ten weeks, who all achieved similar results. *The Food Doctor Diet* has been hailed as a truly sensible, healthy approach to weight loss that really works.

The Food Doctor Diet plan

Ian Marber's Diet weight loss plan is designed to help those people unable to visit Ian for a personal consultation to rebalance their body systems and lose weight healthily and for the long term. The answer lies in identifying your metabolic rate, learning how to choose the right foods and, by doing so, rebalancing your metabolism to increase energy levels, motivation and ultimately weight loss. Yo-yo dieting disrupts the metabolic rate, meaning that the next time you restrict what you eat you tend not to lose the weight you have regained. This is why the Everyday Diet is just that, a diet plan that becomes a way of life as you follow 10 simple principles.

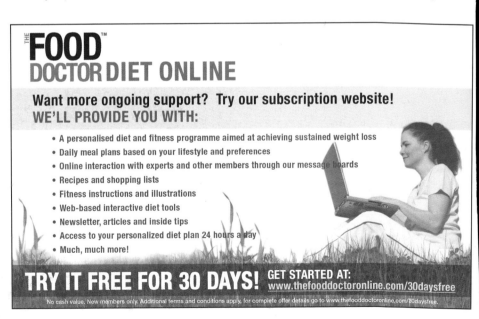